Somatoform and Other Psychosomatic Disorders

Christos Charis • Georgia Panayiotou
Editors

Somatoform and Other Psychosomatic Disorders

A Dialogue Between Contemporary Psychodynamic Psychotherapy and Cognitive Behavioral Therapy Perspectives

Springer

Editors
Christos Charis
Dillenburg, Germany

Georgia Panayiotou
Department of Psychology and Center for Applied Neuroscience
University of Cyprus
Nicosia, Cyprus

ISBN 978-3-030-07750-1 ISBN 978-3-319-89360-0 (eBook)
https://doi.org/10.1007/978-3-319-89360-0

Printed on acid-free paper

This Springer imprint is published by the registered company Springer Nature Switzerland AG
The registered company address is: Gewerbestrasse 11, 6330 Cham, Switzerland

Preface

Cyprus, the island where I (Christos Charis) was born, has been a witness to the seminal events of the world for thousands of years. Germany with its hospitality and openness has been my second home for decades. In order to bring these two worlds together, while working as a psychodynamic psychotherapist in Germany, I worked in cooperation with Associate Professor G. Panayiotou (Ph.D., Clinical Psychologist, trained in the cognitive behavioural [CBT] perspective) of the Department of Psychology/University of Cyprus to organize a seminar on the topic "Somatization, health anxiety and other psychosomatic difficulties: Case formulation and treatment from psychodynamic and cognitive-behavioral perspectives" under the warm sun of Cyprus. Thus, we have all contributed to the growing nationalism of our world today. This book is a synthesis; it represents the result of this conference and the thoughts that were stimulated as a result of the ensuing discussions among attendees and later with additional experts in the field. The conference took place on 24th and 25th October 2016 in Nicosia and served two aims: (a) to bring together psychologists and psychiatrists working with or doing research in areas relevant to somatoform disorders and (b) to provide theory and science-driven clinical training through supervision to a young generation of therapists. The conference was the second in a series of similar meetings, taking place every 2–4 years with a different theme (disorder of interest) each time. Their objective is to initiate a dialogue between different perspectives, enriched with the clinical experience of seasoned clinicians, with the hope to further our understanding of both etiological mechanisms and mechanisms of change in each category of disorders.

It is well documented in psychotherapy research that in addition to the active ingredients of any psychological treatment, psychotherapy, irrespective of perspective, has a significant positive impact due to common non-specific elements such as empathy, giving meaning to difficulties, instilling hope and providing support (Kazdin, 1979; Oei & Shuttlewood, 1996). In our attempt to identify effective elements that different therapeutic approaches including psychoanalytic/psychodynamic traditions and contemporary cognitive behavioural approaches and third-wave therapies have in common, perhaps there is no better place to start than the somatoform disorders, a group of diagnostic categories which psychiatrists, psychologists and researchers have struggled to understand and treat even before the days of Freud.

Patients with functional bodily symptoms (somatization) are commonly seen in primary care. It has been estimated that 20% of primary care patients have a somatoform disorder and these complaints mostly affect the quality of their life and take a chronic course. Treatment of these patients increases health care costs because of their frequent doctor visits and often unnecessary diagnostic procedures. Theirs is typically a complicated and difficult therapy, in part because individuals suffering from these disorders are often unable to express their feelings in words and may be characterized by concrete thinking and low insight.

In spite of differences in conceptualization between the various psychotherapeutic perspectives and the changes in definitions and criteria pertaining to these disorders in DSM-5 (APA, 2013), there is a general understanding among both psychoanalytically/psychodynamically trained professionals and cognitive behavioural therapists that they actually reflect difficulties in dealing with difficult emotions, trauma or stress. Classical psychoanalytic theory posited unacceptable (sexual) desires or repressed trauma as the cause of these symptoms, in individuals whose ego defences were weak or ineffective so that some of the psychic energy failed to be repressed and was converted to physical symptoms to disguise their psychological origin. (For more details about this, see Chap. 2.) In this manner, psychanalytic theory is not at odds with contemporary CBT and acceptance and commitment third-wave approaches, which posit that health anxiety, somatization, medically unexplained symptoms more generally and chronic somatic problems like chronic pain are related to ineffective ways of coping with anxiety and distress and difficulties in emotion regulation. All of the above theoretical approaches, during therapy, in effect aim to aid the patient to acquire increased awareness of his/her emotions and other internal experiences, to increase tolerance and acceptance of them and/or to learn more effective ways of coping.

In this volume we present 11 chapters, which analyse topics that aim to shed light on the aetiology and treatment of somatoform disorders under a psychodynamic and a cognitive-behaviour point of view. There are five chapters representing the psychoanalytic/psychodynamic point of view: Prof. Dr. phil. M. Leuzinger-Bohleber explains why embodied memories are a new pathway to the unconcious. Dr. phil. W. Bohleber makes an intensive study of his subject: the meaning of trauma and its consequences for body and mind. Dr. med. Chr. Charis analyses somatization from a psychodynamic point of view and contributes an additional chapter describing the psychodynamic therapy of a patient with a somatoform disorder. Dr. Schaefer, A., Paar, G., Kriebel, R., and Stäcker, K.H. present a study which examined the influence of a psychodynamic group therapy modified with behaviour and trauma therapy elements on patients with AIDS. For the behavioural/cognitive behavioural view, there are six chapters describing theory and treatment: Dr. C. Leonidou discusses the current state of knowledge on the maintaining mechanisms in illness anxiety, while Dr. G. Panayiotou examines alexithymia as a core trait in psychosomatic disorders. Professor E.C. Karademas provides an overview of theoretical models on the conceptualization and treatment of medically unexplained symptoms, while Dr. E. Constantinou focuses on the role of emotions in the aetiology and maintenance of medically unexplained symptoms. Dr. M. Karekla, with Ms. M. Zacharia and Dr. M. Koushiou, presents on acceptance and commitment therapy for chronic pain, while Drs. Bjorgvinsson, Rutter, Nota, and Yusufov describe the cognitive behavioural treatment of patients with health anxiety. In order to enhance the idea of a dialogue between the two perspectives, chapters are organized across theories: the first two chapters represent an overview of the psychological disorders of interest, Chaps. 3–7 describe theoretical issues on etiological mechanisms and Chaps. 8–11 describe the treatment of various cases, from different theoretical viewpoints.

We would like to thank all our authors, who enrich this book with their interesting contributions. Many thanks also to Mr. G. Styllos (psychoanalyst), who played a decisive role in the planning and organization of the conference, which stimulated the idea for the current volume.

Dillenburg, Germany Christos Charis
Nicosia, Cyprus Georgia Panayiotou

References

American Psychiatric Association. (2013). *Diagnostic and statistical manual of mental disorders (DSM-5®)*. American Psychiatric Pub.

Kazdin, A. E. (1979). Nonspecific treatment factors in psychotherapy outcome research. *Journal of Consulting and Clinical Psychology, 47*, 846–851.

Oei, T. P., & Shuttlewood, G. J. (1996). Specific and nonspecific factors in psychotherapy: A case of cognitive therapy for depression. *Clinical Psychology Review, 16*, 83–103.

Contents

Contributors

Thröstur Björgvinsson, Ph.D., ABPP McLean Hospital, Belmont, MA, USA
Harvard Medical School, Belmont, MA, USA

Werner Bohleber, Ph.D. Frankfurt am Main, Germany

Christos Charis, Dr. med Dillenburg, Germany

Elena Constantinou, Ph.D. Social, Genetic and Developmental Psychiatry Centre, Institute of Psychiatry, Psychology and Neuroscience, King's College London, London, UK

Evangelos C. Karademas, Ph.D. Department of Psychology, University of Crete, Rethymno, Greece

Maria Karekla, Ph.D. Department of Psychology, University of Cyprus, Nicosia, Cyprus

Maria Koushiou, Ph.D. Department of Social Sciences, University of Nicosia, Nicosia, Cyprus

Reinholde Kriebel, Ph.D. Essen, Germany

Chrysanthi Leonidou, Ph.D. Department of Psychology, University of Cyprus, Nicosia, Cyprus

Marianne Leuzinger-Bohleber, Ph.D. Sigmund Freud-Institut, Frankfurt am Main, Germany

Jacob A. Nota, Ph.D. McLean Hospital, Belmont, MA, USA
Harvard Medical School, Boston, MA, USA

Gerhard Paar, Dr. med Essen, Germany

Georgia Panayiotou, Ph.D. Department of Psychology and Center for Applied Neuroscience, University of Cyprus, Nicosia, Cyprus

Lauren Rutter, Ph.D. McLean Hospital, Belmont, MA, USA
Harvard Medical School, Boston, MA, USA

Ann Schaefer, Ph.D. Köln, Germany

Karl-Heinz Stäcker, Ph.D. Department of Psychology, University of Essen-Duisburg, Essen, Germany

Miryam Yusufov, Ph.D. McLean Hospital, Belmont, MA, USA
Harvard Medical School, Boston, MA, USA

Marianna Zacharia, M.Sc. Department of Psychology, University of Cyprus, Nicosia, Cyprus

Chapter 1
Maintaining Mechanisms of Health Anxiety: Current State of Knowledge

Chrysanthi Leonidou and Georgia Panayiotou

Health anxiety (HA), or illness anxiety as currently referred to in the literature, is the distorted preoccupation that the individual has or will acquire a severe medical illness, although medical examinations do not support this belief (Rachman, 2012). Individuals with high levels of HA hold dysfunctional beliefs regarding health and illness that are usually triggered by illness-related information, which may come from an environmental source or bodily sensations (Marcus, Gurley, Marchi, & Bauer, 2007). These dysfunctional beliefs often include an overestimated possibility of having a severe disease or overestimation of the severity of a disease, an increased number of perceived negative consequences and difficulties when facing a health problem (Rachman, 2012) and perceived limited availability of medical and health-care resources in the individual's environment (Hadjistavropoulos et al., 2012). When they experience ambiguous symptoms, health-anxious individuals interpret them as catastrophic and as signs of an illness, which may be fatal if not diagnosed immediately (Fulton, Marcus, & Merkey, 2011). They also believe that serious illnesses are highly prevalent and tend to define good health as a state of being totally symptom-free (Fulton et al., 2011; Rief & Broadbent, 2007). In addition to dysfunctional beliefs, health-anxious individuals experience frequent intrusive thoughts and images either related to past experiences of an illness they or significant others were diagnosed with or linked to a traumatic memory, e.g., maltreatment, as well as images about receiving a diagnosis, suffering from an illness, and dying, and the impact of their death or severe illness on significant others (Muse, McManus, Hackmann, Williams, & Williams, 2010). Depending on the severity of the preoccupation with

C. Leonidou (✉)
Department of Psychology, University of Cyprus, Nicosia, Cyprus
e-mail: leonidou.chrysanthi@ucy.ac.cy

G. Panayiotou
Department of Psychology and Center for Applied Neuroscience, University of Cyprus, Nicosia, Cyprus
e-mail: georgiap@ucy.ac.cy

C. Charis, G. Panayiotou (eds.), *Somatoform and Other Psychosomatic Disorders*,
https://doi.org/10.1007/978-3-319-89360-0_1

health and illness, these beliefs, intrusive thoughts, and images influence the individual's daily functioning.

HA presents on a continuum in the general population, ranging from low to high, pathological levels. Severe HA is a core characteristic of illness anxiety disorder, which is described in the section "Somatic Symptom Disorders" in the fifth edition of the *Diagnostic and Statistical Manual* (American Psychiatric Association, 2013). In addition to excessive levels of anxiety about health, diagnostic criteria include a preoccupation with having or acquiring a serious illness being present for at least 6 months, lower threshold of alarms about personal health status, excessive health-related behaviors such as repeated checks of the body for signs of an illness, and maladaptive avoidance (i.e., of doctors or hospitals). For the diagnosis, these criteria should be met, while somatic symptoms, medical conditions, or high risk of developing a medical condition are absent or if present, they are only mild in intensity or the preoccupation is excessive. This new diagnostic category also proposes two specifiers of the disorder: the care-seeking type, i.e., individuals who frequently seek medical care and the care-avoidant type, i.e., individuals who rarely use medical care because they are too anxious to seek medical attention.

Prevalence and Demographic Characteristics

Since illness anxiety disorder is a new diagnostic category, epidemiological data about its prevalence are based on past studies assessing hypochondriasis or severe HA. These data suggest that the prevalence in medical clinics is 9% (Creed & Barsky, 2004) and 5% in the general population (Asmundson, Taylor, & Cox, 2001), while the epidemiological data presented in DSM-5 refer to an estimation of 1.3–10.0% of illness anxiety disorder in the general population and 3–8% in medical clinic populations (American Psychiatric Association, 2013). Existing evidence on the demographic characteristics of health-anxious individuals is not consistent regarding differences in the prevalence of the disorder related to gender or age. While there was no evidence for gender differences in HA in a series of previous reports (American Psychiatric Association, 2013; Barsky, Wyshak, Klerman, & Latham, 1990; Gureje, Üstun, & Simon, 1997; Leibbrand, Hiller, & Fichter, 2000), there is one study reporting a significant difference between genders, with women reporting higher levels of HA, compared to men (MacSwain et al., 2009). Regarding age, existing evidence linked younger age to hypochondriasis (Magariños, Zafar, Nissenson, & Blanco, 2002), whereas other studies reported nonsignificant correlations between age and hypochondriasis (Barsky, Frank, Cleary, Wyshak, & Klerman, 1991; Leibbrand et al., 2000). Further studies examining the link between demographic characteristics and the prevalence of HA, controlling for factors that may influence these associations, such as presence of medical diagnoses, are needed for more conclusive results.

Impact

Considering the somatic complaints and the constant worry about having or acquiring an illness, it is expected that the daily functioning of these individuals suffers. More specifically, high levels of HA were linked to increased psychological distress (Chaturvedi, Desai, & Shaligram, 2006), interpersonal difficulties, absences from work and unemployment (Terluin, van Rhenen, Anema, & Taris, 2011), lower levels of health-related quality of life (Hyphantis et al., 2009), depression, anxiety, and impact on functionality (Sempertegui, Karreman, van Hout, & Bekker, 2016). In an assessment of the impact of high HA on specific domains of quality of life (Leonidou, Panayiotou, Karekla, & Bati, 2016), it was found that individuals who met HA screening criteria had significantly lower levels of physical and environmental quality of life, as compared to a healthy control group. These findings indicate how health-anxious individuals perceive their functioning in the physical domain and the absence of environmental resources to meet their safety and health-related needs. The above difficulties are often manifested by frequent healthcare visits and excessive healthcare costs (Barsky, Orav, & Bates, 2005; Burton, 2003; Grabe, Baumeister, John, Freyberger, & Völzke, 2009; Kroenke, 2003), which not only affect the individuals but also impact the public healthcare sector and society. In addition to the relatively high prevalence of HA symptomatology, its devastating impact raises the importance of understanding HA symptomatology in order to help health-anxious individuals improve their well-being and to reduce the impact of this category of symptomatology on the societal level.

The Cognitive-Behavioral Conceptualization of Health Anxiety

Following earlier attempts to describe hypochondriasis in psychodynamic terms, the cognitive-behavioral model of HA and hypochondriasis was proposed by Warwick and Salkovskis (1990) to conceptualize the development and maintenance of HA. This model suggests that individuals with high levels of HA form dysfunctional cognitive schemas and beliefs based on previous experiences related to health or illness. These schemas are activated either during health-related critical incidents or when encountering health or illness-related information. The activation of these schemas induces negative automatic thoughts and interacts with mechanisms that seem to maintain HA. These mechanisms can be seen in the domain of cognition, i.e., selective attention, rumination, self-focus, and thinking errors; emotion, i.e., anxiety, depression, and anger; physiology, i.e., increased arousal, bodily sensations, and sleep disturbance; and behavior, i.e., reassurance seeking, avoidance, bodily checking, and safety strategies.

A Brief Overview of Developmental and Predispositional Factors

Although the focus of this chapter will be on factors that were linked to the maintenance of HA, a brief overview of developmental and predispositional factors is provided here as these factors form the basis of the maintenance mechanisms of HA in adulthood. The cognitive-behavioral model described above refers to previous experiences related to illness and health, which based on empirical research, mainly include illnesses during childhood of the individuals themselves or of significant others (Noyes et al., 2002; Thastum et al., 2009). Anxiety about health and related behaviors are therefore developed and reinforced either through instrumental learning, i.e., a reinforced "patient role" and reinforced health-related safety behaviors, indicated by reports of frequently getting sick and more sick leaves from school (Olatunji, Etzel, Tomarken, Ciesielski, & Deacon, 2011; Watt et al., 2000; Watt, O'Connor, Stewart, Moon, & Terry, 2008), or through vicarious learning, i.e., modeling of a reinforced "patient role" (Salkovskis & Warwick, 2001; Watt et al., 2008).

In addition to this, and although the cognitive-behavioral model focuses mostly on previous health-related experiences as predisposing factors of HA, existing literature also describes a range of other developmental and predispositional factors that were linked to high levels of HA. These factors include distressing and traumatic events in childhood, such as childhood maltreatment (Hager & Runtz, 2012; Kim & Cicchetti, 2009; Waldinger, Schulz, Barsky, & Ahern, 2006; Weck et al., 2010), which seems to be related to HA through the mediating role of poor emotion regulation; fearful temperament and behavioral inhibition (Buss & Kiel, 2013); and insecure attachment as proposed by the interpersonal model of HA (Noyes et al., 2003; Sherry et al., 2014; Stuart & Noyes, 1999).

An additional predispositional factor that has both hereditary and environmental roots is anxiety sensitivity, defined as the fear toward anxiety symptoms and their perceived negative consequences, which was found to increase the possibility of anxiety disorder diagnoses. Empirical findings show that anxiety sensitivity is also a risk factor for severe HA (Bravo & Silverman, 2001; Frazier & Waid, 1999; Leonidou, Panayiotou, Bati, & Karekla, 2014b; Olatunji, Deacon, & Abramowitz, 2009; Otto, Pollack, Sachs, & Rosenbaum, 1992). It was positively correlated with the difficulty of health-anxious individuals to disengage their attention from health-threatening stimuli, an indication of hyper-vigilance to threat (Jasper & Witthoft, 2011), and it was predictive of bodily vigilance and emotional avoidance (Zvolensky & Forsyth, 2002). The empirical studies that examine the developmental factors linked to HA are for the most part limited to the studies that were briefly presented here. However, the factors described predispose the development of mechanisms that have been linked to the perpetuation and precipitation of HA, which received more attention in the related research field and are the main focus of this chapter.

Maintenance Mechanisms

The remainder of this chapter focuses on mechanisms that were linked to the maintenance of HA, which have a theoretical basis in the cognitive-behavioral model and have been supported by existing empirical evidence. The maintenance mechanisms are discussed below under the categories that correspond to the cognitive, affective, physiological, and behavioral dimensions of HA.

Cognitive Mechanisms

It was mentioned above that illness-related cognitive schemas, which are developed through early experiences, are activated, in addition to dysfunctional beliefs, and guide information processing. Due to the activation of illness-related schemas, it is tentative that cognitive processes of attention, memory and interpretation employed during processing of health-threatening information are influenced by the content of these schemas, which may result in biased and selective processing of information.

Attentional biases Early literature on hypochondriasis and HA proposed that selective attention toward internal or external health-threatening cues plays an important role in the development and maintenance of HA (Kellner, 1986). The attentional system of health-anxious individuals is particularly sensitive and biased to these cues (Marcus et al., 2007), and this was supported by evidence from studies examining attentional biases using experimental methods (Gropalis, Bleichhardt, Hiller, & Witthöft, 2012; Karademas, Christopoulou, Dimostheni, & Pavlu, 2008; Owens, Asmundson, Hadjistavropoulos, & Owens, 2004; Van Den Heuvel et al., 2005; Witthoft et al., 2016; Witthöft et al., 2013; Witthöft, Rist, & Bailer, 2008). More specifically, health-anxious individuals present an attentional bias toward health-threatening stimuli, characterized by an early focus of attention in short stimulus exposure duration and a slower disengagement of attention from health-threatening cues in long stimulus exposure durations (Jasper & Witthoft, 2011; Kim & Lee, 2014; Lee et al., 2013). These attentional biases were further linked to HA-related behaviors indicating an association between healthcare seeking and a difficulty in disengaging attention from health-threatening words (Kim, Kim, & Lee, 2014; Kim & Lee, 2014) and an association between healthcare avoidance and an avoidant pattern of processing these words, as indicated by the early disengagement of attention (Kim et al., 2014). Other studies also linked these attentional processes to dispositional coping strategies applied during information processing: Monitoring (i.e., vigilance for threatening information throughout the whole processing continuum) was linked to the difficulty in disengaging attention, and blunting (i.e., initial direction of attention to threat and shift of attention away from the threat as soon as threat is identified) was linked to the difficulty in engaging attention to health-threatening stimuli (Kim et al., 2014; Kim & Lee, 2014). This means that health-anxious individuals, by focusing their attention very early on the threat, cannot inhibit unnecessary information processing, and by applying later-onset attentional processes, such as avoidance and maintenance of attention, they cannot process information in a way that will help them to adaptively deal with the health threat.

Memory and interpretation biases In addition to how individuals allocate their attentional resources, biased processing is applied when storing information in memory and during retrieval of this information. It seems that individuals with high levels of HA store and retrieve information in a way that supports their fear about the potential health threat. Although memory biases were not included as a maintaining mechanism in theoretical models of HA, these processes play an important role in perception and interpretation of health-threatening cues (Martin, Buech, Schwenk, & Rief, 2007). Experimental studies reported a faster recognition of words related to health, illness, and bodily pain, compared to other types of words, and this was linked to increased levels of HA (Ferguson, Moghaddam, & Bibby, 2007; Gropalis et al., 2012; Hitchcock & Mathews, 1992; Pauli & Alpers, 2002; Schmidt, Witthöft, Kornadt, Rist, & Bailer, 2013; Witthoft et al., 2016), while future-directed memory seems to be also biased in health-anxious individuals, who tend to report increased number of illness-related events in a future memory task (Sansom-Daly, Bryant, Cohn, & Wakefield, 2014). Considering that these individuals store in their memory health-related information as threatening and that this information is retrieved in situations when the related schema is activated after being triggered by new health-related information, it is expected that interpretation and attribution processes are also influenced by biases. In fact, there is evidence about the link between HA, a biased response to ambiguous phrases with illness-related attributions (Hitchcock & Mathews, 1992), a biased interpretation of information, including health scenarios and bodily symptoms, in a catastrophic way (Bailey & Wells, 2015, 2016; Rief & Hiller, 1998) and a tendency to give more somatic and moderate or severe disease attributions and less normalizing attributions to bodily symptoms (MacLeod, Haynes, & Sensky, 1998; Neng & Weck, 2015). These memory and interpretation biases make health-anxious individuals vulnerable during memorizing, retrieving, and interpreting health-related information accessible in their environment or provided by healthcare professionals and medical examination results, and this seems to maintain and increase HA and related behaviors.

Physiological Mechanisms

Interoceptive awareness The empirical evidence presented above mainly refers to biased processing of health-threatening information coming from the environment. However, similar to other anxiety and somatoform disorders, somatic sensations are a main source of information about their health status for this population. Cognitive processes of attention, memory, and interpretation seem to also be biased during the processing of somatic sensations and bodily changes, resulting in the interpretation of these sensations as signs of a medical disease. To understand this process of misattribution of somatic sensations, it is necessary to look into the concepts of interoception, defined as the perception of sensory events in the body, including visceral perception and representation of changes in physiological reactivity (Cameron, 2002; Craig & Craig, 2002), and interoceptive awareness, the ability to accurately perceive bodily sensations, body condition, and activity. Enhanced interoceptive awareness helps with information processing and in dealing with threats presented in the individual's environment (Pollatos, Matthias, & Schandry, 2007); however, interoceptive awareness seems to suffer in individuals with high HA.

Although health-anxious individuals frequently report a high number of somatic sensations and symptoms, empirical evidence supports that they have lower accuracy in detecting these sensations, such as in the heartbeat tracking task that assesses interoceptive sensitivity, and more false alarms in identifying non-specific skin conductance fluctuations (Krautwurst, Gerlach, Gomille, Hiller, & Witthöft, 2014; Krautwurst, Gerlach, & Witthöft, 2016; Mailloux & Brener, 2002). This is also supported by the finding that habitual somatic symptom reporters self-report increased awareness of somatic sensations (Duddu, Chaturvedi, & Isaac, 2003); however, they are poor performers on objective measures of interoception (Fairclough & Goodwin, 2007). Individuals with high HA levels seem to be characterized by an increased attention toward interoceptive cues, which may be related to frequent symptom reporting and lower threshold for somatic sensations. However, their interoceptive attention seems to be inaccurate and possibly biased due to other processes that take place during interoceptive information processing.

Somatosensory amplification The theory of somatosensory amplification may help to understand the associations described above between attention toward somatic sensations and interoception. Health-anxious individuals generally tend to amplify normal somatic sensations (Bailey & Wells, 2015, 2016; Barsky & Wyshak, 1990; Köteles & Simor, 2014; Köteles, Szemerszky, Freyler, & Bárdos, 2011; Marcus et al., 2007; Rief & Hiller, 1998; Zincir et al., 2016) and are characterized by intolerance of and lower threshold for physical discomfort and heightened attentional focus on somatic sensations, which suggests hyper-vigilance tendencies (Gramling, Clawson, & McDonald, 1996; Katzer, Oberfeld, Hiller, & Witthöft, 2011; Rodic, Meyer, Lieb, & Meinlschmidt, 2016). The somatosensory amplification hypothesis for hypochondriasis (Gramling et al., 1996; Köteles et al., 2011; Marcus et al., 2007; Warwick & Salkovskis, 1990) supports that these individuals are more vigilant to their interoceptive experiences. Body vigilance was found to be a risk factor for anxiety disorders as it enhances perception of bodily sensations that are disorder-relevant and may mimic health problems. It was further linked to avoidant and safety-seeking behaviors, anxiety sensitivity, and healthcare utilization, an association mediated by health-related worries and the feared consequences of having a medical disease (Olatunji, Deacon, Abramowitz, & Valentiner, 2007). This provides evidence for the associations between HA and increased attention to the body. This association between body vigilance and HA may explain the tendency of health-anxious individuals to misinterpret normal and innocuous somatic sensations as signs of a medical disease. As these individuals fear having or acquiring a severe medical disease, this interpretation results in inflated emotional reactivity, something that amplifies the intensity of their somatic sensations. More attention is then focused on confirming the identified signs, leading to even more increased physiological arousal, maintaining the vicious cycle of somatosensory amplification. The maintenance of this cycle seems to also maintain vigilance toward somatic sensations and thus anxiety about health in health-anxious individuals.

Affective Mechanisms

Based on theories of emotion (Damasio, 1994, 1999; James, 1984; Schachter & Singer, 1962), interoception also plays an important role in the experience of emotions, and this may explain why the affective experience of individuals with high levels of HA also influences health-threatening, interoceptive, and environmental information processing. Illness-related cognitive schemas are often developed under distressing conditions; therefore, in addition to other information stored in memory about health and illness, aspects of the emotional experience, such as negative valence and increased arousal, are also stored and then retrieved when these schemas are activated.

Negative affect Memory networks that include both illness-related and affective information may provide some explanation about the link between hypochondriac concerns and increased levels of general trait negative emotionality, in addition to illness-specific anxiety (Hitchcock & Mathews, 1992). Focusing on the affective experience during bodily sensations processing, there is further evidence showing that higher trait negative affectivity is related to lower accuracy in respiratory volume perception, especially during a distressing condition (Bogaerts et al., 2005) and that bodily symptoms within an unpleasant affective content are perceived as more unpleasant (Constantinou, 2014). This may support that both trait and state negative affectivity, and more generally the dimension of negative emotional valence, which was found to be increased in individuals with HA (Jasper & Witthöft, 2013; Schreiber, Neng, Heimlich, Witthöft, & Weck, 2014; Witthoft et al., 2016; Witthöft et al., 2008), influence interoceptive accuracy.

In addition, studies using more objective measures of emotion, focused on the emotional arousal elicited during health-threatening information processing. More specifically, a baseline hypo-reactivity, linked to hyper-vigilance toward somatic sensations among hypochondriacs, and a following increased psychophysiological arousal during the stress-inducing period was recorded in a study looking into the perceptual and cognitive abnormality model of hypochondriasis (Gramling et al., 1996). Evidence from another study further supports increased psychophysiological arousal during illness imagery among hypervigilants, i.e., individuals who pay attention to and report high number of somatic symptoms, which also characterizes health-anxious individuals. However, in contrast to studies that link state negative affect with symptom perception in similar populations, illness imagery and the elicited psychophysiological arousal were not experienced as more unpleasant in this sample (Brownlee, Leventhal, & Balaban, 1992). This shows a discrepancy between components of emotional experience that, as suggested by the authors of this study, may be explained by the tendency of this population to attribute somatic sensations to symptoms or signs of a medical disease, ignoring that these sensations may be part of their emotional experience. Another suggestion is that in an effort to tone down the experienced psychophysiological reactivity, they verbally interpret it as less negative, and this may be reflect an avoidant coping strategy. Both suggestions are relevant to hypotheses about health-threatening information processing that are under investigation in the HA research field.

Emotion regulation and coping The above associations between negative affect, HA and symptom perception are also likely to be influenced by emotion regulation and coping strategies used by health-anxious individuals to regulate negative affect. Emotion regulation techniques regulate behavioral, physiological, and cognitive responses toward threatening cues. When used maladaptively in the long term, they may be dysfunctional and linked to anxiety disorders (Cisler & Koster, 2010). Studies examining emotion regulation among health-anxious individuals, supported the link between high HA and difficulties in emotion regulation, reduced perceived access to effective emotion regulation strategies (Bardeen & Fergus, 2014) and alexithymic characteristics (Zincir et al., 2016), i.e., difficulties in identifying and describing their feelings (Parker, Bagby, & Taylor, 1989; Taylor, Bagby, & Parker, 1997). Avoidant coping and behavioral disengagement as dispositional coping strategies were linked to higher severity of HA symptomatology, and these strategies were found to be increased in groups with high levels of HA and somatization symptomatology, compared to healthy controls (Leonidou et al., 2016). This is in line with existing evidence showing that suppression (Görgen, Hiller, & Witthöft, 2014) and cognitive avoidance (Fergus & Valentiner, 2010) were positively related to HA and illness-related beliefs. This evidence supports the link between the avoidant approach to coping and emotion regulation and HA.

In addition to specific coping and emotional regulation strategies, a more general trait, namely, experiential avoidance, was also linked to HA. Experiential avoidance is the tendency of individuals to avoid experiencing bodily sensations, emotions, thoughts, memories, images, and behavioral predispositions and to change the form or the frequency of these experiences or the triggers of these experiences, especially when they are aversive in nature (Hayes et al., 2004). The findings of a series of studies suggested a strong link between somatization and experiential avoidance (Tull, Gratz, Salters, & Roemer, 2004; Zvolensky & Forsyth, 2002), and this can be explained by the psychological discomfort as a paradoxical effect of the avoidance of negative experiences (Kashdan, Barrios, Forsyth, & Steger, 2006). In line with this evidence, experiential avoidance was found to be a significant positive predictor of HA and a partial mediator in the relationship between anxiety sensitivity and HA (Leonidou, Panayiotou, Bati, & Karekla, 2014a). These two traits seem to be two interrelated factors that play an important role in the onset and maintenance mechanisms of severe HA. The tendency of individuals to avoid internal experiences seems to underlie the link between their fear toward anxiety-related sensations and their level of anxiety about health. In another study (Leonidou & Panayiotou, 2016), the prediction of HA levels by experiential avoidance was replicated, and experiential avoidance was found to mediate the relationship between attentional control and HA. Attentional control is the executive ability to direct attention, and since the impairment in the volitional control of attention is a prominent feature in anxiety disorders (Cisler & Koster, 2010), it was expected to be related to HA. It seems that the tendency to avoid internal experiences also underlies the relationship between low perceived attentional control skills and high levels of HA. Both experiential avoidance and attentional control may be related and exacerbate HA symptoms, as traits relevant to attentional biases in health-related information processing (i.e., vigilance-avoidance hypothesis; Derakshan, Eysenck, & Myers, 2007).

In addition to the avoidant coping and the dispositional tendency to use avoidance when dealing with health-related threats, further strategies that were positively related to cognitive, emotional, and behavioral aspects of HA were rumination, catastrophizing, and blaming others (Görgen et al., 2014). These strategies predicted automatic negative evaluation of ambiguous information, when this follows the presentation of illness-related cues in individuals with high HA (Jasper & Witthöft, 2013; Marcus et al., 2008). Rumination was also linked to retrieval of specific past illness-related memories but predicted generalized and categorical illness-related thoughts about the future (Sansom-Daly et al., 2014), showing that the strategies used to regulate elicited emotion interact with cognitive mechanisms during information processing. The ruminative approach to regulate emotion, in this case, results in the retrieval of past memories, which may remind individuals of their vulnerability to illnesses but at the same time makes them unable to think about strategies that will help them deal with a future illness, resulting in avoidant behaviors. This is also supported by evidence showing that among the most frequent responses to intrusive images about illness were reassurance seeking, checking, distraction, and rumination (Muse et al., 2010). These emotion regulation strategies, which can be seen as HA-related behaviors, seem to perpetuate and precipitate HA.

Behavioral Mechanisms

In addition to the coping responses toward health-related threats presented above, there is also a range of more overt behaviors that were linked to HA and serve as a maintenance mechanism. Maladaptive behavioral responses to health threats prevent the identification of information that contradicts the perceived health threat, giving false safety beliefs or distract attention away from this information (Salkovskis, 1991; Tang et al., 2007). For health-anxious individuals, safety behaviors include avoidance of hospitals, medical centers, patients, and funerals; frequent visits to healthcare professionals, medical examinations, and checks; self-examination; compulsive reassurance seeking by healthcare professionals, the Internet, and books; compulsive searching for information that supports their fear; compulsive checking of body for signs of a disease; and excessive cleaning and excessive concerns about food preparation and intake (Rachman, 2012). There is also evidence from experimental paradigms that during exposure to illness-related conditions, health-anxious participants showed increased avoidance behaviors accompanied by high anxiety and disgust levels (Brady & Lohr, 2014; Goetz, Lee, & Cougle, 2012), while exposure to personally relevant HA triggers provoked anxiety and urges to repeatedly perform safety behaviors, which lasted and were further exacerbated in the long term (Abramowitz & Moore, 2007). All the above behaviors maintain HA through negative reinforcement (Olatunji et al., 2011; Rachman, Radomsky, & Shafran, 2008; Salkovskis, 2003), a mechanism that is also supported by evidence on the effect of health-related safety behaviors on increased HA and hypochondriacal beliefs, selective attention to and more behavioral avoidance of possible health threats (Olatunji et al., 2011). It was also mentioned above that behaviors such as healthcare avoidance and healthcare seeking were linked to attentional processes, something that highlights the interaction between cognitive, affective, and behavioral mechanisms that maintain HA.

To summarize, the mechanisms that seem to underlie the maintenance of HA based on the current state of knowledge include attentional, memory, and interpretation biases during information processing, biased interoceptive awareness, somatosensory amplification, negative affect, and dysfunctional emotional regulation and dispositional coping strategies and HA-related behaviors that aim at reducing distress in the short term but are counterproductive in the long term. Theoretically based and empirically supported knowledge about the mechanisms that seem to maintain HA is important in the conceptualization of HA, since these mechanisms consist of factors that can be modified through prevention and therapeutic interventions that are specifically directed in altering these mechanisms in an effort to effectively reduce the suffering of individuals with HA symptoms.

A Buffering Mechanism

In addition to the maintenance mechanisms of HA, identification of possible buffering mechanisms may also be beneficial in terms of therapeutic effectiveness. Psychological flexibility, defined as the ability to focus on the present moment using a mindful and accepting stance toward the experiences and the capacity to use coping strategies flexibly depending on the context (Bonanno, Papa, Lalande, Westphal, & Coifman, 2004; Karekla & Panayiotou, 2011; Panayiotou, Karekla, & Mete, 2014; Thompson, 1994), is associated with more adaptive functioning, better mental and physical health, life satisfaction, and positive affect (Eftekhari, Zoellner, & Vigil, 2009; Haga, Kraft, & Corby, 2009; Hu et al., 2014), and it also reduces negative emotions, anxiety, and somatization (Masuda & Tully, 2012). And there is, in fact, evidence showing that psychological flexibility buffers the effects of the severity of somatization and HA symptoms on the physical, social, and environmental domains of quality of life (Leonidou et al., 2016). This provides preliminary evidence that a psychological intervention aiming at enhancing psychological flexibility of individuals with high levels of HA may improve their perceived quality of life, as it allows individuals to remain engaged and active in their daily life focusing on their valued goals. Other potential buffering mechanisms, such as social support, need to be investigated in future studies.

Overview of Behavioral and Cognitive Approaches in Therapy

Existing literature suggests theory-based treatment approaches, which are also supported by empirical evidence about their effectiveness in reducing HA levels. Cognitive-behavioral therapy (CBT) is the treatment approach that is more widely examined for its effectiveness in treating HA, supported by randomized controlled trials on individually provided sessions (Tyrer et al., 2014) and on Internet-based sessions (Hedman et al., 2011), while a meta-analysis suggests that CBT is an effective treatment for severe HA (Olatunji et al., 2014). Other treatment approaches for HA stem from the third wave of behavioral therapies and include mindfulness-based cognitive therapy (MBCT) and acceptance and commitment therapy (ACT), and there is preliminary evidence, although mainly from pilot studies, supporting their effectiveness (Eilenberg, Kronstrand, Fink, & Frostholm, 2013; Lovas & Barsky, 2010; McManus, Muse, Surawy, Hackmann, & Williams, 2015; Williams, McManus, Muse, & Williams, 2011). Finally, attentional bias modification training (ABMT) received some attention in the research field of HA; however, results are still limited and contradictory (Lee, Goetz, Turkel, & Siwiec, 2015; Papageorgiou & Wells, 1998). The above treatment approaches for severe HA, and especially those that were only pilot tested, warrant further investigation.

To overview the therapeutic components that seem to be especially helpful in treating HA, these include: (1) Psychoeducation on emotions and emotion regulation, as this may help individuals to understand the aspects of their emotional experience and to learn to apply emotion regulation and coping strategies adaptively. (2) Mindfulness may be useful to practice maintenance of attention on somatic sensations without efforts to control or judgmentally interpret them and focusing on experiencing and accepting them (Hedman et al., 2011; Surawy, McManus, Muse, & Williams, 2015). (3) Interoceptive exposure may help in dealing with anxiety sensitivity, fear, avoidance, and misinterpretation of somatic sensations (Taylor & Asmundson, 2004). (4) Behavioral experiments may be useful to reduce repetitive checking and reassurance and healthcare seeking (Warwick, Clark, Cobb, & Salkovskis, 1996) and may be applied using exposure and response prevention (Asmundson, Abramowitz, Richter, & Whedon, 2010). (5) Challenging illness-related dysfunctional beliefs may be especially helpful when these are linked to experiences of illness (Alberts & Hadjistavropoulos, 2014). Since cognitive and behavioral approaches to therapy aim at modifying specific mechanisms, which are the same mechanisms that underlie the development and maintenance of HA, enriching and tailoring these approaches specifically for this population and further testing their effectiveness will be another step toward treating HA.

Summary

Severe HA is characterized by excessive worry about multiple somatic symptoms and impairs individual's functioning in the psychological, social, professional, and other domains of daily life. This chapter, following the description of this category of symptomatology in terms of epidemiology, predispositional factors, and impact, focuses on reviewing mechanisms that maintain HA, which stem from the cognitive-behavioral conceptualization of HA and existing empirical evidence. It seems evident that cognitive, affective, physiological, and behavioral mechanisms interact during health-threatening information processing in a way that HA and related behaviors are maintained in individuals with high levels of HA. Understanding these maintenance mechanisms in depth, and further identifying possible buffering mechanisms, is crucial for the design of prevention and therapeutic interventions for this population. In conclusion, there is still need for further investigation of some of the mechanisms introduced by the cognitive-behavioral model and the interaction between them and for the examination of possible individual differences in health-threatening information processing among specific groups of health-anxious individuals, e.g., care seekers and care avoiders.

References

Abramowitz, J. S., & Moore, E. L. (2007). An experimental analysis of hypochondriasis. *Behaviour Research and Therapy*, 45(3), 413–424. https://doi.org/10.1016/j.brat.2006.04.005

Alberts, N. M., & Hadjistavropoulos, H. D. (2014). Parental illness, attachment dimensions, and health beliefs: Testing the cognitive-behavioural and interpersonal models of health anxiety. *Anxiety, Stress, and Coping, 27*(2), 216–228. https://doi.org/10.1080/10615806.2013.835401

American Psychiatric Association. (2013). *Diagnostic and statistical manual of mental disorders (DSM-5)* (5th ed.). Washington, DC: American Psychiatric Publishing. https://doi.org/10.1080/09515070801936578

Asmundson, G., Taylor, S., & Cox, B. (2001). *Health anxiety: Clinical and research perspectives on hypochondriasis and related conditions.* New York: Wiley. https://doi.org/10.1348/014466502760379181

Asmundson, G. J. G., Abramowitz, J. S., Richter, A. A., & Whedon, M. (2010). Health anxiety: Current perspectives and future directions. *Current Psychiatry Reports, 12*(4), 306–312. https://doi.org/10.1007/s11920-010-0123-9

Bailey, R., & Wells, A. (2015). Metacognitive beliefs moderate the relationship between catastrophic misinterpretation and health anxiety. *Journal of Anxiety Disorders, 34*, 8–14. https://doi.org/10.1016/j.janxdis.2015.05.005

Bailey, R., & Wells, A. (2016). Is metacognition a causal moderator of the relationship between catastrophic misinterpretation and health anxiety? A prospective study. *Behaviour Research and Therapy, 78*, 43–50. https://doi.org/10.1016/j.brat.2016.01.002

Bardeen, J. R., & Fergus, T. A. (2014). An examination of the incremental contribution of emotion regulation difficulties to health anxiety beyond specific emotion regulation strategies. *Journal of Anxiety Disorders, 28*(4), 394–401. https://doi.org/10.1016/j.janxdis.2014.03.002

Barsky, A. J., Frank, C. B., Cleary, P. D., Wyshak, G., & Klerman, G. L. (1991). The relation between hypochondriasis and age. *The American Journal of Psychiatry, 148*(7), 923–928.

Barsky, A. J., Orav, E. J., & Bates, D. W. (2005). Somatization increases medical utilization and costs independent of psychiatric and medical comorbidity. *Archives of General Psychiatry, 62*(8), 903. https://doi.org/10.1001/archpsyc.62.8.903

Barsky, A. J., & Wyshak, G. (1990). Hypochondriasis and somatosensory amplification. *British Journal of Psychiatry, 157*(3), 404–409. https://doi.org/10.1192/bjp.157.3.404

Barsky, A. J., Wyshak, G., Klerman, G. L., & Latham, K. S. (1990). The prevalence of hypochondriasis in medical outpatients. *Social Psychiatry and Psychiatric Epidemiology, 25*(2), 89–94. https://doi.org/10.1007/BF00794988

Bogaerts, K., Notebaert, K., Van Diest, I., Devriese, S., De Peuter, S., & Van Den Bergh, O. (2005). Accuracy of respiratory symptom perception in different affective contexts. *Journal of Psychosomatic Research, 58*(6), 537–543. https://doi.org/10.1016/j.jpsychores.2004.12.005

Bonanno, G. A., Papa, A., Lalande, K., Westphal, M., & Coifman, K. (2004). The importance of being flexible: The ability to both enhance and suppress emotional expression predicts long-term adjustment. *Psychological Science, 15*(7), 482–487. https://doi.org/10.1111/j.0956-7976.2004.00705.x

Brady, R. E., & Lohr, J. M. (2014). A behavioral test of contamination fear in excessive health anxiety. *Journal of Behavior Therapy and Experimental Psychiatry, 45*(1), 122–127. https://doi.org/10.1016/j.jbtep.2013.09.011

Bravo, I. M., & Silverman, W. K. (2001). Anxiety sensitivity, anxiety, and depression in older patients and their relation to hypochondriacal concerns and medical illnesses. *Aging & Mental Health, 5*(4), 349–357. https://doi.org/10.1080/13607860120080305

Brownlee, S., Leventhal, H., & Balaban, M. (1992). Autonomic correlates of illness imagery. *Psychophysiology, 29*(2), 142–153. https://doi.org/10.1111/j.1469-8986.1992.tb01677.x

Burton, C. (2003). Beyond somatisation: A review of the understanding and treatment of medically unexplained physical symptoms (MUPS). *British Journal of General Practice, 53*(488), 231–239.

Buss, K. A., & Kiel, E. J. (2013). Temperamental risk factors for pediatric anxiety disorders. In R. A. Vasa & A. Krain Roy (Eds.), *Pediatric anxiety disorders: A clinical guide* (pp. 47–68). New York: Springer. https://doi.org/10.1007/978-1-4614-6599-7_3

Cameron, O. G. (2002). *Visceral sensory neuroscience: Interoception*. New York: Oxford University Press.

Chaturvedi, S. K., Desai, G., & Shaligram, D. (2006). Somatoform disorders, somatization and abnormal illness behaviour. *International Review of Psychiatry, 18*(1), 75–80. https://doi.org/10.1080/09540260500467087

Cisler, J. M., & Koster, E. H. W. (2010). Mechanisms of attentional biases towards threat in anxiety disorders: An integrative review. *Clinical Psychology Review, 30*(2), 203–216. https://doi.org/10.1016/j.cpr.2009.11.003

Constantinou, E. (2014). *Affective processing of interoceptive information in persons with medically unexplained symptoms*. Leuven: KU Leuven.

Craig, A. D., & Craig, A. D. (2002). How do you feel? Interoception: The sense of the physiological condition of the body. *Nature Reviews. Neuroscience, 3*(8), 655–666. https://doi.org/10.1038/nrn894

Creed, F., & Barsky, A. (2004). A systematic review of the epidemiology of somatisation disorder and hypochondriasis. *Journal of Psychosomatic Research, 56*(4), 391–408. https://doi.org/10.1016/S0022-3999(03)00622-6

Damasio, A. R. (1994). *Descartes' error: Emotion, reason and the human brain*. New York: Grosset/Putman.

Damasio, A. R. (1999). *The feeling of what happens: Body and emotion in the making of consciousness*. New York: Harcourt Brace.

Derakshan, N., Eysenck, M. W., & Myers, L. B. (2007). Emotional information processing in repressors: The vigilance-avoidance theory. *Cognition & Emotion, 21*(8), 1585–1614. https://doi.org/10.1080/02699930701499857

Duddu, V., Chaturvedi, S. K., & Isaac, M. K. (2003). Amplification and attribution styles in somatoform and depressive disorders: A study from Bangalore, India. *Psychopathology, 36*(2), 98–103. https://doi.org/10.1159/000070365

Eftekhari, A., Zoellner, L. A., & Vigil, S. A. (2009). Patterns of emotion regulation and psychopathology. *Anxiety, Stress & Coping, 22*(5), 571–586. https://doi.org/10.1080/10615800802179860

Eilenberg, T., Kronstrand, L., Fink, P., & Frostholm, L. (2013). Acceptance and commitment group therapy for health anxiety: Results from a pilot study. *Journal of Anxiety Disorders, 27*(5), 461–468. https://doi.org/10.1016/j.janxdis.2013.06.001

Fairclough, S. H., & Goodwin, L. (2007). The effect of psychological stress and relaxation on interoceptive accuracy: Implications for symptom perception. *Journal of Psychosomatic Research, 62*(3), 289–295. https://doi.org/10.1016/j.jpsychores.2006.10.017

Fergus, T. A., & Valentiner, D. P. (2010). Disease phobia and disease conviction are separate dimensions underlying hypochondriasis. *Journal of Behavior Therapy and Experimental Psychiatry, 41*(4), 438–444. https://doi.org/10.1016/j.jbtep.2010.05.002

Ferguson, E., Moghaddam, N. G., & Bibby, P. A. (2007). Memory bias in health anxiety is related to the emotional valence of health-related words. *Journal of Psychosomatic Research, 62*(3), 263–274. https://doi.org/10.1016/j.jpsychores.2007.01.015

Frazier, L. D., & Waid, L. D. (1999). Influences on anxiety in later life: The role of health status, health perceptions, and health locus of control. *Aging & Mental Health, 3*(3), 213–220. https://doi.org/10.1080/13607869956163

Fulton, J. J., Marcus, D. K., & Merkey, T. (2011). Irrational health beliefs and health anxiety. *Journal of Clinical Psychology, 67*(6), 527–538. https://doi.org/10.1002/jclp.20769

Goetz, A. R., Lee, H.-J., & Cougle, J. R. (2012). The association between health anxiety and disgust reactions in a contamination-based behavioral approach task. *Anxiety, Stress & Coping, 26*(4), 1–16. https://doi.org/10.1080/10615806.2012.684241

Görgen, S. M., Hiller, W., & Witthöft, M. (2014). Health anxiety, cognitive coping, and emotion regulation: A latent variable approach. *International Journal of Behavioral Medicine, 21*(2), 364–374. https://doi.org/10.1007/s12529-013-9297-y

Grabe, H. J., Baumeister, S. E., John, U., Freyberger, H. J., & Völzke, H. (2009). Association of mental distress with health care utilization and costs: A 5-year observation in a general population. *Social Psychiatry and Psychiatric Epidemiology, 44*(10), 835–844. https://doi.org/10.1007/s00127-009-0005-9

Gramling, S. E., Clawson, E. P., & McDonald, M. K. (1996). Perceptual and cognitive abnormality model of hypochondriasis: Amplification and physiological reactivity in women. *Psychosomatic Medicine, 58*(5), 423–431. Retrieved from http://www.ncbi.nlm.nih.gov/pubmed/8902894.

Gropalis, M., Bleichhardt, G., Hiller, W., & Witthöft, M. (2012). Specificity and modifiability of cognitive biases in hypochondriasis. *Journal of Consulting and Clinical Psychology, 81*(3), 558–565. https://doi.org/10.1037/a0028493

Gureje, O., Üstun, T. B., & Simon, G. E. (1997). The syndrome of hypochondriasis: A cross-national study in primary care. *Psychological Medicine, 27*(5), 1001–1010.

Hadjistavropoulos, H. D., Janzen, J. A., Kehler, M. D., Leclerc, J. A., Sharpe, D., & Bourgault-Fagnou, M. D. (2012). Core cognitions related to health anxiety in self-reported medical and non-medical samples. *Journal of Behavioral Medicine, 35*(2), 167–178. https://doi.org/10.1007/s10865-011-9339-3

Haga, S. M., Kraft, P., & Corby, E.-K. (2009). Emotion regulation: Antecedents and well-being outcomes of cognitive reappraisal and expressive suppression in cross-cultural samples. *Journal of Happiness Studies, 10*(3), 271–291. https://doi.org/10.1007/s10902-007-9080-3

Hager, A. D., & Runtz, M. G. (2012). Physical and psychological maltreatment in childhood and later health problems in women: An exploratory investigation of the roles of perceived stress and coping strategies. *Child Abuse & Neglect, 36*(5), 393–403. https://doi.org/10.1016/j.chiabu.2012.02.002

Hayes, S. C., Strosahl, K., Wilson, K. G., Bissett, R. T., Pistorello, J., Toarmino, D., … McCurry, S. M. (2004). Measuring experiential avoidance: A preliminary test of a working model. *The Psychological Record, 54*(4), 553–578.

Hedman, E., Andersson, G., Andersson, E., Ljótsson, B., Rück, C., Asmundson, G. J. G., & Lindefors, N. (2011). Internet-based cognitive-behavioural therapy for severe health anxiety: Randomised controlled trial. *British Journal of Psychiatry, 198*(3), 230–236. https://doi.org/10.1192/bjp.bp.110.086843

Hitchcock, P. B., & Mathews, A. (1992). Interpretation of bodily symptoms in hypochondriasis. *Behaviour Research and Therapy, 30*(3), 223–234. https://doi.org/10.1016/0005-7967(92)90068-R

Hu, T., Zhang, D., Wang, J., Mistry, R., Ran, G., & Wang, X. (2014). Relation between emotion regulation and mental health: A meta-analysis review. *Psychological Reports: Measures & Statistics, 114*(2), 341–362. https://doi.org/10.2466/03.20.PR0.114k22w4

Hyphantis, T., Tomenson, B., Paika, V., Almyroudi, A., Pappa, C., Tsifetaki, N., … Creed, F. (2009). Somatization is associated with physical health-related quality of life independent of anxiety and depression in cancer, glaucoma and rheumatological disorders. *Quality of Life Research, 18*(8), 1029–1042. https://doi.org/10.1007/s11136-009-9527-6

James, W. (1984). What is emotion? *Mind, 9*, 188–205.

Jasper, F., & Witthoft, M. (2011). Health anxiety and attentional bias: The time course of vigilance and avoidance in light of pictorial illness information. *Journal of Anxiety Disorders, 25*(8), 1131–1138. https://doi.org/10.1016/j.janxdis.2011.08.004

Jasper, F., & Witthöft, M. (2013). Automatic evaluative processes in health anxiety and their relations to emotion regulation. *Cognitive Therapy and Research, 37*(3), 521–533. https://doi.org/10.1007/s10608-012-9484-1

Karademas, E. C., Christopoulou, S., Dimostheni, A., & Pavlu, F. (2008). Health anxiety and cognitive interference: Evidence from the application of a modified Stroop task in two studies. *Personality and Individual Differences, 44*(5), 1138–1150. https://doi.org/10.1016/j.paid.2007.11.007

Karekla, M., & Panayiotou, G. (2011). Coping and experiential avoidance: Unique or overlapping constructs? *Journal of Behavior Therapy and Experimental Psychiatry, 42*(2), 163–170. https://doi.org/10.1016/j.jbtep.2010.10.002

Kashdan, T. B., Barrios, V., Forsyth, J. P., & Steger, M. F. (2006). Experiential avoidance as a generalized psychological vulnerability: Comparisons with coping and emotion regulation strategies. *Behaviour Research and Therapy, 44*(9), 1301–1320. https://doi.org/10.1016/j.brat.2005.10.003

Katzer, A., Oberfeld, D., Hiller, W., & Witthöft, M. (2011). Tactile perceptual processes and their relationship to medically unexplained symptoms and health anxiety. *Journal of Psychosomatic Research, 71*(5), 335–341. https://doi.org/10.1016/j.jpsychores.2011.03.009

Kellner, R. (1986). *Somatization and hypochondriasis*. Santa Barbara, CA: Praeger.

Kim, J., & Cicchetti, D. (2009). Longitudinal pathways linking child maltreatment, emotion regulation, peer relations, and psychopathology. *Journal of Child Psychology and Psychiatry, 51*(6), 706–716. https://doi.org/10.1111/j.1469-7610.2009.02202.x

Kim, S., Kim, K., & Lee, J.-H. (2014). Effects of dispositional coping strategy and level of health anxiety on attention bias. *Social Behavior & Personality: An International Journal, 42*(7), 1183–1190. https://doi.org/10.2224/sbp.2014.42.7.1183

Kim, S., & Lee, J. H. (2014). Time course of attentional bias for health-related information in individuals with health anxiety. *Journal of Health Psychology, 21*(8), 1527–1535. https://doi.org/10.1177/1359105314557976

Köteles, F., & Simor, P. (2014). Modern health worries, somatosensory amplification, health anxiety, and well-being: A cross-sectional study. *European Journal of Mental Health, 9*(1), 20–33. https://doi.org/10.5708/EJMH.9.2014.1.2

Köteles, F., Szemerszky, R., Freyler, A., & Bárdos, G. (2011). Somatosensory amplification as a possible source of subjective symptoms behind modern health worries. *Scandinavian Journal of Psychology, 52*(2), 174–178. https://doi.org/10.1111/j.1467-9450.2010.00846.x

Krautwurst, S., Gerlach, A. L., Gomille, L., Hiller, W., & Witthöft, M. (2014). Health anxiety: An indicator of higher interoceptive sensitivity? *Journal of Behavior Therapy and Experimental Psychiatry, 45*(2), 303–309. https://doi.org/10.1016/j.jbtep.2014.02.001

Krautwurst, S., Gerlach, A. L., & Witthöft, M. (2016). Interoception in pathological health anxiety. *Journal of Abnormal Psychology, 125*(8), 1179–1184. https://doi.org/10.1037/abn0000210

Kroenke, K. (2003). Patients presenting with somatic complaints: Epidemiology, psychiatric comorbidity and management. *International Journal of Methods in Psychiatric Research, 12*(1), 34–43. https://doi.org/10.1002/mpr.140

Lee, H., Turkel, J. E., Cotter, S. P., Milliken, J. M., Cougle, J., Goetz, A. R., & Lesnick, A. M. (2013). Attentional bias toward personally relevant health-threat words. *Anxiety, Stress & Coping, 26*(5), 493–507. https://doi.org/10.1080/10615806.2012.713474

Lee, H. J., Goetz, A. R., Turkel, J. E., & Siwiec, S. G. (2015). Computerized attention retraining for individuals with elevated health anxiety. *Anxiety, Stress, and Coping, 28*(2), 226–237. https://doi.org/10.1080/10615806.2014.918964

Leibbrand, R., Hiller, W., & Fichter, M. M. (2000). Hypochondriasis and somatization: Two distinct aspects of somatoform disorders? *Journal of Clinical Psychology, 56*(1), 63–72. https://doi.org/10.1002/(SICI)1097-4679(200001)56:1<63::AID-JCLP6>3.0.CO;2-O

Leonidou, C., & Panayiotou, G. (2016). Assessing health anxiety with the Greek SHAI and identifying correlates and predictors. In *Oral presentation at the 30th Annual Conference of the European Health Psychology Society*, Aberdeen, Scotland.

Leonidou, C., Panayiotou, G., Bati, A., & Karekla, M. (2014a). Correlates and predictors of severe health anxiety. In *Poster presented at the 4th Annual Conference of the Centre of Applied Neuroscience*, Nicosia, Cyprus.

Leonidou, C., Panayiotou, G., Bati, A., & Karekla, M. (2014b). Factors associated with the clinical levels of somatization and hypochondriasis: The role of anxiety and panic symptoms. In *Poster presented at the EABCT Congress* (p. 19). Hague, Netherlands: Psychomed.

Leonidou, C., Panayiotou, G., Karekla, M., & Bati, A. (2016). Coping with psychosomatic symptoms: The buffering role of psychological flexibility and impact on quality of life. *Journal of Health Psychology*. https://doi.org/10.1177/1359105316666657

Lovas, D. A., & Barsky, A. J. (2010). Mindfulness-based cognitive therapy for hypochondriasis, or severe health anxiety: A pilot study. *Journal of Anxiety Disorders, 24*(8), 931–935. https://doi.org/10.1016/j.janxdis.2010.06.019

MacLeod, A. K., Haynes, C., & Sensky, T. (1998). Attributions about common bodily sensations: Their associations with hypochondriasis and anxiety. *Psychological Medicine, 28*(1), 225–228. https://doi.org/10.1017/S0033291797005849

MacSwain, K. L. H., Sherry, S. B., Stewart, S. H., Watt, M. C., Hadjistavropoulos, H. D., & Graham, A. R. (2009). Gender differences in health anxiety: An investigation of the interpersonal model of health anxiety. *Personality and Individual Differences, 47*(8), 938–943. https://doi.org/10.1016/j.paid.2009.07.020

Magariños, M., Zafar, U., Nissenson, K., & Blanco, C. (2002). Epidemiology and treatment of hypochondriasis. *CNS Drugs, 16*(1), 9–22. https://doi.org/10.2165/00023210-200216010-00002

Mailloux, J., & Brener, J. (2002). Somatosensory amplification and its relationship to heartbeat detection ability. *Psychosomatic Medicine, 64*(2), 353–357. https://doi.org/10.1097/00006842-200203000-00020

Marcus, D. K., Gurley, J. R., Marchi, M. M., & Bauer, C. (2007). Cognitive and perceptual variables in hypochondriasis and health anxiety: A systematic review. *Clinical Psychology Review, 27*(2), 127–139. https://doi.org/10.1016/j.cpr.2006.09.003

Marcus, D. K., Hughes, K. T., Arnau, R. C., Salkovskis, P., Warwick, H., Salkovskis, P., … Baer, R. (2008). Health anxiety, rumination, and negative affect: A mediational analysis. *Journal of Psychosomatic Research, 64*(5), 495–501. https://doi.org/10.1016/j.jpsychores.2008.02.004

Martin, A., Buech, A., Schwenk, C., & Rief, W. (2007). Memory bias for health-related information in somatoform disorders. *Journal of Psychosomatic Research, 63*(6), 663–671. https://doi.org/10.1016/j.jpsychores.2007.05.005

Masuda, A., & Tully, E. C. (2012). The role of mindfulness and psychological flexibility in somatization, depression, anxiety, and general psychological distress in a nonclinical college sample. *Journal of Evidence-Based Complementary & Alternative Medicine, 17*(1), 66–71. https://doi.org/10.1177/2156587211423400

McManus, F., Muse, K., Surawy, C., Hackmann, A., & Williams, J. M. G. (2015). Relating differently to intrusive images: The impact of mindfulness-based cognitive therapy (MBCT) on intrusive images in patients with severe health anxiety (hypochondriasis). *Mindfulness, 6*(4), 788–796. https://doi.org/10.1007/s12671-014-0318-y

Muse, K., McManus, F., Hackmann, A., Williams, M., & Williams, M. (2010). Intrusive imagery in severe health anxiety: Prevalence, nature and links with memories and maintenance cycles. *Behaviour Research and Therapy, 48*(8), 792–798. https://doi.org/10.1016/j.brat.2010.05.008

Neng, J. M. B., & Weck, F. (2015). Attribution of somatic symptoms in hypochondriasis. *Clinical Psychology and Psychotherapy, 22*(2), 116–124. https://doi.org/10.1002/cpp.1871

Noyes, R., Stuart, S., Langbehn, D. R., Happel, R. L., Longley, S. L., Yagla, S. J., … Goldberg, S. (2002). Childhood antecedents of hypochondriasis. *Psychosomatics, 43*(4), 282–289. https://doi.org/10.1176/appi.psy.43.4.282

Noyes, R., Stuart, S. P., Langbehn, D. R., Happel, R. L., Longley, S. L., Muller, B. A., & Yagla, S. J. (2003). Test of an interpersonal model of hypochondriasis. *Psychosomatic Medicine, 65*(2), 292–300. Retrieved from http://www.ncbi.nlm.nih.gov/pubmed/12651997.

Olatunji, B. O., Deacon, B. J., & Abramowitz, J. S. (2009). Is hypochondriasis an anxiety disorder? *British Journal of Psychiatry, 194*(6), 481–482. https://doi.org/10.1192/bjp.bp.108.061085

Olatunji, B. O., Deacon, B. J., Abramowitz, J. S., & Valentiner, D. P. (2007). Body vigilance in nonclinical and anxiety disorder samples: Structure, correlates, and prediction of health concerns. *Behavior Therapy, 38*(4), 392–401. https://doi.org/10.1016/j.beth.2006.09.002

Olatunji, B. O., Etzel, E. N., Tomarken, A. J., Ciesielski, B. G., & Deacon, B. (2011). The effects of safety behaviors on health anxiety: An experimental investigation. *Behaviour Research and Therapy, 49*(11), 719–728. https://doi.org/10.1016/j.brat.2011.07.008

Olatunji, B. O., Kauffman, B. Y., Meltzer, S., Davis, M. L., Smits, J. A. J. J., & Powers, M. B. (2014). Cognitive-behavioral therapy for hypochondriasis/health anxiety: A meta-analysis of treatment outcome and moderators. *Behaviour Research and Therapy, 58*, 65–74. https://doi.org/10.1016/j.brat.2014.05.002

Otto, M. W., Pollack, M. H., Sachs, G. S., & Rosenbaum, J. F. (1992). Hypochondriacal concerns, anxiety sensitivity, and panic disorder. *Journal of Anxiety Disorders, 6*(2), 93–104. https://doi.org/10.1016/0887-6185(92)90008-U

Owens, K., Asmundson, G., Hadjistavropoulos, T., & Owens, T. (2004). Attentional bias toward illness threat cues in individuals with health anxiety. *Cognitive Therapy and Research, 28*(1), 57–66. https://doi.org/10.1023/B:COTR.0000016930.85884.29

Panayiotou, G., Karekla, M., & Mete, I. (2014). Dispositional coping in individuals with anxiety disorder symptomatology: Avoidance predicts distress. *Journal of Contextual Behavioral Science, 3*(4), 314–321. https://doi.org/10.1016/j.jcbs.2014.07.001

Papageorgiou, C., & Wells, A. (1998). Effects of attention training on hypochondriasis: A brief case series. *Psychological Medicineedicine, 28*(1), 193–200. https://doi.org/10.1017/S0033291797005825

Parker, J. D. A., Bagby, R. M., & Taylor, G. J. (1989). Toronto alexithymia scale, EPQ and self-report measures of somatic complaints. *Personality and Individual Differences, 10*(6), 599–604. https://doi.org/10.1016/0191-8869(89)90219-5

Pauli, P., & Alpers, G. W. (2002). Memory bias in patients with hypochondriasis and somatoform pain disorder. *Journal of Psychosomatic Research, 52*(1), 45–53. https://doi.org/10.1016/S0022-3999(01)00295-1

Pollatos, O., Matthias, E., & Schandry, R. (2007). Heartbeat perception and P300 amplitude in a visual oddball paradigm. *Clinical Neurophysiology, 118*(10), 2248–2253. https://doi.org/10.1016/j.clinph.2007.06.057

Rachman, S. (2012). Health anxiety disorders: A cognitive construal. *Behaviour Research and Therapy, 50*(7–8), 502–512. https://doi.org/10.1016/j.brat.2012.05.001
Rachman, S., Radomsky, A. S., & Shafran, R. (2008). Safety behaviour: A reconsideration. *Behaviour Research and Therapy, 46*(2), 163–173. https://doi.org/10.1016/j.brat.2007.11.008
Rief, W., & Broadbent, E. (2007). Explaining medically unexplained symptoms: Models and mechanisms. *Clinical Psychology Review, 27*(7), 821–841. https://doi.org/10.1016/j.cpr.2007.07.005
Rief, W., & Hiller, W. (1998). Cognitive aspects of hypochondriasis and the somatization syndrome. *Journal of Abnormal Psychology, 107*(4), 587–595. https://doi.org/10.1037/0021-843X.107.4.587
Rodic, D., Meyer, A. H., Lieb, R., & Meinlschmidt, G. (2016). The association of sensory responsiveness with somatic symptoms and illness anxiety. *International Journal of Behavioral Medicine, 23*(1), 39–48. https://doi.org/10.1007/s12529-015-9483-1
Salkovskis, P. M. (1991). The importance of behaviour in the maintenance of anxiety and panic: A cognitive account. *Behavioural and Cognitive Psychotherapy, 19*(1), 6–19.
Salkovskis, P. M. (2003). Cognitive-behavioral treatment for severe and persistent health anxiety (hypochondriasis). *Brief Treatment and Crisis Intervention, 3*(3), 353–368. https://doi.org/10.1093/brief-treatment/mhg026
Salkovskis, P. M., & Warwick, H. M. C. (2001). Meaning, misinterpretations, and medicine: A cognitive-behavioral approach to understanding health anxiety and hypochondriasis. In D. R. Starcevic & V. Lipsitt (Eds.), *Hypochondriasis: Modern perspectives on an ancient malady* (pp. 202–222). New York: Oxford University Press.
Sansom-Daly, U. M., Bryant, R. A., Cohn, R. J., & Wakefield, C. E. (2014). Imagining the future in health anxiety: The impact of rumination on the specificity of illness-related memory and future thinking. *Anxiety, Stress, and Coping, 27*(5), 587–600. https://doi.org/10.1080/10615806.2014.880111
Schachter, S., & Singer, J. E. (1962). Cognitive, social and psychological determinants of emotional state. *Psychological Review, 69*(5), 379–399.
Schmidt, E., Witthöft, M., Kornadt, A., Rist, F., & Bailer, J. (2013). Negative automatic evaluation and better recognition of bodily symptom words in college students with elevated health anxiety. *Cognitive Therapy and Research, 37*(5), 1027–1040. https://doi.org/10.1007/s10608-013-9540-5
Schreiber, F., Neng, J. M. B., Heimlich, C., Witthöft, M., & Weck, F. (2014). Implicit affective evaluation bias in hypochondriasis: Findings from the affect misattribution Procedure. *Journal of Anxiety Disorders, 28*(7), 671–678. https://doi.org/10.1016/j.janxdis.2014.07.004
Sempertegui, G. A., Karreman, A., van Hout, G. C., & Bekker, M. H. (2016). Functional status in patients with medically unexplained physical symptoms: Coping styles and their relationship with depression and anxiety. *Journal of Health Psychology.* https://doi.org/10.1177/1359105316638548
Sherry, D. L., Sherry, S. B., Vincent, N. A., Stewart, S. H., Hadjistavropoulos, H. D., Doucette, S., & Hartling, N. (2014). Anxious attachment and emotional instability interact to predict health anxiety: An extension of the interpersonal model of health anxiety. *Personality and Individual Differences, 56*, 89–94. https://doi.org/10.1016/j.paid.2013.08.025
Stuart, S., & Noyes, R. (1999). Attachment and interpersonal communication in somatization. *Psychosomatics, 40*(1), 34–43. https://doi.org/10.1016/S0033-3182(99)71269-7
Surawy, C., McManus, F., Muse, K., & Williams, J. M. G. (2015). Mindfulness-based cognitive therapy (MBCT) for health anxiety (hypochondriasis): Rationale, implementation and case illustration. *Mindfulness, 6*(2), 382–392. https://doi.org/10.1007/s12671-013-0271-1
Tang, N. K. Y., Salkovskis, P. M., Poplavskaya, E., Wright, K. J., Hanna, M., & Hester, J. (2007). Increased use of safety-seeking behaviors in chronic back pain patients with high health anxiety. *Behaviour Research and Therapy, 45*(12), 2821–2835. https://doi.org/10.1016/j.brat.2007.05.004

Taylor, G. J., Bagby, R. M., & Parker, J. D. A. (1997). *Disorders of affect regulation: Alexithymia in medical and psychiatric illness* (Vol. 7). Cambridge: Cambridge University Press. https://doi.org/10.1002/1099-0879(200007)7:3<240::AID-CPP245>3.0.CO;2-7

Taylor, S., & Asmundson, G. J. G. (2004). What is health anxiety? In *Treating health anxiety: A cognitive-behavioral approach* (pp. 1–18). New York: Guilford.

Terluin, B., van Rhenen, W., Anema, J. R., & Taris, T. W. (2011). Psychological symptoms and subsequent sickness absence. *International Archives of Occupational and Environmental Health, 84*(7), 825–837. https://doi.org/10.1007/s00420-011-0637-4

Thastum, M., Watson, M., Kienbacher, C., Piha, J., Steck, B., Zachariae, R., … Romer, G. (2009). Prevalence and predictors of emotional and behavioural functioning of children where a parent has cancer. *Cancer, 115*(17), 4030–4039. https://doi.org/10.1002/cncr.24449

Thompson, R. A. (1994). Emotion regulation: A theme in search of definition. *Monographs of the Society for Research in Child Development, 59*(2–3), 25–52. https://doi.org/10.1111/j.1540-5834.1994.tb01276.x

Tull, M. T., Gratz, K. L., Salters, K., & Roemer, L. (2004). The role of experiential avoidance in posttraumatic stress symptoms and symptoms of depression, anxiety, and somatization. *The Journal of Nervous and Mental Disease, 192*(11), 754–761. Retrieved from http://www.ncbi.nlm.nih.gov/pubmed/15505519.

Tyrer, P., Cooper, S., Salkovskis, P., Tyrer, H., Crawford, M., Byford, S., … Barrett, B. (2014). Clinical and cost-effectiveness of cognitive behaviour therapy for health anxiety in medical patients: A multicentre randomised controlled trial. *The Lancet, 383*(9913), 219–225. https://doi.org/10.1016/S0140-6736(13)61905-4

Van Den Heuvel, O. A., Veltman, D. J., Groenewegen, D. J., Witter, M. P., Merkelbach, J., Cath, D. C., … Van Dyck, R. (2005). Disorder-specific neuroanatomical correlates of attentional bias in obsessive-compulsive disorder. *Panic Disorder, and Hypochondriasis, 62*(8), 922–933.

Waldinger, R. J., Schulz, M. S., Barsky, A. J., & Ahern, D. K. (2006). Mapping the road from childhood trauma to adult somatization: The role of attachment. *Psychosomatic Medicine, 68*(1), 129–135. https://doi.org/10.1097/01.psy.0000195834.37094.a4

Warwick, H., & Salkovskis, P. (1990). Hypochondriasis. *Behaviour Research and Therapy, 28*(2), 105–117. Retrieved from http://www.sciencedirect.com/science/article/pii/000579679090023C.

Warwick, H. M., Clark, D. M., Cobb, A. M., & Salkovskis, P. M. (1996). A controlled trial of cognitive-behavioural treatment of hypochondriasis. *The British Journal of Psychiatry, 169*(2), 189–195.

Watt, M. C., O'Connor, R. M., Stewart, S. H., Moon, E. C., & Terry, L. (2008). Specificity of childhood learning experiences in relation to anxiety sensitivity and illness/injury sensitivity: Implications for health anxiety and pain. *Journal of Cognitive Psychotherapy, 22*(2), 128–142. https://doi.org/10.1891/0889-8391.22.2.128

Watt, M. C., Stewart, S. H., Asmundson, G., Norton, G., Asmundson, G., Taylor, S., … Costa, P. (2000). Anxiety sensitivity mediates the relationships between childhood learning experiences and elevated hypochondriacal concerns in young adulthood. *Journal of Psychosomatic Research, 49*(2), 107–118. https://doi.org/10.1016/S0022-3999(00)00097-0

Weck, F., Neng, J. M. B., Göller, K., Müller-Marbach, A. M., Witthöft, M., Hiller, W., … Craig, T. K. (2010). Previous experiences with illness and traumatic experiences: A specific risk factor for hypochondriasis? *Psychosomatics, 55*(4), 362–371. https://doi.org/10.1016/j.psym.2013.10.005

Williams, M. J., McManus, F., Muse, K., & Williams, J. M. G. (2011). Mindfulness-based cognitive therapy for severe health anxiety (hypochondriasis): An interpretative phenomenological analysis of patients' experiences. *British Journal of Clinical Psychology, 50*(4), 379–397. https://doi.org/10.1111/j.2044-8260.2010.02000.x

Witthoft, M., Kerstner, T., Ofer, J., Mier, D., Rist, F., Diener, C., … Witthöft, M. (2016). Cognitive biases in pathological health anxiety: The contribution of attention, memory, and evaluation processes. *Clinical Psychological Science, 4*(3), 464–479. https://doi.org/10.1177/2167702615593474

Witthöft, M., Mier, D., Ofer, J., Müller, T., Rist, F., Kirsch, P., … Diener, C. (2013). Neuronal and behavioral correlates of health anxiety: Results of an illness-related emotional Stroop task. *Neuropsychobiology, 67*(2), 93–102. https://doi.org/10.1159/000345545

Witthöft, M., Rist, F., & Bailer, J. (2008). Enhanced early emotional intrusion effects and proportional habituation of threat response for symptom and illness words in college students with elevated health anxiety. *Cognitive Therapy and Research, 32*(6), 818–842. https://doi.org/10.1007/s10608-007-9159-5

Zincir, S. B., Sunbul, M., Sunbul, E. A., Dalkilic, B., Cengiz, F., Kivrak, T., & Durmus, E. (2016). Evaluation of alexithymia, somatosensory sensitivity, and health anxiety levels in patients with noncardiac chest pain health anxiety levels in patients with noncardiac chest pain. *Biomedical Research International, 2014*, 1–6. https://doi.org/10.1155/2014/896183

Zvolensky, M. J., & Forsyth, J. P. (2002). Anxiety sensitivity dimensions in the prediction of body vigilance and emotional avoidance. *Cognitive Therapy and Research, 26*(4), 449–460. https://doi.org/10.1023/A:1016223716132

Chapter 2
Somatoform Disorders from Psychodynamic Point of View

Christos Charis

Introduction

We know the term "Hysteria" and with that connected the specialised concept of "conversion". Besides that there are the terms "dissociation" and "somatisation" (Hoffmann, Eckhardt-Henn, & Scheidt, 2004; Kroll, 1932; Stekel, 1924; Woolfolk & Allen, 2007) (see Table 2.1).

The main function of these theories is to explain psychosomatic symptoms.

The term Hysteria comes from Greek. It was established by Hippocrates. The ancient Greeks (Hippocrates, Plato) believed that Hysteria (the womb) wanders through the body, tries to find semen and in a sense bites the brain and stays there. Because of that this state causes different symptoms. That means Hysteria is a female illness (King, 1993). Today we describe it as a "psychosexual conflict" (Schneider, Sattel, Ronnel, & Henningsen, 2012, p. 11). Charcot and Möbius studied Hysteria systematically. Freud, who spent 6 months with Charcot, was influenced and also studied Hysteria. The former coined the term "conversion" (Breuer & Freud, 1895; Hoffmann et al., 2004).

Hysteria and conversion symptoms represent a conflict between a desire and reality ("defence mechanism"). Therefore, the patient unconsciously represses his/her emotions/wishes/fantasies, because he/she believes that they do not belong to him/her. This phenomenon is termed psychodynamics. Charcot believed that psychosomatic symptoms are due to mental conflicts, which are repressed, and they result in neuromuscle overfunction. In 1859 Briquet described an extreme sensitivity of the nervous system on external stimuli as a cause of psychosomatic symptoms, like pain in the upper abdomen and on the left side of the thorax. Briquet observed that these patients have panic attacks and sensorimotor paralysis too (Hoffmann et al., 2004).

C. Charis (✉)
Dillenburg, Germany

C. Charis, G. Panayiotou (eds.), *Somatoform and Other Psychosomatic Disorders*,
https://doi.org/10.1007/978-3-319-89360-0_2

Table 2.1 Historical background

Hysteria (Charcot, 1825–1893)
Conversion (Freud "Studien der Hysterie", 1895)
Dissociation (Janet, 1859–1947)
Somatisation (Stekel 1924; Kroll, 1932 in the journal: *Psychoanalytische Praxis*)

Dissociation is a description, meaning splitting of the ego because of a trauma. This disturbance begins earlier than Hysteria. Janet used dissociation to describe unintegrated experiences (Hoffmann et al., 2004). The latter term means that the victim is unable verbally to express the associated events and his emotions.

Somatisation: W. Stekel, a physician, psychoanalyst and pupil of Freud, coined the concept somatisation in 1924. Kroll subsequently used that term in the magazine *Psychoanalytische Praxis* (*Psychoanalytical Practice*). It is a process which describes how mental distress is expressed through bodily responses. I am going to discuss later in this chapter the subject of somatisation.

Somatoform disorder is a term established in 1980 in the DSM-3. The ICD adopted that term later. Within that spectrum of disorders, as described in the DSM-3, we find all phenomena I have already mentioned: Hysteria, conversion, dissociation and somatisation.

Definition of Somatoform Disorders

Somatoform disorders are a group of disorders, which includes several clinically significant, physical symptoms, which cannot be fully explained by a general medical cause, and they are not the result of another mental disorder, for example, anxiety. Those patients are very sure that they have a physical illness, and they are worried about these symptoms. They do not accept a mental disorder as the cause of their symptoms. Therefore, there is a complicated interaction between the patient and the physician. The patient insists on more clinical examinations and more physical treatment. The practitioner is afraid that he cannot see a physical cause of the symptoms. If that occurs, the doctor may be afraid that he will be sued. The patient is disappointed, because the physician cannot find a physical cause for his symptoms. Therefore, he/she feels the physician is not taking him seriously, and then he/she changes to another medical practitioner ("doctor shopping", Egle, 1998, p. 95). For example, a patient of mine (Mr P) has had 12 different physicians. At the moment Mr P is back with his first doctor, Mr P is afraid the physicians have made mistakes in their diagnoses. Due to the pressure on the physician routine radiography is excessively promoted. For example, it can lead to harms, and it can alleviate patient anxiety about back pain (Chou, Qaseem, Owens, & Shekelle, 2011).

Table 2.2 Epidemiological data

Somatoform disorders are the third most common mental disorders after addiction and anxiety disorder in lifetime prevalence
"4–10% of the general population and 20% of primary care patients have what are *(is)* called 'non-specific, functional and somatoform bodily complaints'"
Seventeen percent of the population in Germany have chronic pains

Epidemiology

Schaefert et al. (2012) asserted "4–10% of the general population and 20% of primary care patients" have a somatoform disorder (p. 803). Somatoform disorders are the third most common mental disorders after addiction and anxiety disorder in lifetime prevalence (Meyer, Rumpf, Hapke, Dilling, & John, 2000). Seventeen percent of the population in Germany have chronic pains (Nobis, Rolke, Graf-Baumann, 2016) (see Table 2.2).

Epidemiological data show high comorbidities between somatoform and other mental health disorders, which grow with the seriousness of the somatoform condition. The patients suffer from depression, anxiety, post-traumatic stress disorders and personality disorders (Garcia-Campayo, Alda, Sobradiel, Olivan, & Pascual, 2007; Körber & Hiller, 2012). Depression is a very frequent comorbid disorder (mainly with somatisation disorder, reaching up to 47–97%), followed by anxiety disorders (20–70%) and personality disorders (Ebel & Podoll, 1998). My own experience on that subject is that I also see a very high comorbidity in somatoform disorders. Most of my patients have an allergic illness as well, something I cannot fully explain. Perhaps somatoform disorders are more severe illness than we think. My patients with a somatoform disorder have a familial aggregation of approximately 50%. That means that 50% of my patients have one or more brothers/sisters, who have a somatoform disorder, too.

Classification

The ICD-10 describes four groups of somatoform disorders: F 45.0 somatisation disorder and F 45.1 undifferentiated somatoform disorder. In that group we find general symptoms. F 45.2, hypochondriasis and F 45.3, somatoform autonomic dysfunction. In that group there are specific symptoms. F 45.4 includes persistent somatoform pain disorder (WHO ICD-10, 1992) (see Table 2.3).

Somatization disorder is a very rare and severe illness. It is most common in young women. The symptoms last at least 2 years. Mostly the patients have pains which change location. To that disorder category belong: vertigo, symptoms of the gastrointestinal tract, of the respiratory tract, with a tight chest, burning mouth and tongue burning and paraesthesias; sexual and menstrual complaints. Depression (44–100%) and anxiety disorders (20–70%) are very frequent in patients with

Table 2.3 Somatoform disorders in ICD-10

Somatization disorder F 45.0
Undifferentiated somatoform disorder F 45.1
Hypochondriasis F 45.2
Somatoform autonomic dysfunction F 45.3
Persistent somatoform pain disorder F 45.4

Table 2.4 DSM-5: somatic symptom and related disorders

Somatic symptom disorder: includes somatization disorder and undifferentiated somatoform disorder
Illness anxiety disorder: similar to hypochondriasis
Conversion disorder
Psychological factors affecting other medical conditions: attitudes or behaviours adversely influence the course or result of an existing medical illness
Factitious conditions: deliberately created artificial symptoms of a medical illness in order to obtain the sympathy given to people who are really ill, e.g. Munchausen syndrome

somatization. This disorder was previously called Briquet-Syndrom. The difference between persistent somatoform pain disorder and somatization disorder is that in the former, the location of the pain does not change. The patients do not have further symptoms unless they have another illness. In the case that a patient has hypochondria, he/she thinks that he/she is already ill and is worried about that, but he/she is not focused on symptoms, unlike other somatoform patients (Schneider et al., 2012).

In the DSM-5, there is an important change in the definition of the term somatoform disorders compared to what was described in DSM-4. For that diagnostic category, the DSM-5 established the "somatic symptom and related disorders". The category "somatoform disorders" has been abolished. The diagnosis (somatic symptom disorder and related disorders), which includes somatic symptom disorder, illness anxiety disorder, conversion disorder and psychological factors affecting other medical conditions and factitious conditions, represents an important change. This is because it focuses on the reaction of patients about their somatic symptoms (thoughts, emotions and behaviours), which are typically extreme. In patients where somatic symptoms can be medically explained, DSM-5 demands that all other criteria for the disorder should be fulfilled. Factitious disorder and psychological factors affecting other medical conditions have been added to somatic symptom disorder and other disorders. Conversion disorder remains the same as in DSM-4. Hypochondriasis is now called "illness anxiety disorder" (American Psychiatric Association, 2013) (see Table 2.4). Finally DSM-5 did not pay any consideration to the diagnosis of pain disorder, because it is very difficult to find out precisely if psychological factors are implicated in pain complaints (American Psychiatric Association, 2013).

How Do We Explain Somatoform Disorders Today?

A lot of factors affect the course and outcome of somatoform disorders. It is reported that "Current etiopathogenetic models assume complex interactions between psychosocial factors, biological factors, iatrogenic factors or factors related to the medical system and sociocultural factors which can lead to neurobiological changes, and act together in disposition, triggering and maintenance of the complaints" (Schaefert et al., 2012, p. 805).

Biological Aspects

If somebody has a pain in the chest, then his breathing has changed. If somebody has a somatization disorder, then the function of the serotonergic system has altered. If somebody who has a somatoform disorder speaks about stressful topics, then his muscles are stretched. These are examples of the biological factors which need to be considered. Their exact significance is still a matter of debate or speculation (Rief & Boadbrendt, 2007).

Psychological Risk Factors

Divorce of parents, death of parents, the feeling of being rejected by parents and experience of violence and sexual abuse all represent psychological factors. Also parents who have chronic pain themselves can act as models for the patient. Some patients with somatoform disorders develop a tendency to experience physical symptoms as severe, noxious and disturbing, defined as "somatosensory amplification" (Barsky & Wyshak, 1990). These factors are non-specific factors, which make the patient susceptible to developing a somatoform disorder (Schneider et al., 2012). We also know today that insecure attachment styles play an important role in developing somatization, because attachment style affects the interaction between the patient and his environment (DePaulo, 2010; Nickel & Egle, 1999).

Psychodynamic Models That Explain Somatoform Disorders

Psychodynamic therapy tries to verify if somatoform disorders arise out of a mental conflict or structure deficits or both. In this context "structure" means the structure of the personality from a psychodynamic point of view and includes six personality traits, including the capacity of self-perception and self-regulation, communication and bonding. These traits help the individual to regulate his/her self and to regulate one's relationships to the environment. If there are fewer resources in terms of regulating capabilities because the structure is less developed, that state is termed "structure deficits" (Arbeitskreis OPD, 2009). Alternatively somatoform disorders may be due to a trauma (see chapters by Leuzinger-Bohleber and Bohleber; Eckhardt-Henn, Heuft, Hochapfel, & Hoffmann, 2004; Wesiack & Schüßler, 2002; Küchenhoff, 1998). In addition to that, we try to understand if there is a correlation between the complaints of the patient and his mental situation. In other words a pain may, for instance, try to tell us something, and because of that, we try to find out what the pain wants to tell us. The aim of that way of thinking is to adjust the therapy to the problem of the patient. Some patients express a mental conflict symbolically through their symptoms, i.e. through conversion. As I said, Freud established this term. For example, somebody has a wish/fantasy, which is socially unacceptable. He/she may develop physical symptoms, which express the forbidden wish/fantasy. That means his/her unacceptable wish/fantasy is not conscious to him/her any more. Therefore, the patient experiences a relief of tension. We know today that conversion symptoms can arise in any organ system (Engel, 1970), and the complaints affect voluntary motor or sensory function. A famous example for that is the case of Anna O. (Breuer & Freud, 1895). Anna O. was a young German woman. Her father became ill, and she developed a cough while she was looking after her father. After that she spoke only English being unable to express herself in her native language, German. More hysterical symptoms appeared after her father died: she lost the feeling in her hands and feet and developed involuntary spasms, visual hallucinations and tunnel vision. She had dramatic mood swings, and she made multiple suicide attempts. She stopped eating. At night she went into a hypnotic-like state. She fell in love with her therapist (Breuer), and she believed that she was pregnant with his child. Freud explained these hysterical symptoms (this conversion) of Anna O. as unconscious sexual desires because of a childhood sexual abuse by her father. From that point of view, we can better understand why Anna O. had a paralysis whenever she was unconsciously reminded of her feelings towards her father. At the time her father died, she was sitting at his bedside with her arm pressed against the chair at the side of the bed. All these psychosomatic symptoms have a communicative aspect and express symbolically the mental conflict of Anna O. She saw herself as a weak, helpless, little girl through the conversion symptoms and not as an adult woman with sexual desires (Mentzos, 1980). Therefore, Anna O. feels a reduction in tension through her symptoms. That is an important function of psychosomatic complaints. Another paradigm for conversion is the case of some patients with heart neurosis. Most patients with heart neurosis have their symptoms as affect equivalents or affect correlation (see section on "Affect Equivalents"). The symptoms of cardiac neurosis can be very similar to that of a heart disease: shortness of breath, chest pain, exhaustion, palpitations, hyperventilation, dizziness, anxiety, fear and panic attacks. These patients believe that they suffer from a heart disease, but their heart is completely healthy. They unconsciously use their heart to symbolically express a mental message. These patients have not achieved independence from their mothers. They are sometimes said to be still tied to their mother's apron strings (Ermann, 2005; Richter

Table 2.5 Psychodynamic models for somatoform disorders

Conversion: Freud established this term. A famous example for that is the case of Anna O. Another paradigm of conversion is heart neurosis. Somatoform symptoms express symbolically a conflict
Narcissistic mechanism
Psychosomatic symptoms as affect equivalents (Fenichel, 1945). The majority of the psychosomatic symptoms are due to this defence mechanism. In contrast to conversion, there is no desire, no fantasy, which is socially unacceptable and causes these complaints. The psychosomatic symptoms are simply connected to emotions

& Beckmann, 2004). A patient of mine provides another example of converted symptoms, which is explained below.

"Narcissistic Mechanism"

Some patients express their narcissistic problems through chronic pain. We call that "narcissistic mechanism". The patient is in an existential crisis of his self-confidence, which is only just being compensated. Then a trauma or an accident happens by chance, and because of that his symptoms do not cease; they become chronic. The patient concentrates on the symptoms, and so he/she can forget his/her narcissistic crisis, which might have occurred, for example, when his/her partner left him/her (Eckhardt-Henn et al., 2004).

"Affect Equivalents"

As mentioned above, some patients express a mental conflict symbolically through their symptoms. Freud called that "conversion". Freud also realised that some patients have organic complaints without a symbolic meaning that are just connected to the emotions of the patient, for example, the symptoms of some patients with a heart neurosis: shortness of breath, chest pain, exhaustion, palpitations, hyperventilation and dizziness. All these complaints are connected to the emotions of anxiety and fear. Alexander (1951), one of the founders of psychosomatic medicine, suggested the term vegetative neuroses for this type of complaints. Fenichel (1945), a prominent psychoanalyst, called that phenomenon "affect equivalents". These symptoms are usually found in somatic systems not under voluntary control, for example, diarrhoea, sweating and a thumping heart, and are due to activity of autonomic nervous system. For example, when a patient with a somatoform disorder is afraid, he develops diarrhoea. The consequence is anxiety that may be replaced by feelings or sensations in the gastrointestinal tract. It is important to know that symptoms which act as affect equivalents have a communicative aspect. The patient wants to express something unspeakable by an archaic, body-bound language. It is of great influence for the therapy to distinguish between conversion symptoms and affect equivalents. When we realise that the patient converted his conflict on his body, then we must try to make clear the symbolic meaning of these bodily symptoms. If we recognise an affect equivalent, then the therapist must first refer to the affect and attempt to verbalise it; after that the unconscious conflict should be uncovered. This means to bring the unconscious material into the conscious. However it is not always possible to distinguish between affect equivalent and conversion, as, for example, some patients complain of pains. Sometimes patients have both. A case paradigm for that can be found in my other chapter. For severe personality disorders, such as borderline personality disorders, another therapeutical approach is needed (e.g. Fonagy, Gergely, Jurist, & Target, 2002).

Schur's Theory of Psychosomatic Symptoms

Shur, a pioneer of the psychosomatic medicine, has explained psychosomatic symptoms through inadequacies of the personality (mental structure). The development of the personality depends on the quality of the relationship between the child and his/her mother. If the mother validates the somatic experience of the child, then verbalisation and desomatization can take place. That means the child has learnt to put into words the associated facts and his/her emotions. The child has learnt to distinguish between somatic tension (e.g. due to hunger) and an emotional tension (e.g. due to anger). If the mother has failed to validate the bodily experiences of her child, then the child develops a faulty ego integration. If this individual comes later in his/her life in a mental crisis, then it develops psychosomatic symptoms because of the faulty ego. Schur (1955) called this phenomenon resomatization, and it corresponds to a psychological regression. (Regression means the ego reverts to an earlier stage of development.) Parallel to the resomatization of affects, a cognitive change takes place: some of the people with somatoform disorders focus their attention on their bodies and perceive normal physical sensations more intensely and interpret these as signs of a somatic disease (Barsky & Wyshak, 1990, "somatosensory amplification"). This process is, on the one hand, the result of the regression that has taken place, but it is also serves to ward off conflicts (Ermann, 2005).

Rudolf's and Henningsen's Theory of Somatoform Disorders

Further Rudolf (2006), an expert on personality disorders, and his colleague Henningsen, suggested a different concept for somatoform disorders. It focuses on the personality and is based on Fonagy's theory on mentalization (Fonagy et al., 2002). Fonagy describes how the interaction between the caregiver and the child needs to be for the development of the self (as secure and autonomous). This special social relationship (attachment) is the context within which the child learns to regulate its affects. It is important for the development of the child that the mother both mirrors the child's emotions and marks the child's emotional signals by her responses to the baby's behaviour. Acquired experience with violence, operations, traumata or emotional neglect, for example, by the significant persons (primary caregivers), who have been overstrained or ill, can lead to an impairment regarding the body ego, which means that the individual has a false perception of his/her body. In this event it is difficult for the person to distinguish between primarily bodily paraesthesia and emotional tension. Patients such as these develop on that basis psychosomatic symptoms, as Rudolf asserted. These patients feel helpless, when they are under stress because they could not learn how to effectively regulate their feelings. For example, if they are disappointed, they cannot make themselves calm or console themselves, or enlist somebody's assistance. They often try to compensate their personality impairments through being overactive. As a result they can be exploited. In turn they are overextended and frustrated. The aim of therapy is then to help them to learn to regulate their emotions. This therapeutic process was called "containment" by Bion, a famous psychoanalyst.

Diagnostic Issues

At the beginning of therapy during the initial examination, I try to identify the patient's psychodynamics. Does he/she have an unconscious conflict? Does he/she have a moderately/low-integrated structure? Or a mix of both? Does he/she have a psychological trauma? Mostly patients with a somatoform disorder have a conflict and also moderately integrated structure. In that case they have moderate impairments in personality (Rudolf & Henningsen, 2006; Ermann, 2005). The patient, who has an unconscious conflict, represses his/her emotions and develops psychosomatic symptoms because of this repression. Some people with a moderately integrated structure are not able to distinguish and to describe their own emotions. They also may have problems in identifying the emotions of other people. (We call them alexithymic.) These individuals develop psychosomatic symptoms (see Table 2.6).

Table 2.6 Diagnostic issues

Unconscious conflict?
A moderately/low-integrated structure?
Trauma (post-traumatic stress disorder)?
In most cases, there is a combination of conflict and a moderately integrated structure

How Do We Proceed in Practice?

The therapist has to take the time in order to find the descriptions of the patient's complaints and medical history. For this, cooperation with colleagues from other specialist disciplines and/or doctor's reports is necessary. For example, a somatoform pain disorder is not an exclusion diagnosis. This diagnosis includes the recording of a thorough biographical history including traumatization as well as the current mental-social situation of the patient. At this stage of our work, we can also use the operationalised psychodynamic diagnostics (OPD 2), which tries to grasp the psychodynamics: including dysfunctional relationship patterns, prominent conflicts and structure level (Arbeitskreis OPD, 2009). It is important to take care of comorbidity, for instance, if there is a severe depression, which must also be treated with antidepressants. For example, Mr K, a patient, was in a great deal of pain since surgery on a slipped disc in the lower back, which became acute in connection with mental distress. In addition to his persistent somatoform pain disorder (ICD-10 F 45.41), this patient also suffers from severe depression. After treating the depression with antidepressants successfully, we could also effectively influence his pain during the course of the psychotherapy. What should not be done is a repetition of the already existing physical diagnostics in order to soothe the patient. Then with that you achieve exactly the opposite. The physician contributes to the fact that an existing fixation on an organic cause is solidified even more. In practice, frequently morphological findings become manifest, but they do not provide a sufficient explanation for the patients' complaints. The doctor must be careful with those findings; otherwise the patient believes that he has got an organic illness, which causes his/her symptoms (Arbeitskreis PISO, 2012).

Summarising the Aims of the Diagnostic Procedure

We must try to understand what symptoms are present and in which areas of the patient's life they play a limiting role, their emotional significance, and how the patient interacts with the symptoms as well as the resources of the patient that help him/her to relax his/her restrictions. ("What helps you? What do you do to make your pain less severe?") The therapist must try to clarify the current life situation of the patient, in particular trying to grasp what factors contribute to the maintenance of the symptoms in the patient's life. The next step is to try to get a review of the patient's biography (see Table 2.7).

If the therapist is not sure about the diagnosis, then he will also be able to use clinical screening tools, in order to confirm the diagnosis (e.g. in Germany, the test called "Screening für somatoforme Störungen: SOMS 2" (Rief & Hiller, 2003). This psychological tool is validated specifically to measure the concept of somatoform disorders. The Patient Health Questionnaire (PHQ) is a well-known American screening questionnaire for psychiatric conditions, assessing 13 physical symptoms.

Table 2.7 Diagnostic

1. Which symptoms? In which areas of the patient's life do they play a limiting role? Their emotional significance? How does the patient interact with the symptoms? What are the resources of the patient that help him or her to relax his restrictions?
2. Current life situation, what factors contribute to the maintenance of the symptoms in the patient's life?
3. Biography of the patient

If a respondent complaints of significant disturbance from at least three of the symptoms, and there is no evidence of a sufficient medical cause, the therapist should take into account the possibility of a somatoform disorder (Spitzer et al., 1994).

Therapy

The therapy first derives from what the patient addresses. Is he/she fixated on symptoms or does he/she relate to conflicts which burden him? I try to perceive whether he has a conflict or structure deficits or a conflict problem and at the same time structure impairments. Or has he/she got a trauma (PTSD)? I am always mindful of transference and countertransference (Gündel, Kruse, Lahmann, Ronel, & Schneider, 2012).

We then try to establish a viable therapeutic relationship—which applies to all therapies—but what is unique about this therapy is that we make the patient first talk about his physical afflictions and listen to him, in order to establish the relationship. These patients often feel aggrieved because the significant others do not listen. A patient once told me: "I said to my wife I was going to die soon and she answered: I will die sooner than you if things go on like this". He often feels misunderstood and not taken seriously. Many patients have been sent into therapy by others and not by their own choice. Therefore they are wary of the initial therapeutical contact. One has to spare them from confrontations. Another important point is to phrase realistic and reachable therapeutic targets together with the patient to avoid possible disappointments (Gündel et al., 2012).

What follows is an example for a conflict. A female patient with back pain told me: "I do not allow any grief. Of course I feel it when grief surfaces or when I feel sad. But when I was a child this availed to nothing. No one was there. I learnt to be the strong one. I functioned or else I would have drowned". When the patient has a structural problem—and because of that he/she cannot apprehend his/her feelings—I try to make the patient aware of his/her inner psychological processes (Gündel et al., 2012). I explain, as a sample, that there is a connection between body and soul using every day examples: "Imagine, you have a lemon in your mouth". Another technique is to ask questions at the same time: "What did you think in this situation?" Or "What do you feel now as you are talking about it?" A patient once told me: "It seethes in me!" I asked: "What is the feeling behind it?" He could not say. I told him: "When I am seething, I am annoyed". We then tried to understand what made him upset in this situation. So gradually he learnt to make a connection between physical ailments and psychological condition (thoughts, feelings).

We also try to teach the patients that there is a physical contribution to their symptoms, but it is not there without any connection; one has to take the psychic life into consideration to understand the afflictions. To make it conceivable for the patient and to motivate him/her, I tell him/her the tale of the three languages (Grün, 2007). A young man learnt three languages, the language of the quaking frogs, the language of the barking dogs and the one of the birds. One day he came to a forest, and the only option in order not to sleep outside was a castle. He had to sleep in a tower with wild barking dogs that had devoured humans before. Because he could talk to them, he got to know that they guarded a treasure. Therefore they were so aggressive. They led him to the treasure, and he was able to take it with him.

My experience with people that have a structural problem is that they do not have a problem with emotions in general. A patient once said, like shot out his response to my question: “It is rage I feel”. He had a mother who made him livid. The same patient could not recognise his grief as easily. Another quite intelligent female patient, let’s call her Ms X (32 years old, living with a partner), came into therapy because of obsessive thoughts. We concentrated on these obsessive thoughts, and most of them disappeared. Six to 8 weeks before the end of the therapy, her practitioner saw in the EKG a too long QTc time (517 ms); because of that, he stopped giving her medication (Citalopram 10 mg). I talked to the physician who affirmed the cardiological diagnosis: nothing pathological detected. In our last session (100th session), she becomes ill again. She becomes depressive, cries without any reason and says she feels a pressure on her chest which emerged within the last 3–4 weeks and has intensified considerably. Additionally the obsessive thought, which she has had for many years, has increased, too. Later her depression mounts, she cries more, she suffers more and the pressure on her chest lasts longer. She feels hot and cold; at times she suffers from diarrhoea. Apart from that she develops pain in the known BSW in the low back area. During our 100 sessions, neither I did realise the tendency of the patient to somatise nor her separation anxiety. The patient knew that when the therapy has finished, she will have “one appointment less. I am looking forward to that!” Before our 100th session, she was sure that she would not mind the end of the therapy. I should have become suspicious that she had problems with separation because she became depressive during my last vacations. We did not refer to this depressive episode. So we extended the therapy to another 25 sessions. Recently she told me that last Saturday, she did the housework and was full of energy. She was looking forward to spending the evening with friends. In the afternoon she suddenly felt downcast and had a strong pressure on her chest. We are completely in the dark because the patient has no access to her sense of self. For her it is obvious that her state is purely somatic. I feel restless and feel rage. During our talks I stay tenacious and ask her what the “barking dogs” want to tell her. So she experiences having me as “father” who has something to say (transference) and is strict to her, something she does not know of her own father. This time she knows more; she admits: she did the housework on Saturday being full of energy but did far too much, and because of that, her back pain increased considerably. Because of the pain, she could hardly move. As a consequence she has access to her rage and grief. She is aware of the fact that her feelings are related to her high standards. We talk about her perfectionism and follow this up. She remembers: "When I did not get a first at school, hell broke loose".

I also remember a patient who saw the pressure on his chest as purely physical, and I let it pass. He was a patient who did not mourn his wife's death. He had a heart condition, already had a stent, and there was a pressure on his chest that moved from his left chest into his head. I want to call attention to the fact that in some cases, it is difficult to judge whether a symptom is psychosomatic or not. My (personal) experience is that most patients, even if they have a neurotic conflict, have physical symptoms, too, that function as an affect correlative. This means that the symptoms represent an affect/emotion that is close to the patient's consciousness/awareness. When the patient has diarrhoea, he/she is afraid of something. For example, the therapy of patients with a somatoform disorder is difficult, because as a therapist, one often feels bored or irritated because the patients are fixated on their physical symptoms and talk about them in great detail. This behaviour often causes rage or boredom in the therapist. We as therapists have to take great care not to be guarded by negative feelings (countertransference) unreflectively. It is also very important not to start the session with a check-up. To give an example, one patient told me about his stomach symptoms during the session and wanted to show me where it hurts. He likes it best when I examine him during the session. It is therapeutic if one manages to address an emotion that is lying beneath everything. In this case it is the wish of security/safety (Fonagy et al., 2002).

What Is the Transference Like with Somatoform Patients?

It is very often the case that patients with somatoform disorders have been disappointed by their parents because their parents did not answer to them empathetically. These patients rarely experienced their inner life as interesting. Taking this biographical background into consideration, they meet a therapist with a fear that he/she and the parents are inaccessible. In relation to this biographical experience, the somatoform patients try to make the therapist mind them. The patient is looking for attention. The therapist shall actively address the worries of the patient. The therapist should try to give him/her the feeling that he/she is emotionally there, that he/she esteems the patient.

When they then have the experience of being esteemed, they are more likely to want to continue therapy. A patient once said even if he changed his job, he would continue with the therapy (Mr L). Others develop anguish that the therapy could end soon. A patient of mine thanked me that she could still come to the sessions. The extent she looks for attention becomes evident in an observation she made. She said she noticed that if she wanted to attract her mother's attention, she automatically started talking about diseases. She noticed this after some time into therapy. The patient knows that her mother takes up the subject. Her mother (+17) was not accessible to her, and she mainly grew up with her grandparents. I suppose her grandparents could not be empathetic. A memory of the patient might be proof of that. (Screen memory? That means an imagined memory of the childhood which unconsciously hides other very stressful memories.) The 8-year-old patient was lying on the sofa having a fever; her grandmother was working in the kitchen, but the patient felt left alone. The therapist now has to become active—as it is recommended in the specialised literature—and he has to address the worries of the patient (fear/shame). There are patients who have access to their emotions, but they do not talk about them because of fear they will not be taken seriously or of being shamed by the significant other. There are patients, too, who hardly have any feelings or hardly recognise them (as in Alexithymia). These patients feel overwhelmed in a therapeutic situation. This becomes evident for instance in an increase of physical symptoms or the reaction of the patient. In such a situation, one should try to help the patient. This time he/she should have the positive experience of not being left alone with his/her overwhelming emotions. When existing symptoms increase, it is not always a mental overload. Sometimes it means that difficult topics are addressed, and because of that the patient grows.

References

Alexander, F. (1951). *Psychosomatische Medizin*. Berlin: De Gruyter.

American Psychiatric Association. (2013). *Diagnostic and statistical manual of mental disorders* (5th ed.). Arlington: American Psychiatric Association.

Arbeitskreis OPD. (2009). *Operationalisierte Psychodynamische Diagnostik OPD-2. Das Manual für Diagnostik und Therapieplanung* (2nd ed.). Bern: Verlag Hans Huber.

Arbeitskreis PISO. (2012). *Somatoforme Störungen*. Hogrefe, Göttingen: Psychodynamisch-Interpersonelle Therapie (PISO).

Barsky, A. J., & Wyshak, G. (1990). Hypochondriasis and somatosensory amplification. *British Journal of Psychiatry, 157*, 404–409.

Breuer J., & Freud S. (1895). *Studien über Hysterie*. Reprinted (1957) as Studies on Hysteria (J. Strachey (Ed.), Trans.). New York: Basic Books.

Chou, R., Qaseem, A., Owens, D. K., & Shekelle, P. (2011). Diagnostic imaging for low back pain: advice for high-value health care from the American College of Physicians. *Annals of Internal Medicine, 154*, 181–189.

DePaulo D. (2010). *Attachment style and somatization: a multimethod approach to measuring the effect of emotional awareness* (Dissertation. Rutgers University-Graduate School-Newark). https://doi.org/10.7282/T3VQ32GB.

Ebel, H., & Podoll, K. (1998). Komorbidität von somatoformen Störungen mit anderen psychischen Störungen. In G. Rudolf & P. Hennningsen (Eds.), *Somatoforme Störungen. Theoretisches Verständnis und therapeutische Praxis* (pp. 25–38). Stuttgart: Schattauer.

Eckhardt-Henn, A., Heuft, G., Hochapfel, G., & Hoffmann, S. O. (2004). Anhaltende somatofofrme Schmerzstörung. In A. Eckhardt-Henn, G. Heuft, G. Hochapfel, & S. O. Hoffmann (Eds.), *Neurotische Störungen und Psychosomatische Medizin: Mit einer Einführung in Psychosomatik und Psychotherapie* (7. Auflage ed., pp. 287–296). Schattauer: Stuttgart.

Egle, U. T. (1998). Diagnose, Differentialdiagnose und Psycchodynamik der somatoformen Störungen. P. 95. In G. Rudolf & P. Hennningsen (Eds.), *Somatoforme Störungen. Theoretisches Verständnis und therapeutische Praxis* (pp. 89–102). Stuttgart: Schattauer.

Engel, G. L. (1970). Conversion symptoms. In C. M. MacBryde, & R. S. Blacklow (Eds.), *Signs and symptoms. Applied physiology and clinical interpretation* (Chap. 30). Philadelphia: Lippincott.
Ermann, M. (2005). *Herz und Seele*. Stuttgart: W. Kohlhammer.
Fenichel, O. (1945). *The psychoanalytic theory of neurosis*. London: Routledge.
Fonagy, P., Gergely, G., Jurist, E. L., & Target, M. (2002). *Affect regulation, mentalization and the development of the self*. New York: Other Press.
Garcia-Campayo, J., Alda, M., Sobradiel, N., Olivan, B., & Pascual, A. (2007). Personality disorders in somatization disorder patients: A controlled study in Spain. *Journal of Psychosomatic Research, 62*, 675–680.
Grün, A. (2007). *Der Verwandlung trauen. Wie unser Leben heil wird*. Ostfildern: M. Grünewald Verlag.
Gündel, H., Kruse, J., Lahmann, C., Ronel, J., & Schneider, G. (2012). Allgemeine Therapieprinzipien und Phasen der PISO-Intervention. In Arbeitskreis PISO (Ed.), *Somatoforme Störungen Psychodynamisch-Interpersonelle Therapie (PISO)* (pp. 38–62). Göttingen: Hogrefe.
Hoffmann, S. O., Eckhardt-Henn, A., & Scheidt, C. E. (2004). 8. Konversion, Dissoziation und Somatisierung, historische Aspekte und Entwurf eines integrativen Models. In A. Eckhardt-Henn & S. O. Hoffmann (Eds.), *Dissoziative Störungen des Bewußtseins* (pp. 114–130). Stuttgart: Schattauer.
King, H. (1993). One- once upon a text: Hysteria from Hippocrates. In S. L. Gilman, H. King, R. Porter, G. S. Rousseau, & E. Showalter (Eds.), *Hysteria beyond freud* (pp. 3–65). Berkeley: University of California Press.
Körber, S., & Hiller, W. (2012). Medizinisch unerklärte Symptome und somatoforme Störungen in der Primärmedizin. *Journal für Neurologie, Neurochirurgie und Psychiatrie, 13*, 21–28.
Kroll, S. (1932). *Eine ungewöhnliche Somatisation. Eine geheime Todesklausel*. Psychoanalytische Praxis. 2:53.
Küchenhoff, J. (1998). Zur Psychodynamik und Psychotherapie somatoformer Störungen. In G. Rudolf & P. Hennningsen (Eds.), *Somatoforme Störungen. Theoretisches Verständnis und therapeutische Praxis* (pp. 155–168). Stuttgart: Schattauer.
Mentzos, S. (1980). *Hysterie. Zur Psychodynamik unbewusster Inszenierungen*. Fischer Verlag: Frankfurt am Main.
Meyer, C., Rumpf, H. J., Hapke, U., Dilling, H., & John, U. (2000). Lebenszeitprävalenz psychischer Störungen in der erwachsenen Allgemeinbevölkerung – Ergebnisse der TACOS-Studie. *Nervenarzt, 71*, 535–542.
Nickel, R., & Egle, U. T. (1999). *Therapie somatoformer Schmerzstörungen. Manual zur psychodynamisch-interaktionellen Gruppentherapie*. Stuttgart: Schattauer.
Nobis, H. G., Rolke, R., & Graf-Baumann, T. (2016). *Schmerz-Eine Herausforderung*. Heidelberg: Springer.
Richter, H. E., & Beckmann, D. (2004). *Herzneurose* (4th ed.). Gießen: Psychosozial-Verlag.
Rief, W., & Hiller, W. (2003). *Screening für somatoforme Störungen*. Göttingen. Hogrefe.
Rief, W., & Boadbrendt, E. (2007). Explaining medically unexplained symptoms – models and mechanisms. *Clinical Psychology Review, 27*, 821–841.
Rudolf, G., & Henningsen, P. (2006). Somatoforme Störungen. In C. Reimer & U. Rüger (Eds.), *Psychodynamische Psychotherapien* (pp. 311–318). Heidelberg: Springer.
Schaefert, R., Hausteiner-Wiehle, C., Häuser, W., Ronel, J., Herrmann, M., & Henningsen, P. (2012). Non-specific, functional, and somatoform bodily complaints. *Deutsches Ärzteblatt International, 109*(47), 803–813.
Schneider, G., Sattel, H., Ronnel, J., & Henningsen, P. (2012). Störungstheorien und Modelle. P. 11. In Arbeitskreis PISO (Ed.), *Somatoforme Störungen Psychodynamisch-Interpersonelle Therapie (PISO)* (pp. 11–28). Göttingen: Hogrefe.
Schur, M. (1955). Zur Metapsychologie der Somatisierung. In K. Brede (Ed.), *(1971) Einführung in psychosomatische Medizin*. Frankfurt am Main: Fischer Athenäum.
Spitzer, R. L., Williams, J. B., Kroenke, K., Linzer, M., deGruy, F. V., & Hahn, S. R. (1994). Utility of a new procedure for diagnosing mental disorders in primary care. The PRIME-MD 1000 study. *JAMA, 272*, 1749–1756.

Stekel, W. (1924). *Nervöse Angstzustände und ihre Behandlung*. Berlin. Urban und Schwarzenberg.
Wesiack, W., & Schüßler, G. (2002). Psychoanalyse und psychoanalytisch orientierte Therapieverfahren. In T. Von Uexküll (Ed.), *Psychosomatische Medizin* (6th ed., pp. 457–466). München: Urban & Fischer.
Woolfolk, R. L., & Allen, L. A. (2007). *Treating somatization: A cognitive-behavioral approach* (p. 5). New York: Guilford.
World Health Organisation. (1992). *The ICD-10 Classification of Mental and Behavioural Disorders. Clinical descriptions and diagnostic Guidlines*. Geneva: WHO.

Chapter 3
Functional (Medically Unexplained) Physical Syndromes/Symptoms: The Cognitive Behavioral Perspective

Evangelos C. Karademas

The aim of this chapter is to present the cognitive behavioral models and approaches to medically unexplained (functional) physical symptoms and their treatment. A presentation of the entire array of existing models is beyond the scope of this chapter. Here we will try to describe the evolution of these theories/models and briefly present their main aspects.

Medically unexplained physical syndromes and symptoms (MUPS) is rather an umbrella term which refers to a variety of symptoms related to any physical system and contributing to different conditions or syndromes which cannot be explained by a recognized medical illness (Creed, 2016). Such conditions include, but are not limited to, chronic fatigue syndrome, noncardiac and atypical chest pain, fibromyalgia, irritable bowel syndrome, multiple chemical sensitivity, and chronic pelvic pain (Brown, 2007). These symptoms (e.g., pain, dizziness, tiredness) are typically characterized by functional disability (especially the neurological ones, such as sensory loss or paralyses) and thus are experienced by the patients as significantly burdensome.

MUPS is the most frequently reported type of symptoms in general medical practice (Kirmayer & Taillefer, 1997), while it is estimated that almost 50% of new attenders to medical outpatient facilities report at least one MUPS (Nimnuan, Hotopf, & Wessely, 2000). Although 50–75% of patients with MUPS improve over time, many of them (10–30%), and especially those with a more serious condition at baseline, deteriorate (olde Hartman et al., 2009). Hence, MUPS represent a considerable problem for many patients and the healthcare system as well.

MUPS should not be confused with physical symptoms that are the outcome of an anxiety or mood disorder, symptoms or sensations that a person erroneously represents as evidence of a serious illness, or symptoms that cannot be accounted for by one specific medical or psychiatric condition. These are different conditions, despite

E. C. Karademas (✉)
Department of Psychology, University of Crete, Rethymno, Greece
e-mail: karademas@uoc.gr

C. Charis, G. Panayiotou (eds.), *Somatoform and Other Psychosomatic Disorders*,
https://doi.org/10.1007/978-3-319-89360-0_3

the fact that the corresponding symptoms may coexist in several occasions (Kirmayer & Robbins, 1991). Also, it is sometimes difficult to differentiate MUPS from symptoms resulting from a medical or a psychiatric condition, and often the diagnosis follows a large number of clinical referrals and many exams (Brown, 2007).

Medical and mental health professionals use different systems for the classification of MUPS, causing thus much confusion. For example, several MUPS are classified in the somatoform disorder category (F45) of the ICD-10 Version: 16 (WHO, 2016; see, http://apps.who.int/classifications/icd10/browse/2016/en#/F40-F48), whereas they are also classified as "functional somatic syndromes" in general medicine and neurological settings (Picariello, Ali, Moss-Morris, & Chalder, 2015). In addition, as Brown (2007) underlines, the term "MUPS" is rather unsatisfactory as it suggests that there is no explanation for these symptoms, when in fact there are many psychological and/or biobehavioral theories which describe several mechanisms that probably underlie the development and the course of MUPS. Moreover, this term is possible to reinforce dualistic thinking about the causes of illness (i.e., either physical or psychological), while it implies an organic cause, although this is not always correct (IAPT, 2014).

Furthermore, recent studies have found that patients tend to prefer labels containing words like "physical" and "functional" (e.g., persistent physical symptoms, functional symptoms or syndromes). On the contrary, they seem to avoid or even reject terms like "somatization" or "somatoform disorders" (Marks & Hunter, 2015; Picariello et al., 2015). The use of the term "functional somatic syndromes" is also favored by professionals as it seems to be more neutral as far as the medical vs. psychological background of the symptoms is concerned (Creed et al., 2010). Thus, for the purposes of this chapter, in the remainder we will be referring to this cluster of symptoms as functional physical syndromes/symptoms or FPS/S.

Cognitive Behavioral Models for Functional Physical Syndromes/Symptoms

There is not one single cognitive behavioral (CB) model for FPS/S. Instead, there is a number of them, and although they share many similarities, they also differ in several ways. For instance, some of these models focus solely on psychosocial factors and processes, whereas others emphasize the interaction between psychological and biological (e.g., neuroendocrinological) factors. The number of factors probably involved in the development and maintenance of FPS/S, as described by the several CB models, is quite large. Therefore, the aim of this section is to comprehensively present only the main aspects of the major cognitive behavioral models in the field.

In general, the CB models for FPS/S adopt the typical distinction between predisposing, precipitating, and perpetuating factors (Deary, Chalder, & Sharpe, 2007). Fundamental to these models is also the notion that there is not a single specific mechanism but rather a series of feedback loops and interactions between several factors in different domains which lead to the development and maintenance of FPS/S. Although each model puts more emphasis on different aspects of these interactions (e.g., certain models emphasize the role of attentional processes, whereas others focus on dysfunctional beliefs and representations), all models suggest that there is multifactorial self-maintaining ("autopoietic") cycle which is central for the development of FPS/S (Deary et al., 2007).

A further fundamental aspect of the CB models is that they include not only psychological but also physiological variables in their effort to explain the onset and maintenance of FPS/S. As Deary et al. (2007, p. 788) underlined, "...[the CB model] is in many ways a meta-model, providing a skeleton structure to join the dots of whatever factors each patient presents." Thus, important factors that are not strictly cognitive or behavioral (e.g., the role of health professionals and physiological arousal) can easily be included in these models as predisposing or perpetuating factors. In addition, although the general CB model can largely describe the development of FPS/S, at the same time it gives room for the development of more specific models that may apply to different conditions as well as for more individualized models for each particular patient.

In general, the CB models assume that the key process to the development of FPS/S is the interpretation of bodily sensations in a catastrophic way. The environment seems to have a decisive impact on the genesis of FPS/S, as a significant event (or events) may trigger the entire process. These "events" may be physical, such as a symptom, a disease or an injury, or psychological, such as a negative life event or other stressor. In any case, a trigger may lead, under certain conditions, to a prolonged activation of stress reactions which, in turn, facilitate the development of more physical symptoms. These symptoms, due to a cohort of factors that will be described later, can be interpreted in a negative way, increase physical arousal, and, consequently, lead to the generation of even more sensations and symptoms which are again misinterpreted as harmful or be attributed to an illness (Witthöft & Hiller, 2010). This is probably the starting point of an autopoietic cycle that finally leads to the maintenance of functional physical symptoms. The CB models point out four clusters of factors that are responsible for the development and maintenance of FPS/S (Deary et al., 2007), namely, cognitive factors (including, attention and perception), psychobiological factors (such as prolonged physiological arousal), behavior (e.g., help and reassurance seeking), and social factors (e.g., reinforcement from family and health professionals). It is worth noting that, although the latter cluster of factors (i.e., social) is not emphasized in certain CB models, it seems to be important for the precipitation and perpetuation of the FPS/S.

Deary et al. (2007) and Rief and Broadbent (2007) have reviewed a significant number of predisposing, precipitating, and perpetuating factors which are important for the development of FPS/S. According to these two reviews, the predisposing factors include negative affectivity, incorrect concepts about health and illness, possible genetic influences as well as early experience (e.g., abuse or other traumas; vicariously learned illness behaviors), and personality characteristics (e.g., neuroticism).

A family history of chronic illness as well as other family-related factors (e.g., attachment) may also be important precursors of FSS/S.

There is also a long list of perpetuating psychological factors that interact with physical factors. These are:

- Sensitization to symptom- and health-related stimuli due to prior exposure to them (e.g., prior illness)
- Stress-related physical reactions (e.g., the hypothalamus pituitary adrenal (HPA) axis downregulation; immune system dysregulation)
- Attentional and cognitive biases (e.g., excessive focus on physical sensations; selective attention to bodily processes; beliefs about personal vulnerability)
- Misattribution of bodily sensations or symptoms to a disease
- Dysfunctional illness beliefs (e.g., overestimation of the link between felt symptoms and negative consequences; incorrect beliefs about the potential symptoms of a disease)
- High expectations of experiencing physical symptoms, illness worries, and health anxiety
- Negative interactions with health professionals
- Development of "symptoms cognitive schemata"
- Behavioral responses (e.g., help-seeking, increased healthcare use, avoidance of activity)
- Dysfunctional social response/social reinforcement of symptoms (e.g., validation of patient's dysfunctional illness beliefs and behaviors, continuous provision of reassurance from family members)

These factors reinforce the cognitive and emotional reactions toward physical symptoms or sensations and, through continuous feedback loops (i.e., autopoietic cycles), may produce a functional physical syndrome/symptom.

Rief and Broadbent (2007) and Deary et al. (2007) highlighted the considerable evidence that exists for the importance of almost all of the above factors in the onset and perpetuation of FPS/S. The research findings also provide support to the more generic assumption of the CB models regarding the role of autopoietic processes in the development of FPS/S (Deary et al., 2007). Next, we will synoptically present some of the most salient CB models for FPS/S so as to highlight the processes and factors included in the genesis of FPS/S.

The Basic CB Models for FPS/S

Although there is now evidence that the processes behind the development of hypochondriasis and FPS/S are different (Witthöft & Hiller, 2010), the first CB models did not make such a differentiation. One of the first influential approaches, the "somatosensory amplification" model, was developed for hypochondriasis by Barsky and Wyshak (1990) and emphasized the role of attention and perception. According to this model, people with hypochondriasis attribute usually benign somatic sensations to a serious disease.[1] Consequently, they focus their attention on these sensations or their body function in general. This in turn results to an augmented perception of sensations (which are now perceived as "symptoms") and complaints. As the anxiety rises, and through a vicious cycle, the person perceives more and more disturbing physical signals which they attribute to a disease. Although this model was formulated for hypochondriasis, it served later as a basis for new models which were developed to also explain FPS/S.

A more elaborated model based on the previous one was developed by Kirmayer and his collaborators (Kirmayer & Taillefer, 1997; Looper & Kirmayer, 2002). This model emphasized the role of behavioral and social factors, as well as the importance of feedback loops in addition to the significance of somatosensory amplification. According to this model, the existence of new or chronic health problems or strong physical sensations, or the presence of significant emotional arousal, may cause a heightened attention to body and somatic functions. However, the more the attention focused on the body, the greater becomes the awareness of possible physical sensations. When sensations come into awareness, the evaluation of their severity is likely to be amplified as a result of their attribution to illness, cognitive distortions (e.g., catastrophizing), and personal vulnerability cognitions (e.g., I am a weak person) which are based on past experience (including past illnesses or traumas).

These reactions initiate behaviors that are related to illness, such as help-seeking (e.g., visiting a doctor, frequent medical examinations) and avoidance behaviors (e.g., resting, avoiding exposure to "pathogens"), which in turn affect social and occupational life. The social environment (family, friends, health professionals) may also play a crucial role in the entire process, as it may reinforce patient's dysfunctional responses and thus impede recovery. This mechanism, through a feedback loop, intensifies both the physiological reactivity and the emotional arousal of the person, resulting in additional attention to physical sensations and illness worry and, eventually, to the development of functional physical syndromes/symptoms.

[1] At this point we should underline that, despite the fact that most CB models emphasize the role of misattribution of physical sensations to physical causes or a physical illness, more recent theoretical approaches and research findings question the importance of misattribution (Henningsen & Creed, 2010). Rief and Broadbent (2007) concluded that the relationship between causal attributions and FPS/S is more complicated than expected. For example, high scores in psychological illness attributions (besides attribution to a physical condition) have been reported in patients with FPS/S in several studies. Also, Knoop, Prins, Moss-Morris, and Bleijenberg (2010) showed that the effect of CB therapy on chronic fatigue was related to changes in illness-related beliefs as well as to changes in the tendency to focus attention on physical sensations. The attribution of symptoms to a physical illness did not change as a result of the intervention but also did not have any effect on the outcome.

Brown's Integrative Conceptual Model for FPS/S

Another multicomponent model, called the "integrative conceptual model," which emphasized the role of the cognitive system and tried to integrate different theoretical concepts in a single framework regarding FPS/S, was developed by Brown (2004). This model tried to specify the vague details of the previous CB models regarding the development and continuation of FPS/S.

As several other cognitive researchers, Brown distinguishes two attentional control systems: a primary attentional system (PAS) and a secondary one (SAS). The first is an effortless and (semi)automatic mode of information processing, whereas the latter is a controlled, effortful, and deliberate mode of processing available (new and older) information. Brown's model explicitly suggests that "unexplained physical symptoms" are "real" to the individual reporting them (in distinction to malingering). FPS/S is the final result of alterations in the ways persons perceive their body which are based on information from their cognitive system (perception and memory). Brown used the term "*rogue representations*" to label the inappropriate information on which the altered body image is based.

To this model, bodily sensations (as any other perception) may be interpreted in various ways depending on previous personal experience (including personal knowledge, beliefs, and wishes). However, PAS selects the most active interpretation of the stimulus (i.e., body sensation), which is then uses to organize sensory information and activate further thoughts and behavior. In the case of FPS/S, PAS selects rogue representations or, in other words, inappropriate information concerning the nature of the physical symptoms. This results in a misinterpretation of the initial sensation and the activation of more thoughts and actions that correspond to this misinterpretation.

According to the model, rogue representations may be acquired from different sources. Exposure to illness and physical symptoms, several emotion conditions and emotional arousal, and traumatic experiences (especially the physical experience of these conditions) leave their traces in memory and provide the sources for the development of rogue representations. A frequent similar source is the exposure to the physical symptoms of others, especially family members. Also, the sociocultural conceptions of illness and symptoms (e.g., popular, but often inaccurate, beliefs of what is a "genuine" symptom or which symptoms corresponds to each illness) often form the basis of rogue representations. Finally, rogue representations may be the result of verbal autosuggestions (e.g., "I feel ill, so I must be ill") or heterosuggestions (e.g., being told by significant others or health professionals that "This symptom might be serious").

Yet, according to the model, rogue representations do not always lead to a chronic problem. A number of other factors are also involved in this process. For example, high levels of introspection (i.e., paying more attention to self and personal thoughts and feelings), boring vs. stimulating environments, and attending to the body have been identified as factors facilitating the development of FPS/S. However, according to Brown, the most significant factor for the maintenance of the problem is the high degree of high-level attention allocated by SAS to symptom perception and the associated rogue representations.

In other words, the experience of FPS/S is the result of the recurrent redirection of attention onto symptoms. Focusing on the symptom (e.g., whether it is still present or not; when it is present and when not; how it feels) intensifies the activation of rogue representations and, at the same time, renders them even more accessible in the future. According to Brown, if the symptom-focused attention is continued long enough, then the activation of the rogue representations is strong enough to ensure their constant selection by PAS over time.

Anything that facilitates and increases symptom-focused attention indirectly contributes to the onset and maintenance of FPS/S. The model names five such crucial factors:

(a) Misattribution of symptoms to a serious medical condition.
(b) Negative emotional states, which may increase the catastrophic misinterpretation of physical symptoms and trigger or perpetuate rumination, as well as cause the narrowing of attention on physical sensations and lead to a continuous selection of rogue representations.
(c) Illness worry and rumination, accompanied by self-focused attention and constant monitoring of the body state that maintains the allocation of attention to rogue representations and increase negative affect, symptom misinterpretation, and illness behaviors.
(d) Illness behaviors that usually direct attention toward physical symptoms while increasing anxiety and doubt (e.g., seeking for medical help; avoidance; symptom checking; looking for information through the internet or other resources).
(e) Personality factors. There is evidence that traits, such as negative affectivity, increase vulnerability to the development of functional physical symptoms.
(f) Attention to symptoms and the associated coping strategies and illness behaviors (like the adoption of a sick-role) may also bring about secondary gains for the individual (e.g., greater attention from significant others) reinforcing, subsequently, the maintenance of FPS/S.

Finally, this model emphasizes the role of traumatic experiences (e.g., physical, sexual, and emotional abuse) as frequent underlying factors in the development of FPS/S. Brown (2004) adopts the notion that the use of body-focused attention helps traumatized persons to avoid thoughts and emotions associated with the traumatic experience. In addition, a traumatic event may cause harm to cognitive and emotional self-regulation increasing thus the possibility of using rogue representations (for further discussion about the role of trauma in FPS/S and the relevant CB models, see Roelofs & Spinhoven, 2007).

Overall, Brown's integrative conceptual model describes functional physical syndromes/symptoms as false alarms of a highly sensitized information processing system (Witthöft & Hiller, 2010) in combination with the existence of prior maladaptive ("rogue") representations. Several aspects of this model have not been tested empirically, and future studies are warranted to examine the several parts of this very interesting theoretical framework.

Other CB Models Focusing on the Perception Process and Memory

A key aspect of the processes leading to the development and maintenance of FPS/S, as depicted by the CB models, is perception, that is, how individuals perceive physical sensations and "translate" them into "symptoms" and disease. Two models have explicitly focused on this topic, Pennebaker's and the signal-filter model developed by Rief and Barsky.

Pennebaker (1982) suggested that there is a constant sensory stimulation of the brain as the organs, the skin, and the different body parts continuously send neural impulses to the higher cortical structures. Typically, the neural system has learned to prevent the overstimulation of the perceptual system by filtering irrelevant information or "sensory noise." Pennebaker has shown that an individual may focus on a physical sensation when either the sensory signals are amplified or when any distracting external stimulation is reduced.

Rief and Barsky (2005), in their psychobiological model, also proposed that FPS/S and relevant problems are the result of two interrelated processes: an increase in physical sensations and signals due to several potential factors (both biological and psychological) and a deficient filter system which magnifies instead of inhibiting or selecting these sensations and signals. In this respect, their model is similar to the gate-control theory for pain (Melzack & Wall, 1965). Rief and Barsky also provided a summary of the factors that may distort this filtering process leading to the development of FPS/S. Overarousal, chronic stimulation of the HPA axis, and sensitization to specific stimuli are some of the factors that increase the impact of the sensory signals, while selective attention, health anxiety, depressive mood, and infections may decrease the capability of the filter system. Also, memory and previous experiences, expectations, previous traumas, as well as neuronal plasticity and neurotransmission-related factors may increase the cortical perception of the sensations. In their model, Rief and Barsky (2005) have incorporated previous models and evidence regarding the psychobiological processes that impact perception, including the potential role of the interactions between the immune and the neuroendocrine systems in the perception of bodily sensations, as well as the development of sickness behavior patterns (e.g., repeated use of coping strategies/behaviors that originally aimed to deal with the health threat but eventually become dysfunctional, such as activity avoidance).

It is worth mentioning here another model which, although not developed for the explanation of FPS/S, provides a very useful framework for the understanding of symptom perception. The model was developed by Kolk and Gijsbers van Wijk (Gijsbers van Wijk & Kolk, 1997; Kolk, 2000; Kolk, Hanewald, Schagen, & Gijsbers van Wijk, 2003) and brings together the works of Pennebaker, Kirmayer, and Cioffi. According to this model, the perception of physical symptoms is preceded by physiological changes that may be the result of normal bodily processes, an organic disease, emotional state, or environmental conditions and stimuli. These changes trigger receptors and generate information about the body state and function. Not all this information comes into awareness, as a selective process takes place. Attention regulation holds the gates of which information will be further processed. Attention to and processing of physical sensations depend on several factors, including negative mood, selective attention to normal conditions, physiological processes, as well as the ratio of information coming from the body to information from the environment.

Negative mood, selective attention to the body and its functions, and low external information (e.g., a boring environment) can lower the detection threshold for bodily sensations. The environmental stimuli may also augment attention to and awareness of bodily sensations when they act as stressors generating a negative emotional state. From that moment, whether a physical sensation will be labeled as a physical symptom or not is a matter of interpretation which is based on personal cognitive structures (i.e., cognitive schemata and beliefs) regarding illness. The model suggests that healthy individuals tend to alternate between a physical and a psychological "explanation" of the symptom, whereas clinical populations ("somatizers" as they call them) are more likely to show a more extreme preference for either physical or psychological attribution (it is the extremeness of preference toward one of the possible cluster of causes and not the attribution itself that characterizes this group of persons; Kolk et al., 2003).

A Transdiagnostic/Problem-Specific Approach

Recently, P. Salkovskis and his collaborators (Salkovskis et al., 2016) combined new and old concepts and presented a new approach in the understanding of FPS/S. The model also focuses on therapy and suggests that, as far as the understanding and treatment of FPS/S is concerned, there is need to take into account both problem/syndrome specific issues and a "transdiagnostic" perspective for FPS/S in general.

The model accepts the general CB thesis that it is the way a person appraises a condition that elicits emotional and behavioral responses, and this applies to FPS/S as well. Based on Salkovskis's (1996) previous work, the model suggests that people may misinterpret bodily sensations and medical issues based on a combination of prior beliefs and experience and the formation of currently unhelpful cognitions. In the case of FPS/S, the trigger is most likely the perception of a bodily variation or symptom (e.g., pain, fatigue) or a current or previous (physical or psychological) health problem. This trigger may cause an emotional and behavioral response, the extent of which depends on the details of the meaning attributed to the trigger. The response is determined, specifically, by the perceived likelihood of an illness or disability associated with the symptoms (i.e., the perception of a more severe or burdensome disease), the perceived "awfulness" of this condition (i.e., the severity of consequences), the perceived coping ability (i.e., how capable the person is to cope with the illness they believe they have and its consequences), and perceived rescue factors (i.e., factors that might reduce the severity of illness/consequences or enhance coping abilities, such as medical treatment and social support). Next, several key appraisals and misinterpretations (especially catastrophizing of felt symptoms or sensations), in interaction with dysfunctional cognitions and beliefs (e.g., thinking errors, like "all or nothing" thinking) and behavior (especially avoidance of activity and safe keeping), are involved in the maintenance of the psychological distress and disability in FPS/S.

A continuous negative (catastrophic) interpretation of the initial and current symptoms or sensations and fear about the future course of this condition underlie the perpetuation of FPS/S. This interpretation is based on and reinforced by feedback loops/vicious cycles of avoidance or erratic patterns of activity, cognitive and physiological changes, in the core of which is negative thinking. These feedback loops include specific and also generalized FPS/S maintenance factors. The specific factors are numerous and refer to mood changes (especially, anxiety and depression, which contribute to mood-appraisal spirals), attentional processes (both automatic, e.g., selectively attend to information that seems to confirm the existence of a disease and disregard information that points toward a good health, and purposeful, e.g., looking for symptoms), emotional avoidance, safety-keeping behaviors (e.g., frequent searching for information in the internet) and activity avoidance, rumination as a form of catastrophizing and worry, autonomic arousal which is further perceived as evidence of a physical disease, increased health anxiety, intrusive memories, interpersonal difficulties (e.g., bitterness toward others), physiological factors, etc. There are also several generalized factors and processes that may lead to additional vulnerability, including psychological inflexibility (i.e., adopting only a particular perspective on personal physical condition), unrelentingly high personal standards and concerns about possible mistakes, and negative generalized beliefs about self (e.g., nothing good is ever going to happen to me; there is a history of severe illnesses in my family) and/or the environment (e.g., No one understands how I really feel).

The critical point of this theory is the constant feedback loops (vicious cycles) between specific and generalized factors in the maintenance of functional physical symptoms. For example, in one of these cycles, the initial trigger might be a felt symptom (like, nausea) that, in combination with a preexisting negative belief about personal vulnerability to health problems, is appraised as a sign of a potential severe disease which the person is not really able to manage. In turn, this interpretation may lead to attentional biases toward the felt symptom as well as fear and other negative emotions which may cause further physical arousal. The spiral effects between negative appraisals, mood, and attentional biases reinforce a catastrophic interpretation of the condition and a series of behavioral reactions, such as continuous checking for more symptoms. The interaction between these factors leads to the perpetuation of symptoms. As Salkovskis et al. (2016) underline, rarely a single vicious cycle may lead to the maintenance of FPS/S. More such cycles are usually involved in this complicated process. Based on this theoretical formulation, Salkovskis et al. made certain suggestions about a possible psychological treatment of FPS/S, to which we will refer later in this chapter (see section "A Hybrid Transdiagnostic/Problem Specific Approach").

The Common Sense Model of Self-Regulation in Illness

A theory well known in the field of health psychology which describes the processes of adaptation to illness is the Common Sense Model of Self-Regulation (CSM; Leventhal, Diefenbach, & Leventhal, 1992; Leventhal, Meyer, & Nerenz, 1980), which has received significant empirical support (e.g., Dempster, Howell, & McCorry, 2015; Hagger, Koch, Chatzisarantis, & Orbell, 2017; Hudson, Bundy, Coventry, & Dickens, 2014). Although this model has not been developed for FPS/S, it may be helpful for further understanding this phenomenon from a broader CB/social cognitive perspective as recent studies suggest (see, e.g., Schroeder et al., 2012; Webster, Thompson, & Norman, 2015). The model provides suggestions regarding the ways patients understand/represent their symptoms, the relationship of illness representations to information processing, as well as the link between these factors and illness-related behavior. Therefore, it may be useful for the clarification of certain processes that, according to the overall CB model, are important for precipitating and perpetuating FPS/S (De Gucht & Maes, 2006).

According to the CSM, when a person comes across a symptom or illness, they develop a constellation of dynamic representations (i.e., subjective beliefs and emotions) of their experience in order to make sense of and manage it. Specifically, illness representations refer to the identity of symptom/illness (e.g., the label of the disease and the symptoms associated with it), cause (i.e., causal attributions of the symptom/disease), consequences of the symptom/disease, timeline (i.e., perceptions about the course of the symptom/disease), cure/control (what they or the medical personnel or others can do to cure or manage the symptom/disease), as well as emotional reactions to the symptom/disease, including fear, anxiety, depression, or anger (Leventhal et al., 1992). Illness representations guide short- and long-term action plans and coping procedures in order to manage symptoms and regulate the negative emotions. Illness representations are based on a variety of information resources, including personal knowledge and experience, and input from others and health professionals. For example, a recent study has shown that when primary care providers discuss with patients with FPS/S their illness and treatment representations, then patients' adherence to treatment and adherence intentions improves (Phillips, McAndrew, Laman-Maharg, & Bloeser, 2017).

The illness representations developed and the behaviors adopted by the patients are typically considered by them as accurate and proper, even when actually they are not. Illness representations are guided by the personal ways an individual understands their condition as well as by several habitual and other (semi-)automatic processes (Breland, Fox, Horowitz, & Leventhal, 2012) which the individual trusts. Therefore, the representations that are based on these "trusted" processes are "psychologically correct" to this individual. This process may also explain how a functional physical symptom may be perpetuated through the interplay between maladaptive cognitive illness representations (e.g., a representation of symptom as indicative of a serious condition and beyond personal control; see also Brown's concept of rogue representations, section "The Brown's Integrative Conceptual

Model for FPS/S"), negative emotional representations (e.g., fear and sadness), and action plans (e.g., continuous visits to health professionals, avoiding activity), which are perceived by the patient as "psychologically correct" and, consequently, with no need to change.

The CSM suggests that the cognitive-emotional (i.e., illness representations) and behavioral reactions to a symptom are greatly determined by the activation of an illness-related prototype (a memory structure about illness) that is based on personal or family history, knowledge, and beliefs about the symptom or the disease. Each "prototype" includes representations about both the nature of the symptom (e.g., "This sensation comes and goes. There must be something really wrong"), potential action plans (e.g., "I need a doctor now"), and expected outcomes (e.g., "The doctor will make the sensation disappear"). Furthermore, according to the CSM, through the "symmetry rule," a perceptual event (e.g., the perception of a symptom or sensation) creates a pressure for a corresponding conceptual event (e.g., labeling of the symptoms and causal attribution) and vice versa (e.g., a person seeks for symptoms when one is diagnosed with or believes that suffers from a disease; Leventhal et al., 1992). The use of prototypes together with the symmetry rule may explain how an initially benign sensation or symptom becomes significant for the patient. The physical sensation is translated into a conceptual event (e.g., it gets a "name") which is compared against a prior prototype of illness. If there is some degree of matching, then the patient is convinced that they are probably dealing with a disease. This belief may not be subject to easy amendments (e.g., as a result of a consultation with a physician) as it is based on a complex symptom-related belief system generated by extensive personal experience and vicarious learning and encoded in the corresponding illness prototype.

Another aspect of the model, which might be relevant as a perpetuating factor of FPS/S, is "coherence." It refers to the consistency among illness representations and action plans and the patients' experience that their behavior usually succeeds in fulfilling their expectations (Phillips, Leventhal, & Leventhal, 2013). A coherent system leads to stable cognitive-emotional and behavioral responses providing, thus, the patient with a sense of control and securing the continuation of these responses (Phillips, Cohen, Burns, Abrams, & Renninger, 2016), even if maladaptive in the long-term.

Cognitive Behavioral Therapy for Functional Physical Syndromes/Symptoms

Although there is some evidence that other psychological therapies, such as the interpersonal therapy and the acceptance and commitment therapy, are also beneficial in the management of functional physical syndromes/symptoms, cognitive behavioral therapy (CBT) and graded exercise therapy (GET, which is also based on the greater CB tradition) seem to be the most effective treatment for FPS/S (IAPT, 2014). A typical CBT for FPS/S is based on the acceptance of symptoms as real and distressing for the patient (Witthöft & Hiller, 2010). The case formulation for each patient puts equal emphasis on the conditions and factors that trigger, intensify, and perpetuate FPS/S, as well as on the cognitive-emotional and behavioral reactions that accompany these symptoms.

As in the more classical CBTs (e.g., Beck, 1976), the treatment typically includes psychoeducational elements (e.g., regarding the relationship between the factors that seem to initiate and amplify reactions for a particular patient, or about the association between thoughts, emotions, and behavior, and the relation of physical reactions to psychological phenomena), homework, cognitive restructuring of catastrophizing representations and cognitions, stress management (e.g., biofeedback, relaxation training), and problem-solving. It also includes an array of behavior modification techniques, such as controlling excessive safety-seeking and body-checking behaviors, gradual exposure, gradual increase of physical activity (pacing), goal planning, reinforcement and behavioral experiments, attention control strategies, etc.

In general, both older and recent reviews and meta-analyses of controlled clinical trials have revealed small- to medium-sized and lower to those found for anxiety and affective disorders but, in any case, clinically significant effects of CBT-based interventions as far as the reduction of physical symptoms and psychological reactions (e.g., anxiety and depression) is concerned (Deary et al., 2007; Witthöft & Hiller, 2010). In their review of controlled clinical trials, Kroenke and Swindle (2000) concluded that CBT-based interventions were effective mostly for the management of functional physical symptoms (in more than 70% of cases) than psychological distress (in less than 50% of the cases). Also, a recent Cochrane meta-analysis of randomized clinical trials showed that CBT reduced somatic symptoms more effectively in comparison to standard (but not enhanced) care and waiting list conditions (van Dessel et al., 2014). Interestingly, another meta-analysis (Kleinstäuber, Witthöft, & Hiller, 2011) showed that CBT-based interventions designed for and delivered by physicians (e.g., reattribution training; Goldberg, Gask, & O'Down, 1989) are also effective and, in certain cases, may be even more effective than the traditional CBT delivered by mental health professionals.

Next, we will present in more detail three specific treatment approaches, as examples of the CBT-based interventions for FPS/S.

Looper and Kirmayer's Intervention Approach

Earlier we presented Kirmayer and his collaborators' model of processes that contribute to somatic distress (see section "The Basic CB Models for FPS/S"). Based on this model, Looper and Kirmayer (2002) proposed a multimodal treatment approach which includes a variety of CB treatment strategies that correspond to the different aspects of their model and are expected to interrupt the feedback loops that maintain the problem.

Specifically, Looper and Kirmayer suggested that medical treatments focusing on symptom management as well as psychological interventions, such as biofeedback and stress management, may form the first steps in addressing the physiological disturbance and the emotional arousal that initiate the development of functional physical syndromes/symptoms. At a second step, attention training, distraction, hypnosis, and/or environmental manipulations may be useful for managing the perceptual and attentional processes that result in excessive attention to body and physical sensations. At the next level, psychoeducation and cognitive techniques, such as restructuring of automatic thoughts and cognitive errors, may be useful for dealing with the misattributions of sensations to an illness, catastrophizing, maladaptive beliefs about illness, and personal cognitive schemata that contribute to the maintenance of the problem. In addition, behavior modification techniques, including reinforcement, pacing, graded exposure to potential threat signals (e.g., physical sensations), behavioral experiments, and response prevention to maladaptive reactions (e.g., continuous help-seeking) can address dysfunctional behaviors, such as avoidance and the need for continuous reassurance.

Finally, at the social environment level and given its role in the maintenance and perpetuation of the symptoms, the use of corresponding treatment strategies is probably crucial. For example, consultation to healthcare professionals about the needs of these patients and the potentially best ways to deal with them, the involvement of family members and significant others in the treatment plan, couple or family therapy, and the use of support groups may help toward the direction of modifying those social responses that contribute to FPS/S. Furthermore, Looper and Kirmayer suggested that interventions in the compensation social system and the disability policies, which may reinforce the adoption of a sick role, could be helpful and should, therefore, be considered (e.g., taking actions to increase the system flexibility so as to allow and facilitate gradual return to work).

A Hybrid Transdiagnostic/Problem-Specific Approach

Salkovskis et al. (2016; see also section "A Transdiagnostic/Problem Specific Approach," this chapter) strongly suggest that there is need for the treatment plan for functional physical syndromes/symptoms to be at the same time both transdiagnostic (i.e., to apply to FPS/S in general) and problem specific (i.e., to also employ specific strategies/techniques so as to address the specific difficulties of each patient or type of problem). The authors consider the CB model of health anxiety (see, Salkovskis & Warwick, 1986) as the appropriate core of their treatment approach for FPS/S. This core is "invested" with CB treatment approaches for depression, given that many patients with FPS/S suffer not only from anxiety but also from depressive symptoms, as well as other "syndrome-specific" elements/treatment strategies and techniques that correspond to each particular problem/patient.

The model has certain principles. The main principle is that intervention aims at helping the patient identify their problem and not to reassure or convince them that there is nothing wrong. The symptoms are real, even though a psychological approach is needed to fully understand their existence and discover ways to manage them. In all important aspects, the treatment of FPS/S follows the typical steps and method of the cognitive behavioral therapy models. For example, the emphasis on proper assessment leading to an accurate case formulation, collaborative work, and time-limited and agreed contract-based intervention and the emphasis on the strong relationships between thoughts, emotion, and behavior are all parts of this intervention. According to Salkovskis et al. (2016), the central components and stages of CB therapy for FPS/S are similar to those used in mental health problems. There are, however, differences in the attention that professionals should pay to engagement issues as well as the use of specific strategies/techniques so as to match patients' precise difficulties and different patterns of symptoms (e.g., chronic fatigue vs. atypical chest pain).

The treatment starts with a full general assessment concerning personal history, the development of the problem, current pattern of symptoms, other difficulties, etc. It continues with a more focused assessment which includes a complete evaluation of (a) the symptom-related initiating and maintaining factors and (b) patient's appraisals and thoughts about their condition. Salkovksis et al. also provide a list of assessment tools for FPS/S, divided into transdiagnostic measures (e.g., regarding anxiety and depression, disability, general symptoms), symptom-specific measures (e.g., sleep problems, fatigue), and process measures (e.g., catastrophizing, rumination). Liaison with healthcare professionals may be part of this intervention phase.

The next step is the development of a formulation of the symptoms based on assessment. This formulation will be presented to the patient so as to provide them with an explanation of their symptoms and, through discussion, to lead to an agreed model of how the interaction between physical and psychological factors contribute to the development of the patient's particular symptoms. The formulation can be adjusted to new information throughout the intervention. Through the use of techniques, such as self-monitoring, behavioral experiments, and detailed discussions with the professional, patients are helped to understand their condition using a psychological perspective that always refers to the current formulation of the symptoms.

As treatment progresses, dysfunctional and inaccurate beliefs and representations are challenged, and behavior is modified. Treatment may be directed on the complex nature of patients' concerns (like the perceived likelihood of an illness or disability, the perceived severity of the symptoms, and the perceived coping ability and potential rescue factors; see also section "A Transdiagnostic/Problem Specific Approach" of this chapter) and their behavior (e.g., excessive medical consultation, excessive focusing on bodily sensations). Finally, intervention may focus on issues regarding patient's self-esteem, cognitive styles (e.g., catastrophizing and black-and-white thinking), attitudes about health and illness, perfectionism, etc. Of course, strategies directed at each patient's particular pattern of symptoms are deployed throughout the intervention. This is a very promising CB intervention approach for functional symptoms, but its effectiveness is still to be proved in future studies (some of which are already under way; Salkovskis et al., 2016).

Reattribution Techniques

This intervention program was developed for use by family doctors/general practitioners and not mental health professionals and does not include highly specialized techniques. Nevertheless, it is an interesting approach for involving physicians in the management of FPS/S, and it also underlines the importance of the social environment in the development as well as the treatment of these symptoms. The program was initially described by Goldberg et al. (1989). Its aim was for physicians to help patients reattribute FPS/S and relate these symptoms to psychosocial processes.

Originally, the reattribution intervention consisted of three stages, but later a fourth one was added (Morriss et al., 2006). These four stages are feeling understood, broadening the agenda, making the link, and negotiating further treatment. The first stage (feeling understood) aims in getting the patient feel understood and accepted by the physician as well as help the latter achieve a better understanding of patient's experience and beliefs. Typically, this stage includes a full history and clarification of symptoms, exploration of the social and family factors possibly contributing to patient's experience, as well as patient's health beliefs, thoughts about the symptoms, and emotional reactions. The second stage (changing the agenda) includes feedback to the patient regarding the results of the physical examinations and acknowledgment that symptoms are real, reframing patient's complaints by summarizing other symptoms and linking them to psychosocial factors. The third step (making the link) refers to making a link between symptoms and potential psychosocial causes. The physician is urged to discuss with the patient and make explicit alternative possible explanations for the development of symptoms (i.e., regarding causes/triggers and mechanisms), including the role of anxiety, depression, tension and stress, lifestyle, patient's beliefs, and family influences, one at a time. In the final stage (negotiating further treatment), the physician explores patient's personal understanding, worries, and concerns about treatment. The physician also negotiates the appropriate treatment (which may include a psychological intervention as well) and makes specific plans for follow-ups, if necessary. A detailed teaching package for physicians, including instructional videos, microteaching, role-playing, and feedback of videotaped actual clinical performance, has been developed as part of this intervention (Goldberg et al., 1989; Morriss et al., 2006).

A recent review of the studies using the reattribution intervention model (Gask, Dowrick, Salmon, Peters, & Morriss, 2011) showed that its impact on clinical outcomes is mixed. The authors suggested that the reattribution intervention model is probably too simplistic in its current form to have an impact on patients with complex FPS/S, while the reattribution of symptoms, as a sole target for intervention, might not always be helpful. Thus, models such as this one should probably be part of a more composite intervention plan, for example, as a "first step" in a "stepped care," intervention program that will also include psychological treatment and/or pharmacotherapy, if needed (Gask et al., 2011). In any case, this model is a good example of how healthcare professionals could be involved in a multi-facet CB intervention strategy that will include, besides the more traditional psychological treatment delivered by specialized professionals, other forms of consultation in order to better address patients' needs.

Synthesis and Conclusion

As noted at the beginning of this chapter, there is not a single cognitive behavioral model for functional physical syndromes and symptoms. There are several of them, while new and more elaborate ones are continuously presented. These models share several similarities, especially regarding their cognitive and behavioral background, but also differ as a result of their effort to highlight different aspects of the development of FPS/S and incorporate new research findings and theoretical developments. Still, all CB models for FPS/S adopt two core notions: (a) different physiological, social, and psychological factors are involved in the development, maintenance, and, finally, perpetuation of the symptoms; (b) not a single but rather a sequence of processes and feedback loops between these factors and their interactions underlie the development and maintenance of FPS/S. The CB perspective is in many ways a meta-model (Deary et al., 2007) which provides an overview of the overall processes underlying the genesis and perpetuation of FPS/S. With the addition of more specific factors and processes, this fundamental model can apply to different specific conditions and the unique experience of each patient.

Figure 3.1 presents a summary of the factors that have been proposed by several CB models as involved in the development and maintenance of FPS/S. This schematic depiction begins with some examples of potential triggers of the process; continues with emphasizing the importance of attentional and cognitive factors, emotional arousal, and catastrophizing; and goes on highlighting the role of dysfunctional behavior, the activation of maladaptive cognitive schemata, and the significant impact of the social environment and the healthcare system. The figure ends with a description of FPS/S as a chronic condition characterized by the adoption of a sick role (e.g., persistent complaining, self-pity), possible physical alterations (as a potential result of the chronic activation of physical systems, such as the autonomic nervous system), and the emergence of a (rather stable) pattern of reactions toward symptoms (e.g., constant representation of symptoms as harmful, anxiety and depression, habitual inactivity, frequent visits to physicians).

There is ample and strong evidence for the importance of several of these factors in the development of FPS/S (e.g., about attentional processes; for reviews, see Deary et al., 2007; Rief & Broadbent, 2007; Witthöft & Hiller, 2010). Still, for some factors, such as the attribution of symptoms to a physical illness, recent research findings question their importance (e.g., Henningsen & Creed, 2010). This fact, in combination with the need to incorporate the impact of biological processes and mechanisms (e.g., immunological activities) into the existing models, as well as the need to describe in more detail how symptoms and correspondent reactions become

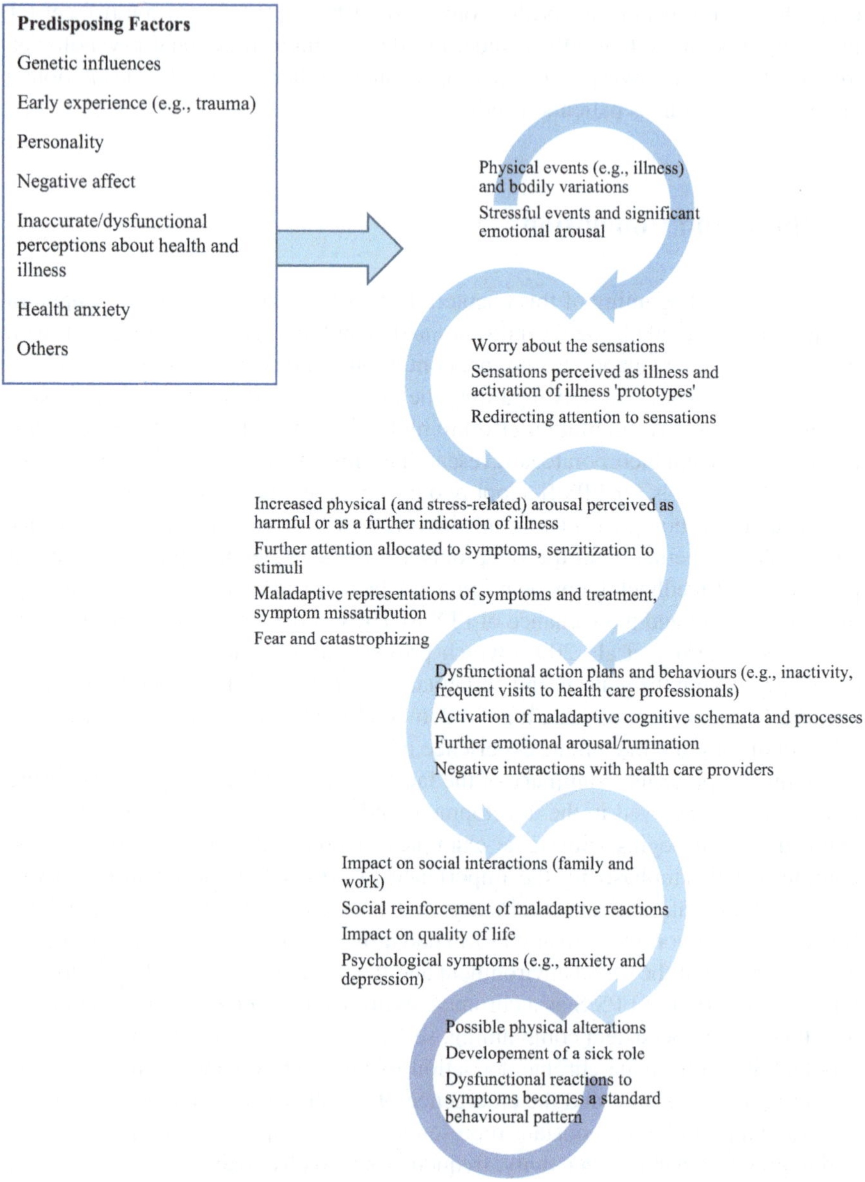

Fig. 3.1 The spiral of feedback loops and interactions between factors generating and perpetuating functional physical syndromes/symptoms according to the general cognitive behavioral approach

chronic (e.g., the role of the environment and social reinforcement; Rief & Broadbent, 2007), points to the necessity for further theoretical advancement and empirical validation of the CB models. The addition of approaches that may not directly refer to functional physical symptoms but rather to the overall illness experience, such as the Common Sense Model (Leventhal et al., 1980, 1992), as well as models that address both general and specific problems, such as the hybrid transdiagnostic/problem-specific approach developed by Salkovskis et al. (2016), will probably enrich the CB approach to functional physical syndromes and symptoms and will open new ways in understanding this complicated phenomenon.

In turn, this effort will lead to more effective psychological interventions for FRS/S. So far, the CB treatment modes for FPS/S have used, more or less, the intervention strategies and techniques of a typical cognitive behavioral therapy, including psychoeducation, cognitive restructuring, attention regulation techniques, problem-solving and emotion regulation, an array of behavior modification techniques, etc. Overall, there is evidence suggesting that CBT for functional physical syndromes/symptoms is indeed effective (Deary et al., 2007; Kroenke & Swindle, 2000; van Dessel et al., 2014; Witthöft & Hiller, 2010).

However, as Deary et al. (2007) highlighted, CBT-based treatments vary greatly in content and method of delivery, while it is still unknown which strategies and mechanisms of change are the most effective and for which particular problem and population. Also, there is no adequate data on the cost-effectiveness of treatment. In addition, little is known about the effectiveness of CBT in the "front line," that is, not when delivered by mental health professionals but by physicians or other healthcare providers (e.g., nurses) who come in direct contact with all patients suffering from FPS/S (e.g., in primary care). Such interventions might be very helpful considering the importance of the physician—patient relationship in the establishment of functional physical syndromes/symptoms. Such efforts have been developed in the past (e.g., Fink, Rosendal, & Toft, 2002; Kennedy et al., 2005), while much attention has gained the relevant reattribution treatment approach (Goldberg et al., 1989; Morriss et al., 2006). In the future, the delivery of combined standard medical and functional symptom-specific CB interventions by a specialized physician might prove to be the appropriate treatment, at least in primary care and for the less complicated cases (e.g., before a FPS/S evolves into a chronic condition).

Of course, much more work is needed toward this direction, and much more research is warranted to answer the many questions about the use of CBT-based intervention programs in FPS/S. Still, we may overall assert that, currently, CBT is probably the most effective psychological treatment for the management of such symptoms (IAPT, 2014), while the development of new ideas and approaches will continue to enhance the effectiveness of CB treatments for functional physical syndromes and symptoms.

Acknowledgments Funding: This work was supported by the University of Crete Special Account for Research under Grant 4953.

References

Barsky, A. J., & Wyshak, G. L. (1990). Hypochondriasis and somatosensory amplification. *British Journal of Psychiatry, 157*, 404–409.

Beck, A. T. (1976). *Cognitive therapy and the emotional disorders*. New York, NY: International Universities Press.

Breland, J. Y., Fox, A. M., Horowitz, C. R., & Leventhal, H. (2012). Applying a common-sense approach to fighting obesity. *Journal of Obesity, 2012*, 710427.

Brown, R. J. (2004). Psychological mechanisms of medically unexplained symptoms: An integrative conceptual model. *Psychological Bulletin, 130*, 793–812.

Brown, R. J. (2007). Introduction to the special issue on medically unexplained symptoms: Background and future directions. *Clinical Psychology Review, 27*, 769–780.

Creed, F. (2016). Exploding myths about medically unexplained symptoms. *Journal of Psychosomatic Research, 85*, 91–93.

Creed, F., Guthrie, E., Fink, P., Henningsen, P., Rief, W., Sharpe, M., & White, P. (2010). Is there a better term that "medically unexplained symptoms"? *Journal of Psychosomatic Research, 68*, 5–8.

De Gucht, V., & Maes, S. (2006). Explaining medically unexplained symptoms: Toward a multidimensional, theory-based approach to somatization. *Journal of Psychosomatic Research, 60*, 349–352.

Deary, V., Chalder, T., & Sharpe, M. (2007). The cognitive behavioural model of medically unexplained symptoms: A theoretical and empirical review. *Clinical Psychology Review, 27*, 78–797.

Dempster, M., Howell, D., & McCorry, N. K. (2015). Illness perceptions and coping in physical health conditions: A meta-analysis. *Journal of Psychosomatic Research, 79*, 506–513.

Fink, P., Rosendal, M., & Toft, T. (2002). Assessment and treatment of functional disorders in general practice: The extended reattribution and management model—An advanced educational program for nonpsychiatric doctors. *Psychosomatics, 43*, 93–131.

Gask, L., Dowrick, C., Salmon, P., Peters, S., & Morriss, R. (2011). Reattribution reconsidered: Narrative review and reflections on an educational intervention for medically unexplained symptoms in primary care settings. *Journal of Psychosomatic Research, 71*, 325–334.

Gijsbers van Wijk, C. M. T., & Kolk, A. M. (1997). Sex differences in physical symptoms: The contribution of symptom perception theory. *Social Science and Medicine, 45*, 231–246.

Goldberg, D., Gask, L., & O'Down, T. (1989). The treatment of somatization: Teaching techniques of reattribution. *Journal of Psychosomatic Research, 33*, 689–695.

Hagger, M. S., Koch, S., Chatzisarantis, N. L. D., & Orbell, S. (2017). The common-sense model of self-regulation: Meta-analysis and test of a process model. *Psychological Bulletin, 143*(11), 1117–1154.

Henningsen, P., & Creed, F. (2010). The genetic, physiological and psychological mechanisms underlying disabling medically unexplained symptoms and somatization. *Journal of Psychosomatic Research, 68*, 395–397.

Hudson, J. L., Bundy, C., Coventry, P. A., & Dickens, C. (2014). Exploring the relationship between cognitive illness representations and poor emotional health and their combined association with diabetes self-care. A systematic review with meta-analysis. *Journal of Psychosomatic Research, 76*, 265–274.

Improving Access to Psychological Therapies (IAPT). (2014). *Medically unexplained symptoms/functional symptoms. Positive practice guide*. London: IAPT, National Health System.

Kennedy, T., Jones, R., Darnley, S., Seed, P., Wessely, S., & Chalder, T. (2005). Cognitive behaviour therapy in addition to antispasmodic treatment for irritable bowel syndrome in primary care: Randomized clinical trial. *British Medical Journal, 331*(7514), 435.

Kirmayer, L. J., & Robbins, J. M. (1991). Three forms of somatization in primary care: Prevalence, co-occurrence, and sociodemographic characteristics. *Journal of Nervous and Mental Diseases, 179*, 647–655.

Kirmayer, L. J., & Taillefer, S. (1997). Somatoform disorders. In S. M. Turner & M. Hersen (Eds.), *Adult psychopathology and diagnosis* (3rd ed., pp. 333–383). New York, NY: Wiley.

Kleinstäuber, M., Witthöft, M., & Hiller, W. (2011). Efficacy of short-term psychotherapy for multiple medically unexplained physical symptoms: A meta-analysis. *Clinical Psychology Review, 31*, 146–160.

Knoop, H., Prins, J., Moss-Morris, R., & Bleijenberg, G. (2010). The central role of cognitive processes in the perpetuation of chronic fatigue syndrome. *Journal of Psychosomatic Research, 68*, 489–494.

Kolk, A. M. M. (2000). Women and somatic distress. In J. Ussher (Ed.), *Women's health: Contemporary international perspectives* (pp. 507–516). Leicester: The British Psychological Society.

Kolk, A. M., Hanewald, G. J. F. P., Schagen, S., & Gijsbers van Wijk, C. M. T. (2003). A symptom perception approach to common physical symptoms. *Social Science & Medicine, 57*, 2343–2354.

Kroenke, K., & Swindle, R. (2000). Cognitive-behavioral therapy somatization and symptoms syndromes: A critical review of controlled clinical trials. *Psychotherapy and Psychosomatics, 69*, 205–215.

Leventhal, H., Diefenbach, M., & Leventhal, E. A. (1992). Illness cognition: Using common sense to understand treatment adherence and affect cognition treatment. *Cognitive Therapy and Research, 16*, 223–230.

Leventhal, H., Meyer, D., & Nerenz, D. (1980). The common-sense representations of illness danger. In S. Rachman (Ed.), *Medical psychology* (Vol. 2, pp. 7–30). New York: Pergamon.

Looper, K. J., & Kirmayer, L. J. (2002). Behavioral medicine approaches to somatoform disorders. *Journal of Consulting and Clinical Psychology, 70*, 810–827.

Marks, E. M., & Hunter, M. S. (2015). Medically unexplained symptoms: An acceptable term? *British Journal of Pain, 9*, 109–114.

Melzack, R., & Wall, P. D. (1965). Pain mechanisms: A new theory. *Science, 150*, 971–978.

Morriss, R., Dowrick, C., Salmon, P., Peters, S., Rogers, A., Dunn, G., ... & Gask, L. (2006). Turning theory into practice: Rationale, feasibility and external validity of an exploratory randomized controlled trial of training family practitioners in reattribution to manage patients with medically unexplained symptoms (the MUST). *General Hospital Psychiatry, 28*, 343–351.

Nimnuan, C., Hotopf, M., & Wessely, S. (2000). Medically unexplained symptoms: How often and why are they missed? *Quarterly Journal of Medicine, 93*, 21–28.

olde Hartman, T. C., Borghuis, M. S., Lucassen, P. L. B. J., van de Laar, F. A., Speckens, A. E., & van Weel, C. (2009). Medically unexplained symptoms, somatization disorder and hypochondriasis: Course and prognosis. A systematic review. *Journal of Psychosomatic Research, 66*, 363–377.

Pennebaker, J. W. (1982). *The psychology of physical symptoms*. New York, NY: Springer.

Phillips, L. A., Cohen, J., Burns, E., Abrams, J., & Renninger, S. (2016). Self-management of chronic illness: The role of 'habit' versus reflective factors in exercise and medication adherence. *Journal of Behavioral Medicine, 39*, 1076–1091.

Phillips, L. A., Leventhal, H., & Leventhal, E. A. (2013). Assessing theoretical predictors of long-term medication adherence: Patients' treatment-related beliefs, experiential feedback and habit development. *Psychology and Health, 28*, 1135–1151.

Phillips, L. A., McAndrew, L., Laman-Maharg, B., & Bloeser, K. (2017). Evaluating challenges for improving medically unexplained symptoms in US military veterans via provider communication. *Patient Education and Counseling, 100*, 1580–1587.

Picariello, F., Ali, S., Moss-Morris, R., & Chalder, T. (2015). The most popular terms for medically unexplained symptoms: The views of CFS patients. *Journal of Psychosomatic Research, 78*, 420–426.

Rief, W., & Barsky, A. J. (2005). Psychobiological perspectives on somatoform disorders. *Psychoneuroendocrinology, 30*, 996–1002.

Rief, W., & Broadbent, E. (2007). Explaining medically unexplained symptoms-models and mechanisms. *Clinical Psychology Review, 27*, 821–841.
Roelofs, K., & Spinhoven, P. (2007). Trauma and medically unexplained symptoms. Towards an integration of cognitive and neuro-biological accounts. *Clinical Psychology Review, 27*, 798–820.
Salkovskis, P. M. (1996). The cognitive approach to anxiety: Threat beliefs, safety-seeking behavior, and the special case of health anxiety and obsessions. In P. M. Salkovskis (Ed.), *Frontiers of cognitive therapy* (pp. 48–74). New York, NY: Guilford.
Salkovskis, P. M., Gregory, J. D., Sedgwick-Taylor, A., White, J., Opher, S., & Ólafsdóttir, S. (2016). Extending cognitive-behavioral theory and therapy to medically unexplained symptoms and long-term physical conditions: A hybrid transdiagnostic/problem specific approach. *Behavior Change, 33*, 172–192.
Salkovskis, P. M., & Warwick, H. M. (1986). Morbid preoccupations, health anxiety and reassurance: A cognitive-behavioral approach to hypochondriasis. *Behavior Research and Therapy, 24*, 597–602.
Schroeder, S., Achenbach, S., Körber, S., Nowy, K., de Zwaan, M., & Martin, A. (2012). Cognitive-perceptual factors in noncardiac chest pain and cardiac chest pain. *Psychosomatic Medicine, 74*, 861–868.
van Dessel, N., den Boeft, M., van der Wouden, J., Kleinstäuber, M., Leone, S. S., Terluin, B., … & van Marwijk, H. (2014). Non-pharmacological intervention for somatoform disorders and medically unexplained physical symptoms (MUPS) in adults. *Cochrane Database of Systematic Reviews, 11*, CD011142.
Webster, R., Thompson, A. R., & Norman, P. (2015). 'Everything's fine, so why does it happen?' A qualitative investigation of patients' perceptions of noncardiac chest pain. *Journal of Clinical Nursing, 24*, 1936–1945.
Witthöft, M., & Hiller, W. (2010). Psychological approaches to origins and treatments of somatoform disorders. *Annual Review of Clinical Psychology, 6*, 257–283.
World Health Organization (WHO). (2016). *International statistical classification of diseases and related health problems. 10th Revision* (5th ed.). Geneva: WHO.

Chapter 4
Negative Affect and Medically Unexplained Symptoms

Elena Constantinou

The idea that medically unexplained symptoms (MUS), i.e. physical symptoms that cannot be attributed to or adequately explained by an identifiable organic cause, are linked to our emotional lives is definitely not new. As a matter of fact, the most stereotypical cases of MUS that come into one's mind are probably Freud's hysteria-suffering Victorian women, who experienced a series of physical symptoms as manifestations of suppressed or unresolved emotional memories. About 130 years later, unexplained physical symptoms still constitute a debilitating and puzzling phenomenon, with epidemiology studies indicating that about 12% of the general population (Rief, Hessel, & Braehler, 2001) and one third of primary care patients (Kroenke, 2003; Toft et al., 2005) report MUS. Importantly, affective processes are still considered to play a key role in the development and maintenance of such symptomatology. James W. Pennebaker's seminal work in *The Psychology of Physical Symptoms* (1982) laid the foundation stone of modern cognitive-perceptual theories of symptom perception (Brown, 2004; Deary, Chalder, & Sharpe, 2007; Rief & Barsky, 2005), which focus on the perceptual process underlying the experience of physical symptoms and the psychological factors that can bias this process leading to MUS. Among others, affective processes are seen by current conceptualizations as one of these factors biasing symptom perception toward overperception of symptoms (i.e., the presence of MUS).

The following chapter aims to discuss the role of affective processes in biased symptom perception as observed in MUS. I first summarize evidence that supports

E. Constantinou (✉)
Social, Genetic and Developmental Psychiatry Centre, Institute of Psychiatry, Psychology and Neuroscience, King's College London, London, UK
e-mail: elena.constantinou@kcl.ac.uk

C. Charis, G. Panayiotou (eds.), *Somatoform and Other Psychosomatic Disorders*,
https://doi.org/10.1007/978-3-319-89360-0_4

the link between negative affect[1] and MUS, then I describe the mechanisms proposed to explain this relationship and the evidence that supports them, and finally I discuss questions still to be explored, as well as the importance of studying emotions in the context of MUS.

Biased Symptom Perception: Medically Unexplained Symptoms (MUS)

Throughout history "unexplained" physical complaints have been described using various labels like hysteria, somatization, psychosomatic or psychogenic phenomena, somatoform symptoms, or more recently in the medical world functional somatic symptoms. Medically unexplained symptoms (MUS) is an alternative term, which, contrary to the rest, does not allude to a certain theoretical conceptualization of these symptoms. It serves, thus, as a theory-neutral umbrella term that encompasses a range of physical symptoms that may stem from different processes, like somatization, somatosensory amplification, and hypochondriasis. Additionally, MUS can vary in severity, from mild physical complaints in everyday life in the general population to clinically severe symptoms as seen in functional syndromes (e.g., irritable bowel syndrome, chronic fatigue syndrome, fibromyalgia) or somatoform disorders. Despite the heterogeneity of all these conditions, cognitive-perceptual theorists tend to "lump" them together focusing on their common characteristics (Wessely, Nimnuan, & Sharpe, 1999) and consider them as different manifestations of biases in the symptom perception process. This view is also reflected in the recent change in DSM-V, which groups all these phenomena under the somatic symptom disorder category (Rief & Martin, 2014).

Association Between MUS and Negative Affect

Neurobiological findings Initial evidence for the link between negative affect and symptom perception comes from neurobiological findings indicating common and intertwined neural pathways involved in emotional processing and interoception, i.e., the perception of all signals generated by our body (Bechara & Naqvi, 2004). Interoception encompasses a series of processes leading to the subjective experience of bodily sensations: the central representation of afferent signals from various organs, their affective evaluation and integration with situational cues, and the activation of previous somatic experiences stored in memory, which are used to interpret the incoming signals (Craig, 2002).

[1] The term "negative affect" is used as a generic term referring to both emotions, i.e., intense, short-term reactions toward certain stimuli or contexts, as well as moods, i.e., more long-lasting diffuse affective states (feeling good or bad; Forgas, 1995), as research findings from studies using either emotions or moods are reported here.

Affective processes have been closely linked to interoception quite early in the history of psychology, as autonomic bodily changes were viewed as necessary elements that give rise to emotional experiences (James, 1884). James' views regained attention in contemporary theories of emotion based on neuroimaging findings. In his highly influential theory, Damasio (1994) proposed that the subjective experience of emotion is the outcome of a hierarchical representation of bodily state, which is perceived and integrated with environmental or situational cues. This hierarchical representation is mirrored in brain activity (see Critchley, 2005; Critchley, Mathias, & Dolan, 2001). During an emotional experience, emotional cues (real or imaginary) are perceived by first-order structures (sensory-motor structures, amygdala) and produce a series of bodily changes (muscular, chemical, visceral, etc.). These changes are then signaled back to the brain via interoceptive pathways (brainstem, thalamus, hypothalamus, limbic structures, somatosensory cortices). Second-order structures integrate the representation of these bodily changes with mental representations in memory activated by the emotional stimulus (cingulate and prefrontal cortex). The juxtaposition of bodily changes and the activated representation of the situation/stimulus produce the subjective experience of emotion (Damasio, 1994).

Similarly, neurobiological theories of interoception (Craig, 2002) also point to a link between affective processes and interoception. According to A.D. Craig (2002), interoceptive signals serve a homeostatic function and as such involve both a sensory and an affective-motivational aspect. Unpleasant bodily signals, like pain, reflect a disturbance in the body that requires an adaptive response by the organism to recover the necessary balance (Craig, 2002; Damasio & Carvalho, 2013). Brain imaging studies show that during interoception, afferent signals are firstly represented in the CNS at regions related to homeostasis, i.e., the lamina I system, and then combined with efferent parasympathetic activity in the thalamocortical pathways to form a representation of the bodily state. This bodily state representation is projected to the insular cortex, where it is re-represented from posterior to anterior insula resulting to the subjective experience of feelings (Craig, 2002).

Thus, it seems that second-order structures linked to human awareness, like the anterior insula (Craig, 2009), can form the link between the conscious experience of physical symptoms (Wiech & Tracey, 2009) and that of affect (Zaki, Davis, & Ochsner, 2012). Recent findings suggest that activation in anterior insula is associated with the biasing effects of negative affect on the perception of painful stimuli (Orenius et al., 2017). Even more, increased attention to and perception of interoceptive signals has been associated with increased activity in anterior insula (Critchley, Wiens, Rotshtein, Öhman, & Dolan, 2004), while both the ACC and the insular cortex have been associated with the experience of "unexplained" physical symptoms (Landgrebe et al., 2008), suggesting that these areas are implicated in overperception of physical symptoms and MUS.

Correlational findings Another important source of evidence for the role of negative affect in MUS comes from correlational studies indicating a strong association in the general population between trait characteristics related to negative affect, like trait negative affectivity (NA) and neuroticism, and elevated symptom reports, especially vague and systemic physical symptoms, like dizziness and fatigue (Rosmalen, Neeleman, Gans, & de Jonge, 2007; Van Diest et al., 2005; Watson & Pennebaker, 1989; Williams

& Wiebe, 2000). While trait NA has been linked to the subjective experience of especially ambiguous physical symptoms, no such associations have been found in regard to actual health status in nonclinical samples (Kolk, Hanewald, Schagen, & Gijsbers van Wijk, 2002; Watson & Pennebaker, 1989), thus suggesting that trait NA is associated with biased symptom perception. Using a longitudinal design, de Gucht, Fischler, and Heiser (2004) further showed that an increase in negative affectivity over time and a decrease in positive affectivity predict an increase in reported MUS at a 6-month follow-up, thus suggesting that the presence of negative affect (and the lack of positive affect) precedes the experience of MUS.

The association between negative affect and MUS is also supported by clinical findings indicating comorbidity between clinical levels of MUS and both anxiety and depression. Epidemiological data from various countries have shown that a high percentage of depressed patients (30–60% in some countries) report multiple unexplained physical symptoms (Simon, VonKorff, Piccinelli, Fullerton, & Ormel, 1999), while patients with functional syndromes (Henningsen, Zimmermann, & Sattel, 2003) or somatoform disorder (Steinbrecher, Koerber, Frieser, & Hiller, 2011) tend to also suffer from major depression or an anxiety disorder. A recent meta-analysis of longitudinal studies has shown that pre-existing levels of depression and anxiety double the risk of developing IBS, a gastrointestinal functional syndrome, suggesting that negative affect is a predisposing factor for the development of clinical MUS (Sibelli et al., 2016).

Experimental findings A crucial finding of correlational studies is the observation that trait characteristics, e.g., neuroticism or trait NA, influence symptom perception indirectly via their effects on increasing state negative affect (Brown & Moskowitz, 1997; de Gucht et al., 2004; Williams & Wiebe, 2000), which seems to be even more strongly linked to physical symptom reports (Charles & Almeida, 2006; Leventhal, Hansell, Diefenbach, Leventhal, & Glass, 1996; Watson & Pennebaker, 1989). The role of state negative affect in symptom perception is more clearly illustrated by experimental studies manipulating state affect.

Typically, such studies involve the presentation of affective stimuli along with a laboratory challenge that creates bodily sensations (e.g., pain, respiratory, or gastrointestinal sensations) to examine biases in symptom perception. These studies overall show an augmenting effect of state negative affect (state NA) on the perception of physical symptoms. For example, the brief presentation of unpleasant stimuli (like affective pictures or emotional faces) has been found to result in reduced pain tolerance during a cold pressor task (de Wied & Verbaten, 2001; Meagher, Arnau, & Rhudy, 2001), increased pain perception during the delivery of electric shocks (Rhudy, Williams, McCabe, Russell, & Maynard, 2008), more discomfort during esophageal distension (Phillips et al., 2003), and more perceived unpleasantness of dyspnea sensations (Von Leupoldt, Mertz, Kegat, Burmester, & Dahme, 2006). Pleasant stimuli, on the other hand, that induce positive affect, result in reduced physical symptoms in these studies. Similar findings have been reported with other affective stimuli like odors (Villemure, Slotnick, & Bushnell, 2003), imagery

(Rietveld, Everaerd, & Van Beest, 2000) or hypnosis (Houghton, Calvert, Jackson, Cooper, & Whorwell, 2002).

The emotional modulation of symptom perception has been replicated multiple times, but importantly experimental studies have also shown that the level of modulation depends on individual differences. Specifically, this emotional modulation seems to be more pronounced in patients with clinical levels of MUS. Montoya et al. (2005), for example, showed that unpleasant stimuli augmented pain perception for fibromyalgia patients but not for patients with musculoskeletal (organically explained) pain. Similarly, Van Den Houte et al. (2017) found increased symptom perception after showing unpleasant pictures in patients with fibromyalgia or chronic fatigue syndrome but not in healthy controls. On the other hand, some studies have shown an inability of pleasant cues to reduce symptom experiences in fibromyalgia patients (Kamping, Bomba, Kanske, Diesch, & Flor, 2013; Rhudy et al., 2013). Similarly, Elsenbruch et al. (2010) showed that for patients with IBS stress had a stronger effect on cortical responses to rectal distensions in comparison with healthy controls, but also relaxation had a diminished effect. Hence, for individuals with clinical MUS, negative affect seems to have a pronounced effect leading to excessive symptom reporting, while the dampening effect of positive affect on symptom experiences is absent or minimal.

Furthermore, research suggests that these moderating effects extent to nonclinical levels of MUS. Bogaerts et al. (2008), for example, showed that the effects of unpleasant cues on the perception of respiratory symptoms were especially pronounced in healthy individuals reporting frequent symptoms in daily life (a group seen as a nonclinical proxy for MUS individuals; Bogaerts et al., 2008). Additionally, work from the same group (Bogaerts, Janssens, De Peuter, Van Diest, & Van den Bergh, 2010) indicated that merely presenting unpleasant cues can result in the expected augmented experience of physical symptoms even without any laboratory challenge, but importantly, this was only observed in individuals who tended to report frequent symptoms.

To further delineate these individual differences, we used the same paradigm, i.e., we presented pleasant and unpleasant pictures without any laboratory challenge to healthy individuals that reported frequent symptoms in daily life and controls, and we assessed symptom experiences after picture viewing but also their physiological reactions to the emotional pictures (heart rate and skin conductance; Constantinou, Bogaerts, Van Diest, & Van den Bergh, 2013). We found that, frequent symptom reporters did not differ in their subjective experience of unpleasantness or in physiological reactivity to the pictures, but they experienced more physical symptoms after watching unpleasant pictures, especially highly arousing unpleasant pictures than controls. Thus, the augmented emotion modulation of physical symptoms observed in this group is not due to them experiencing more negative affect or having more physiological reactions toward unpleasant cues. This is in line with studies showing that individuals with clinical MUS do not differ from controls in actual autonomic arousal (Houtveen, Rietveld, & de Geus, 2003; Houtveen & Van Doornen, 2007; Van Middendorp et al., 2013). Furthermore, these findings suggest that the effects of emotion on symptom perception is not the outcome of increased bottom-up physiological input accompanying highly arousing conditions, which would naturally lead to increased symptom experiences. Thus, emotional influences on symptom reporting cannot be reduced to a mere somatization process, i.e., the interpretation of emotional arousal as symptoms (Kirmayer & Taillefer, 1997). Rather, it seems that state negative affect triggers symptom experiences in a top-down manner for individuals prone to experience MUS.

Summing up, findings from experimental studies provide further evidence for the augmenting effects of negative affect on symptom experiences. However, they also provide evidence for moderators of this effect, as it seems that trait characteristics, like a tendency to experience physical symptoms in daily life, interact with state negative affect. Examining these interactions can be crucial in delineating the mechanisms, through which emotions influence symptom perception.

How Negative Affect Leads to MUS: Proposed Mechanisms

While the link between negative affect and symptom overreporting as seen in MUS has been replicated multiple times, the mechanisms underlying this relationship have not yet been fully understood. Understanding how negative affect leads to symptom overreporting may have important implications for our conceptualization and dealing with MUS. In the following sections, I will discuss three mechanisms previously proposed to explain the effects of emotion on health and illness in general (Salovey, O'Leary, Stretton, Fishkin, & Drake, 1991) and will attempt to link them to MUS more specifically.

Hypothesis 1: Negative affect influences immune function and actual health The first hypothesis suggests that negative affect induces a series of bodily changes including immunological changes, which can in turn influence actual health status (and not just what is subjectively experienced). This hypothesis has been mainly driven by research on stress and its direct effects on the HPA axis and autonomic nervous system function (see review by Glaser & Kiecolt-Glaser, 2005). The stress-induced deregulation of the immune system can make individuals more susceptible to infectious diseases but also impair their immune response toward pathogens, thus prolonging illness episodes (Glaser & Kiecolt-Glaser, 2005). Research findings overall support this link between negative affect and immune function (Denson, Spanovic, & Miller, 2009). Especially, chronic stressors, like unemployment, have been found to suppress immune function (Segerstrom & Miller, 2004), while similar suppression has been linked to depression and anxiety (Kiecolt-Glaser, McGuire, Robles, & Glaser, 2002). However, the immunosuppressive effects of negative affect are less consistent when looking at acute experimentally induced stressors. In their review, Segerstrom and Miller (2004) suggest that acute stressors seem to downregulate specific immunity but upregulate natural immunity, as an adaptive response to the stressor. A more recent review (Marsland, Walsh, Lockwood, & John-Henderson, 2017), though, concludes that there are reliable effects of acute stress on inflammatory markers, but these effects were mainly observed between 30 and 90 min after stress. Therefore, while this mechanism may be important in delineating how affect influences susceptibility to disease and health outcomes in the long term, it cannot adequately explain the immediate effects of state affect (e.g., as induced by presenting emotional pictures for a few seconds) on physical symptoms presented above.

Importantly, research with individuals with either clinical (Elsenbruch et al., 2006) or nonclinical (Houtveen & Van Doornen, 2007) levels of MUS shows similar autonomic and neuroendocrine responses to negative affect in these groups in comparison with controls. Although differences in the function of the HPA axis and the immune system in general have been hypothesized to play a role in the etiology of MUS, overall research has provided inconsistent findings in regard to such biological differences in MUS individuals (Tak et al., 2011). Some studies do suggest differential effects of acute stress in the immune function of patients with clinical levels of MUS (Gaab et al., 2005), but again these changes seem to emerge within a larger time window than the immediate emotion effects mentioned above. Thus, while individuals that frequently experience MUS seem to be more influenced by negative affect in their experience of physical symptoms, this does not seem to be fully accounted for by consistently observed differences in biological reactivity to stress in this group.

Hypothesis 2: Negative affect induces self-focused attention The second proposed mechanism suggests that negative affect influences symptom perception via the changes it induces in self-focused attention (see review by Mor & Winquist, 2002). Thus, state negative affect leads to increased symptom reports because it induces more self-focus.

This is the most prominent hypothesis stemming from cognitive-perceptual theories of symptom perception (Pennebaker, 1982; Rief & Barsky, 2005), which focused on the selective mechanism of attention, as a main source of bias in symptom perception. A cornerstone for these theories is the view that at any given moment, our central nervous system receives information both from outside and inside the body, which compete for limited attentional resources. Hence, whether bodily signals will be attended to and consciously perceived depends on whether the intensity of these signals exceeds the amount and intensity of other competing stimuli (Pennebaker, 1982). Most of the time bodily signals are thus filtered out by attentional processes as non-important information to enter consciousness compared to other ongoing activities.

Biased symptom perception in these models is the result of deficient attentional filtering, which allows non-important bodily signals to gain awareness. This deficient filtering may occur for several reasons, e.g., the intensity of the bodily signals, the amount of other competing external information, beliefs and prior expectations, but also an individual's tendency for introspection or selective attention to the body (Rief & Barsky, 2005). Watson and Pennebaker (1989) in their influential symptom perception hypothesis were the first to explicitly propose a link between introspection/heightened self-focus and the influence of negative affect on symptom perception. They pointed out that people with high trait negative affectivity (trait NA) tend to be more introspective, while they tend to focus more on negative aspects of themselves and the world and interpret stimuli in a negative way (Watson & Clark, 1984). These core characteristics of people with high trait NA, especially their introspective/self-focused nature, make them more prone to notice even minor unpleasant bodily signals, so that the chances for these signals to enter consciousness are increased (Watson & Pennebaker, 1989). Furthermore, once consciously experienced, bodily signals are more likely to be interpreted as threatening, i.e., as physical symptoms, under the negativistic prism characterizing high trait NA (Watson & Pennebaker, 1989). The same mechanism is suggested to apply for state NA, as it is also considered to lead to momentary increases in self-focus (Palfai & Salovey, 1992).

Although limited, correlational studies provide some support for this hypothesis. Kolk, Hanewald, Schagen, and Van Wijk (2003), for example, showed that high trait NA predicted increased daily symptom reports indirectly via increased selective attention to the body in a primary care patient sample. Similar findings were reported by Williams and Wiebe (2000) in a student sample, although the mediating effect of self-focused attention was only seen for women and only partially, that is, trait NA also had a direct effect on symptom reports that was not mediated by self-focus. This partial mediation has been replicated by Goodwin, Fairclough, and Poole (2013), while, to the contrary, Kolk et al. (2002) did not find a relationship between trait NA and selective attention at all; rather trait NA predicted symptom reports directly. Thus, findings from correlational studies assessing NA and self-focus in a trait-like fashion seem to support Watson and Pennebaker' s hypothesis to some extent but also suggest that this is not the only pathway of affective influences on symptom reporting.

Despite the popularity of this hypothesis, few experimental studies have explored the introspection/self-focus hypothesis in more depth. Aronson, Feldman Barrett, and Quigley (2006) examined the association of trait NA with hypervigilance toward bodily signals, as assessed by a heartbeat detection task, and found that although trait NA predicted daily symptom reports, it did not do so via a heightened sensitivity to bodily signals. In fact, NA did not correlate with people's performance on the task, a finding that comes in line with studies that failed to show increased performance in such a task in individuals with MUS (Mussgay, Klinkenberg, & Ruddel, 1999; Schaefer, Egloff, & Witthöft, 2012). It should be noted, though, that when interoceptive stimuli are more threatening than resting heartbeats, e.g., dyspnea sensations, people high in trait NA seem to be indeed more vigilant to and less able to shift attention away from such threatening internal sensations (Stegen, Van Diest, Van de Woestijne, & Van den Bergh, 2001), providing some support for the role of attention in the NA-symptom reporting link. This finding comes in line with earlier work from the group of Omer Van den Bergh on interoceptive fear conditioning, which showed that healthy individuals could learn to experience physical symptoms only when bodily signals were combined with unpleasant stimuli (state NA) and when people attended to their bodies rather than when distracted (Van den Bergh, Stegen, & Van de Woestijne, 1998). These findings suggest that a combination of self-focused attention with state NA is a necessary condition for bodily signals to be perceived and stored in memory as symptom episodes (Van den Bergh et al., 1998).

This combination was further emphasized in the work of Gendolla, Abele, Andrei, Spurk, and Richter (2005), who proposed, instead of a mediation relationship, a joint impact effect of negative affect and self-focused attention on symptom experiences. They specifically showed in a series of correlational and experimental studies that self-focused attention augments symptom experiences only when combined with negative affect but has no effect under positive affect (Gendolla et al., 2005). Likewise, negative affect can lead to increased symptom reporting only when people are simultaneously focused to the self, e.g., in front of a mirror. They further showed that the combination of NA and self-focus promotes the accessibility of symptom schemata in memory, as seen by people's performance during a Stroop or lexical decision task (Gendolla et al., 2005). This finding suggests that both self-focused attention and NA may activate other processes that in turn account for the augmented symptom reports.

Findings from brain imaging studies seem to corroborate this hypothesis suggesting independent effects of attention and emotion, since negative affect and attentional focus have been found to modulate pain perception independently via separate neural pathways, with affective modulation being focused mostly at the ACC, while attentional modulation induced changes in the anterior insula (Villemure & Bushnell, 2009). Thus, while emotional and attentional influences may have similar behavioral effects (increased symptom reports), these may stem from different mechanisms. EEG data, for example, have shown that unpleasant stimuli modulate pain perception at later stages of processing and at areas linked to working memory and the integration of perceptual inputs with long-term memory, like the right DLPFC, temporo-occipital junction, and temporal pole, which suggests that emotional influences on pain perception are more linked to memory than attentional processes (Godinho, Magnin, Frot, Perchet, & Garcia-Larrea, 2006).

Overall, although the effects of trait and state NA on symptom reporting have been traditionally attributed to the introspective features of negative affect, research findings suggest that self-focused attention can account for the influences of trait negative affect only partially, while experimental findings point toward independent effects of emotion and self-focused attention on the experience of physical symptoms. Additionally, there is no evidence so far to suggest that MUS individuals become more introspective under negative emotional states (rather the opposite may hold, see, e.g., Brown, Brunt, Poliakoff, & Lloyd, 2010). Therefore, self-focused attention cannot adequately explain why MUS individuals tend to be more influenced by negative affect in their symptom reports. Research findings, rather, suggest that other processes beyond self-focused attention initiated by or related to negative affect may better or additionally explain such emotional influences. This points out to the third proposed mechanism, i.e., mood-congruent recall, which is described below.

Hypothesis 3: Negative affect induces mood-congruent schematic activations The third mechanism proposed by Salovey et al. (1991) to underlie affective influences on symptom perception is mood-congruent recall, i.e. the automatic activation of memories that are consistent or congruent in affective value with an individual's current affective state. Negative affective states are more possible to activate symptom/illness memories, which inherently have a congruent unpleasant affective value, thus when people experience ambiguous bodily sensations in an unpleasant context, they may be more prone to interpret them in a mood-congruent negative way, i.e. as symptoms. On the other hand, positive affect is less likely to activate symptom memories (it even inhibits the activation of such memories), as they are affectively incongruent, thus reducing the possibility of a symptomatologic interpretation of bodily signals under a positive affective context (as ingeniously illustrated in the roller coaster study by Rietveld & Van Beest, 2007).

Although the mood congruency hypothesis has not been systematically examined in the area of symptom perception, mood congruency effects have been observed and discussed extensively in regard to other cognitive processes like attention, perception, memory, and judgment (see reviews by Rusting, 1998; Clore & Huntsinger, 2007). One of the most prominent theories trying to delineate mood congruency effects is the network theory of affect developed by Gordon H. Bower (1981). Bower's model was based on the principles of associative network theories, which suggest that semantic knowledge is organized and stored in memory as nodes within a semantic network (Anderson, 1983; Collins & Loftus, 1975). Semantic processing is viewed as a spread of activation within this semantic network initiated by incoming sense data (Anderson, 1983; Collins & Loftus, 1975). Data from the senses are analyzed at various levels and eventually activate the representations of relevant concepts in memory. Once a node is activated, the activation spreads to its closest connections, i.e., to other related concepts, according to the strength of their association (Collins & Loftus, 1975).

Bower's network theory of affect poses that, similarly to other semantic knowledge, emotion categories are represented in the brain within a network of nodes (Bower, 1981, 1991). Affective contexts or stimuli activate the corresponding emotional nodes in memory (e.g., fear node) while at the same time inhibit the activation of unrelated nodes (e.g., joy node). Once an emotion node is activated, the activation is spread within the memory network to other related nodes (Bower, 1991) that may represent, for example, physiological reactions, facial expressions, and memories of prior experiences that have been associated with that emotion. In that way being in a specific emotional state primes or brings into increased readiness congruent concepts, perceptual categories, and ways of interpreting the world and inhibits incongruent ones, a process that influences cognitive processes like perception, memory, and judgment (Bower, 1991).

This priming process suggested by the network model of affect can explain mood-congruency phenomena at all stages of information processing. Specifically, people tend to selectively attend to and encode in a richer way stimuli congruent with their current mood; they evaluate and interpret stimuli according to their mood and remember with more ease mood-congruent material (Bower, 1981). Although most initial work focused on memory recall paradigms (see review by Singer & Salovey, 1988), possibly the best instantiation for the network model of affect has been the sequential affective priming paradigm, which assesses the influence of briefly presented pleasant or unpleasant primes on the processing of subsequent targets (Fazio, Sanbonmatsu, Powell, & Kardes, 1986). A plethora of studies using such a paradigm has shown mood congruency effects in the encoding of information (Fazio, 2001; Hermans, de Houwer, & Eelen, 1994). Brain imaging data have also mapped these effects as they show that limbic areas, like the amygdala, are activated at early stages of processing of emotional stimuli, and once activated they provide feedback and alter the readiness of regions involved in perception and memory processes (Pourtois, Schettino, & Vuilleumier, 2013; Winkielman, Knutson, Paulus, & Trujillo, 2007). Additionally, processing affectively incongruent stimuli has been associated with activations of areas related to inhibition of emotional information, like dorsomedial and ventrolateral prefrontal cortex (Bhanji & Beer, 2012), which further confirms an automatic activation of congruent emotional networks that needs to be inhibited.

Although not explicitly explored in the context of MUS, this proposed process of affective priming within a semantic network comes in line with contemporary theories of symptom perception in general (Pennebaker, 1982) and MUS more specifically (Brosschot, 2002; Brown, 2004), which focus on the top-down influences of symptom schemata on symptom perception. Symptom schemata are cognitive structures used to organize and cluster the mental representations of various bodily sensations into broader categories (Pennebaker, 1982), e.g., sensations of chest tightness, and respiratory sensations like respiratory effort and air hunger, can be grouped together under the experience of dyspnea. The activation of such symptom schemata in memory can influence the perception of bodily signals in a top-down manner, as they can result in selective encoding of information in the environment that confirms the schema or in the interpretation of incoming afferent bodily signals in a way congruent to the schema (as illness-related) or even in the inference of symptoms without any afferent input (Pennebaker, 1982). According to Brown (2004) the excessive activation of such symptom schemata is a central process in the development of MUS. Due to various environmental and idiosyncratic factors, maladaptive symptom schemata are created and become overactivated in some individuals (Brown, 2004). This overactivation of symptom schemata is suggested to stem from body-focused attentional bias (Brown, 2004), since increased body-focused attention leads to recurrent activation of symptom schemata, and the more they are activated, the more strength they gain in memory, so that they are activated more easily in the future (less amount of activation is required). The excessive activation or sensitization (Brosschot, 2002) of symptom schemata leads to biased symptom experiences, since information related to symptom schemata will tend to attract attention over other information in the environment (attentional bias) and be better remembered (memory bias), while ambiguous information will tend to be interpreted as physical symptoms (interpretation bias). Although not specified in these models of MUS, one could hypothesize that for individuals with MUS, these sensitized symptom schemata may also be more easily activated in the presence of mood-congruent (unpleasant) stimuli, resulting in the observed affective modulation of symptom perception in MUS.

Mood congruency and MUS This hypothesis stemming from theories of MUS corresponds with mood congruency theories, which posit that people differ in how strong or rich their associations are with certain emotion nodes, thus leading to individual differences in mood congruency effects (Clark & Teasdale, 1985). For example, people high in trait NA, i.e., individuals who tend to experience negative emotions frequently, probably have a more elaborate and enriched network for negative emotions, with more interconnections and stronger links, so when people high in trait NA experience state negative affect, they may activate the mood-congruent semantic memory network more easily compared to those low in NA (Rusting, 1998). Rafienia, Azadfallah, Fathi-Ashtiani, and Rasoulzadeh-Tabatabaiei (2008), for example, showed that individuals high in neuroticism show more pronounced mood congruency effects after negative but not after positive mood induction, while similar findings have been observed for individuals high in trait anxiety (Egloff & Hock, 2001; Gasper & Clore, 1998).

Similarly, people with a history of repeated symptom experiences (e.g., clinical or nonclinical levels of MUS) have more elaborated and extended symptom schemata (Brown, 2004), which are probably also more strongly connected with negative emotion structures in memory. It can be, therefore, hypothesized that for these people, negative affect can activate symptom schemata more easily or more profoundly, resulting in biased symptom experiences. To examine this assumption, we asked individuals who report frequent symptoms in daily life and controls (low symptom reporters) to complete a semantic priming task twice, once after positive and once after negative mood induction (Constantinou, Bogaerts, Van Diest, & Van den Bergh, 2015). During the semantic priming task, participants were asked to classify a target word, which was preceded briefly by either a congruent or incongruent prime word. The task included words from four categories: (a) neutral body-related words (body parts), (b) neutral body-unrelated words (kitchen utensils), (c) unpleasant body-related words (physical symptoms), and (d) unpleasant body-unrelated words (weapons). Results indicated a nonsignificant tendency for negative mood to result in pronounced semantic priming effects for the high symptom reporters but not the low symptom reporters. This was only seen for neutral body-related words (see Fig. 4.1).

Although this is just a trend based on a small sample, it is the first evidence that negative affect results in increased schematic processing of body-relevant information differentially in individuals with frequent symptom experiences. Gendolla et al. (2005) also showed increased activation of symptom schemata under conditions of unpleasant mood and self-focus, but our findings suggest that this process is pronounced in individuals prone to MUS. Furthermore, in our study the effects of emotion were found only for neutral body-related words, suggesting that frequent symptom reporters do not have a general tendency to engage in schematic processing or use more schematic (top-down) information under unpleasant conditions, but rather this occurs only when the schemata involved are body-relevant. Importantly, the group difference was observed for neutral body-related words rather than symp-

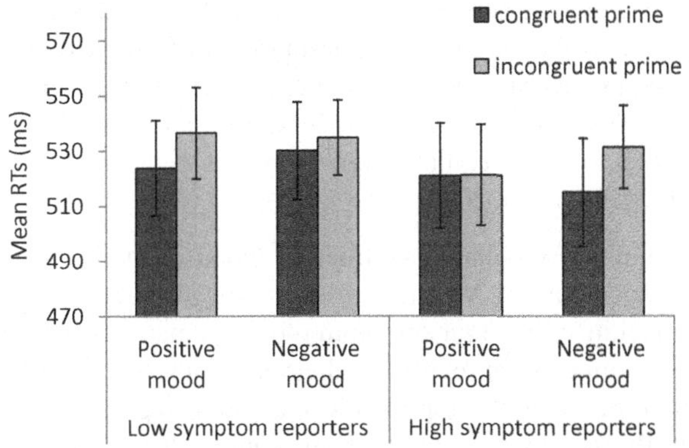

Fig. 4.1 Semantic priming effects indicated by faster reaction times (RTs) during congruent than incongruent trials, for high ($N = 18$) and low ($N = 22$) symptom reporters when target words were neutral body words (body parts): mood × congruency × group interaction: $F(1,38) = 2.48$, $p = .12$, partial $\eta^2 = .06$. (Figure taken from Constantinou, Bogaerts, Van Diest, et al., 2015)

tom words, suggesting that even nonthreatening body-related information is represented in a semantic network in connection to unpleasantness for high symptom reporters (while symptoms are most likely linked to negative affect for everyone).

It must be noted of course that the findings of this study have not yet been replicated, therefore should be treated with caution. In addition, it is not clear from current findings what drives this differential effect. The pronounced priming effects observed in frequent symptom reporters under negative affect may be due to the strength and structure of body-relevant schemata in this group but may also be due to a reduced ability to inhibit such activations from spreading under conditions of negative affect. The following section will focus more on this aspect.

Mood congruency, emotion regulation, and MUS Isen (1985) was the first to point out to the moderating role of emotion regulation on mood congruency effects. Emotion regulation is an umbrella term encompassing all processes employed either intentionally or incidentally by individuals to "influence which emotions they have, when they have them, and how they experience and express these emotions" (Gross, 1998, p. 275). As such, emotion regulation processes can play a vital role in whether and to what extent emotions can influence other psychological processes. Following the network theory of affect, emotion regulation processes can result in structural differences in the affective networks in memory, as emotion regulation involves individuals typically trying to maintain positive affect by thinking of positive events and associations and reduce negative affect by focusing away from negative events and associations (Isen, 1985). Hence, habitual effective use of emotion regulation will eventually lead to restricted negative emotion networks in memory and extended positive ones (Isen, 1985; Rusting & DeHart, 2000), which result in restricted spread of activation after processing unpleasant stimuli. Conversely, people who are less able to regulate their emotions efficiently may have extended negative emotion networks in memory and less elaborate or less accessible positive ones; thus they are less able to inhibit or counteract a pervasive spread of activation from unpleasant cues (Rusting & DeHart, 2000). Studies have shown, for example, that dysphoric individuals exhibit a pronounced difficulty to activate pleasant memories to downregulate unpleasantness (Joormann & Siemer, 2004; Joormann, Siemer, & Gotlib, 2007).

The role of emotion regulation abilities in mood congruency may be of high importance in the context of MUS, as research suggests that people who tend to report MUS (nonclinical habitual symptom reporters, patients with functional syndromes) are less competent in regulating their emotions. Specifically, patients with functional syndromes seem to report lower emotion regulation skills in general (Schwarz, Rief, Radkovsky, Berking, & Kleinstäuber, 2017) and use more emotion avoidance strategies, like suppression (Van Middendorp et al., 2008), while among patients those who inhibit their negative emotions tend to experience more daily symptoms compared to those who express them (Van Middendorp et al., 2010). Furthermore, patients with MUS seem to be deficient in identifying and differentiating their feelings (de Gucht et al., 2004; Pedrosa Gil et al., 2009; Montoro et al., 2016; Waller & Scheidt, 2004), a necessary component for efficient emotion regulation (Barrett, Gross, Conner Christensen, & Benvenuto, 2001). Finally, even in nonclinical samples, reduced ability to regulate emotions has been associated with increased symptom reports (Keefer, Parker, & Saklofske, 2009; Mattila et al., 2008; Salovey, Stroud, Woolery, & Epel, 2002).

At the same time, a series of studies has shown that the effective use of emotion regulation strategies (either intentional or incidental) depends heavily on core higher-order processes, like executive functions, as neuroimaging studies show involvement of ventrolateral and dorsolateral prefrontal areas in emotion regulation (see review by Berkman & Lieberman, 2009). Executive functioning seems to also be compromised in patients with functional syndromes (Aizawa et al., 2012; Correa, Miró, Martínez, Sánchez, & Lupiáñez, 2011), while brain imaging studies have shown deficient employment of prefrontal areas by functional syndrome patients, both during cognitive tasks requiring executive control (Aizawa et al., 2012; Glass et al., 2011) and during unpleasant bodily stimulation (Tillisch, Mayer, & Labus, 2011). Thus, findings suggest a deficiency in inhibitory control networks for people with MUS, which may contribute to their observed poor emotion regulation capacities.

Overall, prior research suggests a diminished ability to employ appropriate emotion regulation strategies, as well as compromised executive control in people with a tendency toward MUS. Their inability to efficiently regulate negative affect may result in extensive and uninhibited activations within a negative emotion network in memory, thus resulting in pronounced mood congruency effects and the augmented symptom reporting observed in individuals with a tendency toward MUS after the presentation of unpleasant pictures (Bogaerts et al., 2010; Constantinou et al.,

2013). A recent study from the Van den Bergh group using the same picture paradigm provides some support for this notion (Van Den Houte et al., 2017), as they showed that among patients with MUS, those with difficulty in identifying their emotions showed a larger increase in symptom experiences after viewing unpleasant pictures.

A crucial implication of this notion is the hypothesis that training MUS individuals in emotion regulation may eliminate the biasing effects of negative affect on symptom experiences. To explore this assumption, we conducted two studies, one with a nonclinical sample with varied levels of daily symptom reporting (Constantinou, Van Den Houte, Bogaerts, Van Diest, & Van den Bergh, 2014) and one with patients with irritable bowel syndrome (IBS) and healthy controls (Constantinou, Bogaerts, Van Diest, et al., 2015), which incorporated an emotion regulation task, namely, affect labeling (Lieberman et al., 2007), in the picture viewing paradigm. Specifically, participants were asked to rate their experienced physical symptoms after viewing either pleasant or unpleasant pictures under three conditions: (a) merely view the pictures (control condition), (b) affective labeling (i.e., select a label to match the emotion depicted in the picture, e.g., excited, content, sad, afraid), and (c) non-affective labeling (i.e., select a label to match the content of the picture, e.g., human, animal, landscape, or object). Previous research has shown that affective labeling results in a reduction of experienced negative affect when compared to non-affective labeling or control condition (Lieberman et al., 2007). Results from our studies showed that individuals with MUS, whether healthy individuals reporting frequent symptoms in daily life or patients with IBS, tended to be more influenced by affective cues, that is, they reported more symptoms after unpleasant pictures compared to pleasant ones, as previously found. Importantly, these affective influences tended to diminish after the application of an emotion regulation strategy (either affective or non-affective labeling of the pictures; see Fig. 4.2).

These findings suggest that regulating experienced affect can attenuate the effects of negative affect on symptom reporting. Symptom overreporting is linked to the amount of experienced negative affect, and when this is somehow downregulated, the bias seems to disappear. Even though the effects of affect labeling were less robust for the patient sample and restricted to general arousal-related symptoms, but not IBS-relevant symptoms, results still provide initial experimental evidence for the possible usefulness of emotion regulation tasks in reducing the biasing effects of negative affect on physical symptoms in those people who are most influenced by it (individuals with MUS).

Prior research has shown that interventions targeting emotion regulation, like guided expressive writing of personal emotional experiences, can have important health benefits, including reduced symptom reports, for various clinical and nonclinical groups (reviews by Baikie & Wilhelm, 2005; Pennebaker, 1997). Clinical trials provide some indications about the efficacy of such interventions for patients with MUS (Broderick,

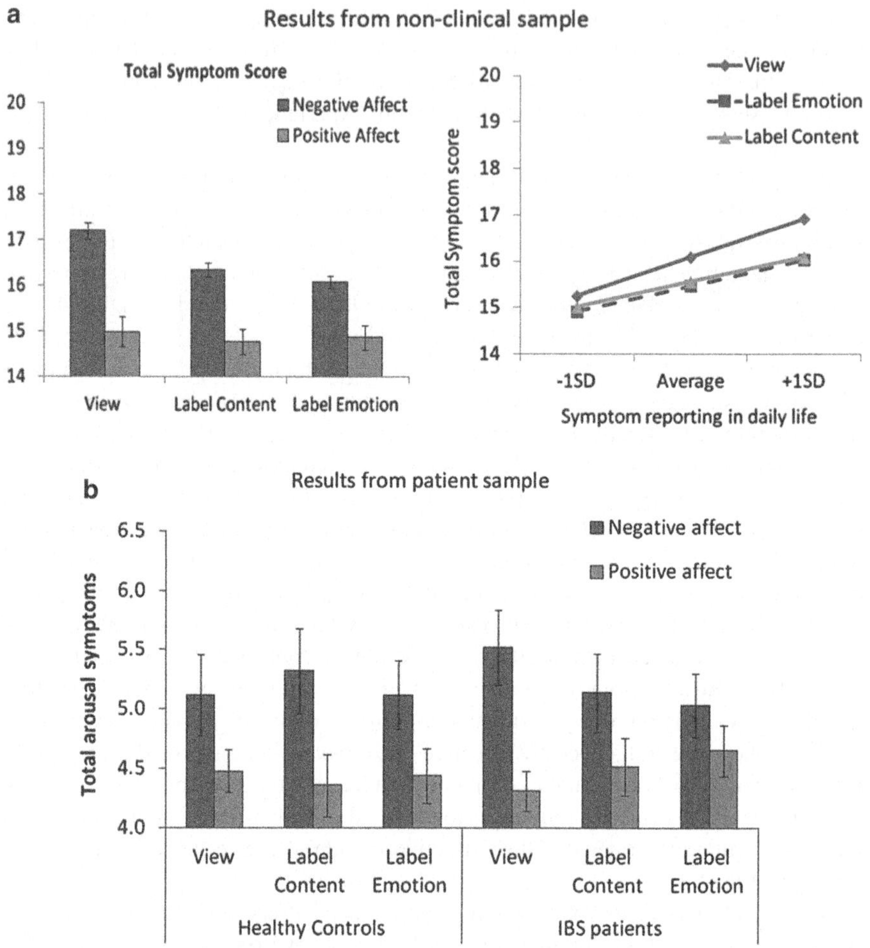

Fig. 4.2 (**a**) Findings from the nonclinical sample on the total symptom score reported at the end of each picture series. Graphs represent the effect of the labeling task for positive and negative pictures (left) and the effect of the labeling task at different levels of symptom reporting in daily life (right). (**b**) Findings from the clinical study on the general arousal symptoms only for IBS patients and healthy controls for negative and positive pictures (Figures taken from Constantinou et al., 2014; Constantinou, Bogaerts, Van Oudenhove, et al., 2015)

Junghaenel, & Schwartz, 2005; Halpert, Rybin, & Doros, 2010), while the usefulness of incorporating emotion regulation training with standard CBT therapy for patients with MUS is being currently explored (Kleinstäuber et al., 2016). Nevertheless, more controlled experimental work is needed to delineate the mechanisms behind such interventions and specifically investigates emotion regulation as a way to reduce affective biases on symptom perception.

Summary

Traditional views among cognitive-perceptual approaches to MUS regarding how negative affect in linked to symptom perception emphasized self-focused attention as the mediator of this relationship, suggesting that negative affect induces self-focus, which in turn results in more bodily signals being inappropriately attended to and reported as symptoms (Kolk et al., 2002; Watson & Pennebaker, 1989). Hence, negative affect has been assumed to increase the amount of bottom-up information being perceived, leading consequently to symptom overreporting.

However, a substantial set of findings suggests that this mechanism cannot adequately explain the effects of negative affect on symptom overreporting, especially for individuals with MUS. Rather, findings presented above provide support for an alternative mechanism proposed to explain affective influences on symptom reporting (mood congruency hypothesis; Salovey et al., 1991), which suggests that negative affect primes symptom schemata in memory as they are affectively congruent and that these schemata are used to organize incoming bodily information and categorize them as symptoms. Based on this hypothesis, negative affect relates more to top-down, rather than bottom-up, sources of symptom misperception.

This notion is in line with recent theoretical (Brosschot, 2002; Brown, 2004) and neurobiological accounts (Edwards, Adams, Brown, Pareés, & Friston, 2012) of MUS, which emphasize the role of prior symptom experiences and memory representations in the development of MUS. These views assume that biased symptom perception stems from the excessive reliance on maladaptive prior experiences over sensory data, during the integration of top-down and bottom-up information (Edwards et al., 2012), a bias that can be triggered by contextual cues activating symptom schemata. Prior research has shown that making symptom schemata salient, by memory recall of prior symptom episodes (Skelton, Loveland, & Yeagley, 1996; Williams et al., 2003), by instructions directing attention to symptoms (Bogaerts et al., 2008; Crane & Martin, 2003), or by priming tasks (Meerman, Verkuil, & Brosschot, 2011; Skelton & Strohmetz, 1990), induces a susceptibility toward increased symptom reporting, especially in people most prone to MUS (Bogaerts et al., 2008), who have more elaborate and easily activated symptom schemata (Brosschot, 2002; Brown, 2004). The current chapter provides evidence that negative affect serves as another contextual cue that activates such symptom schemata in memory and modulates the process of symptom perception leading to symptom overreporting as seen in MUS.

Figure 4.3 illustrates an attempt to map the effects of negative affect along the symptom perception process.[2] Afferent signals from the body indicating a physiological change initiate a symptom perception process, although other cues may also serve as triggers, like instructions, expectations, cues, or contexts previously connected with symptoms. Incoming stimuli, whether physiological changes

[2] This process is depicted in Fig. 4.3 and described hereafter in a linear fashion for simplicity purposes. It should not be assumed that the various processes occur necessarily one after the other.

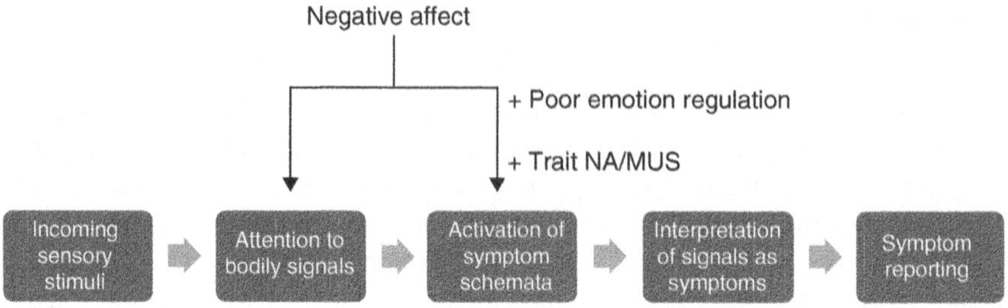

Fig. 4.3 Effects of negative affect during symptom perception and moderating factors

or other cues, may draw attention to the body and bodily sensations. Although numerous factors determine whether attention will be allocated to the bodily signals (Cioffi, 1991; Pennebaker, 1982), unpleasant affect may additionally contribute to an increased focus to the body at this early stage of processing (Watson & Pennebaker, 1989). If bodily signals receive attention, then they are further processed at various levels along the interoceptive pathways in the brain (Craig, 2009) and are integrated with environmental cues. At the same time, relevant prior experiences and concepts in memory are activated as possible interpretations of the incoming stimuli (Brown, 2004). If symptom schemata are activated during this process, and especially if they receive greater activation than other possible interpretations (Brown, 2004; Cioffi, 1991), incoming bodily signals will be interpreted within this framework, i.e., they will be categorized as symptoms, resulting in the conscious experience of a symptom. In cases where no actual physiological change has occurred, but rather certain cues have created the expectation of symptoms, then symptom schemata are activated directly by the cues, which in turn influence in a top-down manner the perception of normal noise in the sensory systems toward symptom reporting (Edwards et al., 2012) or create somatosensory illusions (Brown et al., 2010).

Negative affect has an effect at this stage as it can contribute to the activation and selection of symptom schemata over other possible interpretations of incoming stimuli. If the perceiver is experiencing negative affect, symptom schemata will tend to be activated, as they are affectively congruent with perceiver's current emotional state. The influence of negative affect becomes even stronger when individuals have poor emotion regulation abilities, while more reliance on schematic information and stronger mood congruency effects are expected in individuals with extended negative affect networks in memory (e.g., high trait NA individuals), as well as in individuals with extended symptom schemata (e.g., individuals that experience frequently MUS).

Future Research Directions

The main conclusion stemming from the findings above is that affective influences in the context of symptom reporting seem to relate more to memory recall processes and to the activation of top-down information during symptom perception, rather than attentional processes as traditionally assumed (Watson & Pennebaker, 1989). Nevertheless, these are not mutually exclusive or incompatible mechanisms. Rather it may be that attentional and schematic processes explain different dimensions of affective biases in symptom reporting. There are, for example, studies suggesting that negative affect can have independent effects on the encoding of concurrent symptoms and recall of prior symptom experiences (Larsen, 1992; Suls & Howren, 2012). Nevertheless, more research is needed to delineate how a mood congruent schema activation hypothesis relates to the one of self-focused attention.

Another important issue for further exploration is the concept of maladaptive or sensitized symptom schemata and how to assess such schematic processes in the context of symptom perception. Future studies could combine tasks like semantic priming, sentence completion, or memory recall tasks, as ways to assess symptom schemata, with symptom reporting and mood induction procedures. Additionally, such tasks could be used to examine in which ways are symptom schemata maladaptive in individuals with MUS (see, e.g., Hermans et al., 2010, for the usage of a priming procedure to assess maladaptive panic schemata). This would provide more information on the exact nature of these schemata, their relation to unpleasantness and their influence on symptom perception. Finally, further research could examine the effects of manipulating such symptom schemata, especially mitigating the affective component of such schemata, to reduce biased symptom overreporting (see, e.g., Walentynowicz, Van Diest, Raes, & Van den Bergh, 2017).

Some Implications of Investigating Emotional Influences in MUS

Delineating the mechanisms underlying the emotional influences on symptom experiences can have not only theoretical significance but also important clinical implications regarding the management of MUS. The connection between negative affect and symptom overreporting as seen in MUS has been repeatedly observed in clinical settings (Henningsen et al., 2003) and acknowledged by health professionals treating patients with MUS. The assessment of comorbid emotional problems, like anxiety and depression, is an integral part of assessing functional syndromes, while management of MUS in primary care includes at least some form of psychoeducation about the link between physical symptoms and psychosocial factors (Barsky & Borus, 1999; Drossman et al., 1999; Sharpe, 2002). In addition, the importance of dealing with negative affect has been recognized and incorporated into psychological therapies for the treatment of MUS (Kleinstäuber, Witthöft, & Hiller, 2011, 2016).

Determining how negative affect influences symptom reporting can assist in optimization and better tailoring of psychological treatments (Kleinstäuber et al., 2011) as it would allow identifying people most prone to these influences and most importantly the processes that may reduce such influences. Specifically, findings presented above point to the possible usefulness of reducing the amount of schematic processing during symptom perception, especially under conditions of negative affect. Recent work, for example, has shown that mindfulness, a strategy that involves purposeful allocation of attention to current sensory experiences in a neutral, nonevaluative way, can increase sensory processing of bodily signals and lead to a more objective representation of the signals, with less top-down influences and less interference of the emotional aspects of these signals (Gard et al., 2012). Focusing on the way bodily signals are represented may be more useful in eliminating biased symptom reporting in individuals with MUS rather than trying to reduce the signals themselves. Thus, strategies like mindfulness can be incorporated in the management of MUS (Reiner, Tibi, & Lipsitz, 2013).

Additionally, examining negative affect in symptom reporting highlights the importance of emotion regulation in the management of MUS. We have showed (Constantinou et al., 2014; Constantinou, Bogaerts, Van Oudenhove, et al., 2015) that patients with functional syndromes, who are assumed to spontaneously use ineffective ways to cope with affect (Van Middendorp et al., 2008), can benefit from procedures that somehow engage them in affect regulation processes. Thus, therapeutic interventions aiming at regulating affect can be vital in helping patients become more resistant to stressful events in life and diminish the effects of negative events on patients' symptomatology.

Finally, an important conclusion from this line of research is that individuals with MUS do not always show biased symptom overreporting. Rather, their biased symptom experiences emerge under certain conditions (one of them being contexts or periods with negative affect). Thus, trait characteristics interact with situational factors to produce MUS. This is crucial to keep in mind, as these patients often struggle to be credible, receive little empathy for their symptoms in their interactions with doctors (Ring, Dowrick, Humphris, Davies, & Salmon, 2005), and are categorized as "difficult" by their physicians (Reid, Whooley, Crayford, & Hotopf, 2001). Investigating further the situational factors that can influence the presence of biased symptom reporting may help in eliminating the dualistic thinking of symptoms as "psychological" or "imaginary," "organic" or "real," and the stigma against a group of patients that experience what can be rather debilitating symptomatology.

Acknowledgements This chapter relies greatly on the PhD thesis of Dr. Elena Constantinou, which was obtained at the Health Psychology Group, Department of Psychology, KU Leuven (Belgium), under the supervision of Prof. Dr. Omer Van den Bergh (co-supervisors: Dr. Ilse Van Diest & Dr. Katleen Bogaerts).

References

Aizawa, E., Sato, Y., Kochiyama, T., Saito, N., Izumiyama, M., Morishita, J., … Fukudo, S. (2012). Altered cognitive function of prefrontal cortex during error feedback in patients with Irritable Bowel Syndrome, based on fMRI and dynamic causal modeling. *Gastroenterology, 143*(5), 1188–1198.

Anderson, J. R. (1983). A spreading activation theory of memory. *Journal of Verbal Learning and Verbal Behavior, 22*, 261–295.

Aronson, K. R., Feldman Barrett, L., & Quigley, K. (2006). Emotional reactivity and the over-report of somatic symptoms: Somatic sensitivity or negative reporting style? *Journal of Psychosomatic Research, 60*, 521–530.

Baikie, K. A., & Wilhelm, K. (2005). Emotional and physical health benefits of expressive writing. *Advances in Psychiatric Treatment, 11*(5), 338–346.

Barrett, L. F., Gross, J., Conner Christensen, T., & Benvenuto, M. (2001). Knowing what you're feeling and knowing what to do about it: Mapping the relation between emotion differentiation and emotion regulation. *Cognition & Emotion, 15*(6), 713–724.

Barsky, A. J., & Borus, J. F. (1999). Functional somatic syndromes. *Annals of Internal Medicine, 130*(11), 910–921.

Bechara, A., & Naqvi, N. (2004). Listening to your heart: Interoceptive awareness as a gateway to feeling. *Nature Neuroscience, 7*, 102–103.

Berkman, E. T., & Lieberman, M. D. (2009). Using neuroscience to broaden emotion regulation: Theoretical and methodological considerations. *Social and Personality Psychology Compass, 3*, 475–493.

Bhanji, J. P., & Beer, J. S. (2012). Unpacking the neural associations of emotion and judgment in emotion-congruent judgment. *Social Cognitive and Affective Neuroscience, 7*(3), 348–356.

Bogaerts, K., Janssens, T., De Peuter, S., Van Diest, I., & Van den Bergh, O. (2010). Negative affective pictures can elicit physical symptoms in high habitual symptom reporters. *Psychology & Health, 25*(6), 685–698.

Bogaerts, K., Millen, A., Wan, L., De Peuter, S., Van Diest, I., Vlemincx, E., … Van den Bergh, O. (2008). High symptom reporters are less interoceptively accurate in a symptom-related context. *Journal of Psychosomatic Research, 65*(5), 417–424.

Bower, G. H. (1981). Mood and memory. *American Psychologist, 36*, 129–148.

Bower, G. H. (1991). Mood congruity of social judgments. In J. P. Forgas (Ed.), *Emotion and social judgments* (pp. 31–54). Oxford: Pergamon Press.

Broderick, J. E., Junghaenel, D. U., & Schwartz, J. E. (2005). Written emotional expression produces health benefits in fibromyalgia patients. *Psychosomatic Medicine, 67*, 326–334.

Brosschot, J. F. (2002). Cognitive-emotional sensitization and somatic health complaints. *Scandinavian Journal of Psychology, 43*, 113–121.

Brown, R. J. (2004). Psychological mechanisms of medically unexplained symptoms: An integrative conceptual model. *Psychological Bulletin, 130*(5), 793–812.

Brown, R. J., Brunt, N., Poliakoff, E., & Lloyd, D. M. (2010). Illusory touch and tactile perception in somatoform dissociators. *Journal of Psychosomatic Research, 69*(3), 241–248.

Brown, K. W., & Moskowitz, D. S. (1997). Does unhappiness make you sick? The role of affect and neuroticism in the experience of common physical symptoms. *Journal of Personality and Social Psychology, 72*, 907–917.

Charles, S. T., & Almeida, D. M. (2006). Daily reports of symptoms and negative affect: Not all symptoms are the same. *Psychology and Health, 21*(1), 1–17.

Cioffi, D. (1991). Beyond attentional strategies: A cognitive-perceptual model of somatic interpretation. *Psychological Bulletin, 109*(1), 25–41.

Clark, D. M., & Teasdale, J. D. (1985). Constraints on the effects of mood on memory. *Journal of Personality and Social Psychology, 48*(6), 1595–1608.

Clore, G., & Huntsinger, J. R. (2007). How emotions inform judgment and regulate thought. *Trends in Cognitive Sciences, 11*(9), 393–399.

Collins, A. M., & Loftus, E. F. (1975). A spreading-activation theory of semantic processing. *Psychological Review, 82*(6), 407–428.

Constantinou, E., Bogaerts, K., Van Diest, I., & Van den Bergh, O. (2013). Inducing symptoms in high symptom reporters via emotional pictures: The interactive effects of valence and arousal. *Journal of Psychosomatic Research, 74*(3), 191–196.

Constantinou, E., Bogaerts, K., Van Diest, I., & Van den Bergh, O. (2015). Influences of mood on information processing styles in high and low symptom reporters. *Health Psychology Report, 3*(4), 300–311.

Constantinou, E., Bogaerts, K., Van Oudenhove, L., Tack, J., Van Diest, I., & Van den Bergh, O. (2015). Healing words: Using affect labeling to reduce the effects of unpleasant cues on symptom reporting in IBS patients. *International Journal of Behavioral Medicine, 22*(4), 512–520.

Constantinou, E., Van Den Houte, M., Bogaerts, K., Van Diest, I., & Van den Bergh, O. (2014). Can words heal? Using affect labeling to reduce the effects of unpleasant cues on symptom reporting. *Frontiers in Psychology, 5*, 807.

Correa, Á., Miró, E., Martínez, M. P., Sánchez, A. I., & Lupiáñez, J. (2011). Temporal preparation and inhibitory deficit in fibromyalgia syndrome. *Brain and Cognition, 75*(3), 211–216.

Craig, A. D. (2002). How do you feel? Interoception: The sense of the physiological condition of the body. *Nature Reviews Neuroscience, 3*(8), 655–666.

Craig, A. D. (2009). How do you feel now? The anterior insula and human awareness. *Nature Reviews Neuroscience, 10*(1), 59–70.

Crane, C., & Martin, M. (2003). Illness schema and level of reported gastrointestinal symptoms in irritable bowel syndrome. *Cognitive Therapy and Research, 27*(2), 185–203.

Critchley, H. D. (2005). Neural mechanisms of autonomic, affective, and cognitive integration. *Journal of Comparative Neurology, 493*(1), 154–166.

Critchley, H. D., Mathias, C. J., & Dolan, R. J. (2001). Neuroanatomical basis for first and second-order representations of bodily states. *Nature Neuroscience, 4*, 207–212.

Critchley, H. D., Wiens, S., Rotshtein, P., Öhman, A., & Dolan, R. J. (2004). Neural systems supporting interoceptive awareness. *Nature Neuroscience, 7*, 189–195.

de Gucht, V. M. J., Fischler, B., & Heiser, W. J. (2004). Personality and affect as determinants of medically unexplained symptoms in primary care. A follow up study. *Journal of Psychosomatic Research, 56*(3), 279–285.

de Wied, M. A., & Verbaten, M. N. (2001). Affective pictures processing, attention, and pain tolerance. *Pain, 90*, 163–172.

Damasio, A. R. (1994). *Descartes' error: Emotion, reason, and the human brain*. New York: Grosset/Putnam.

Damasio, A., & Carvalho, G. B. (2013). The nature of feelings: Evolutionary and neurobiological origins. *Nature Reviews Neuroscience, 14*(2), 143–152.

Deary, V., Chalder, T., & Sharpe, M. (2007). The cognitive behavioural model of medically unexplained symptoms: A theoretical and empirical review. *Clinical Psychology Review, 27*(7), 781–797.

Denson, T. F., Spanovic, M., & Miller, N. (2009). Cognitive appraisals and emotions predict cortisol and immune responses: A meta-analysis of acute laboratory social stressors and emotion inductions. *Psychological Bulletin, 135*(6), 823–853.

Drossman, D. A., Creed, F. H., Olden, K. W., Svedlund, J., Toner, B. B., & Whitehead, W. E. (1999). Psychosocial aspects of the functional gastrointestinal disorders. *Gut, 45*(Suppl. 2), II25–II30.

Edwards, M. J., Adams, R. A., Brown, H., Pareés, I., & Friston, K. J. (2012). A Bayesian account of 'hysteria'. *Brain, 135*(11), 3495–3512.

Egloff, B., & Hock, M. (2001). Interactive effects of state anxiety and trait anxiety on emotional Stroop interference. *Personality and Individual Differences, 31*(6), 875–882.

Elsenbruch, S., Lucas, A., Holtmann, G., Haag, S., Gerken, G., Riemenschneider, N., … Schedlowski, M. (2006). Public speaking stress-induced neuroendocrine responses and circulating immune cell redistribution in irritable bowel syndrome. *The American Journal of Gastroenterology, 101*(10), 2300–2307.

Elsenbruch, S., Rosenberger, C., Bingel, U., Forsting, M., Schedlowski, M., & Gizewski, E. R. (2010). Patients with irritable bowel syndrome have altered emotional modulation of neural responses to visceral stimuli. *Gastroenterology, 139*(4), 1310–1319.

Fazio, R. H. (2001). On the automatic activation of associated evaluations: An overview. *Cognition & Emotion, 15*(2), 115–141.

Fazio, R. H., Sanbonmatsu, D. M., Powell, M. C., & Kardes, F. R. (1986). On the automatic activation of attitudes. *Journal of Personality and Social Psychology, 50*, 229–238.

Forgas, J. P. (1995). Mood and judgment: The affect infusion model (AIM). *Psychological Bulletin, 117*(1), 39–66.

Gaab, J., Rohleder, N., Heitz, V., Engert, V., Schad, T., Schürmeyer, T. H., & Ehlert, U. (2005). Stress-induced changes in LPS-induced pro-inflammatory cytokine production in chronic fatigue syndrome. *Psychoneuroendocrinology, 30*(2), 188–198.

Gard, T., Hölzel, B. K., Sack, A. T., Hempel, H., Lazar, S. W., Vaitl, D., & Ott, U. (2012). Pain attenuation through mindfulness is associated with decreased cognitive control and increased sensory processing in the brain. *Cerebral Cortex, 22*(11), 2692–2702.

Gasper, K., & Clore, G. L. (1998). The persistent use of negative affect by anxious individuals to estimate risk. *Journal of Personality and Social Psychology, 74*, 1350–1363.

Gendolla, G. H. E., Abele, A. E., Andrei, A., Spurk, D., & Richter, M. (2005). Negative mood, self-focused attention, and the experience of physical symptoms: The joint impact hypothesis. *Emotion, 5*, 131–144.

Glaser, R., & Kiecolt-Glaser, J. K. (2005). Stress-induced immune dysfunction: Implications for health. *Nature Reviews Immunology, 5*(3), 243–251.

Glass, J. M., Williams, D. A., Fernandez-Sanchez, M. L., Kairys, A., Barjola, P., Heitzeg, M., … Schmidt-Wilcke, T. (2011). Executive function in chronic pain patients and healthy controls: Different cortical activation during response inhibition in fibromyalgia. *The Journal of Pain, 12*(12), 1219–1229.

Godinho, F., Magnin, M., Frot, M., Perchet, C., & Garcia-Larrea, L. (2006). Emotional modulation of pain: Is it the sensation or what we recall? *The Journal of Neuroscience, 26*(44), 11454–11461.

Goodwin, L., Fairclough, S. H., & Poole, H. M. (2013). A cognitive–perceptual model of symptom perception in males and females: The roles of negative affect, selective attention, health anxiety and psychological job demands. *Journal of Health Psychology, 18*(6), 848–857.

Gross, J. J. (1998). The emerging field of emotion regulation: An integrative review. *Review of General Psychology, 2*, 271–299.

Halpert, A., Rybin, D., & Doros, G. (2010). Expressive writing is a promising therapeutic modality for the management of IBS: A pilot study. *The American Journal of Gastroenterology, 105*, 2440–2448.

Henningsen, P., Zimmermann, T., & Sattel, H. (2003). Medically unexplained physical symptoms, anxiety, and depression: A meta-analytic review. *Psychosomatic Medicine, 65*(4), 528–533.

Hermans, D., De Cort, K., Noortman, D., Vansteenwegen, D., Beckers, T., Spruyt, A., & Schruers, K. (2010). Priming associations between bodily sensations and catastrophic misinterpretations: Specific for panic disorder? *Behaviour Research and Therapy, 48*(9), 900–908.

Hermans, D., de Houwer, J., & Eelen, P. (1994). The affective priming effect: Automatic activation of evaluative information in memory. *Cognition & Emotion, 8*(6), 515–533.

Houghton, L., Calvert, E. L., Jackson, N. A., Cooper, P., & Whorwell, P. (2002). Visceral sensation and emotion: A study using hypnosis. *Gut, 51*, 701–714.

Houtveen, J. H., Rietveld, S., & de Geus, E. J. (2003). Exaggerated perception of normal physiological responses to stress and hypercapnia in young women with numerous functional somatic symptoms. *Journal of Psychosomatic Research, 55*(6), 481–490.

Houtveen, J. H., & van Doornen, L. J. (2007). Medically unexplained symptoms and between-group differences in 24-h ambulatory recording of stress physiology. *Biological Psychology, 76*(3), 239–249.

Isen, A. M. (1985). Asymmetry of happiness and sadness in effects on memory in normal college students: Comment on Hasher, Rose, Zacks, Sanft, and Doren. *Journal of Experimental Psychology: General, 114*(3), 388–391.

James, W. (1884). What is an emotion? *Mind, 9*, 188–205.

Joormann, J., & Siemer, M. (2004). Memory accessibility, mood regulation, and dysphoria: Difficulties in repairing sad mood with happy memories? *Journal of Abnormal Psychology, 113*(2), 179–188.

Joormann, J., Siemer, M., & Gotlib, I. H. (2007). Mood regulation in depression: Differential effects of distraction and recall of happy memories on sad mood. *Journal of Abnormal Psychology, 116*(3), 484–490.

Kamping, S., Bomba, I. C., Kanske, P., Diesch, E., & Flor, H. (2013). Deficient modulation of pain by a positive emotional context in fibromyalgia patients. *Pain, 154*(9), 1846–1855.

Keefer, K.V., Parker, J.D.A., & Saklofske, D.H. (2009). Emotional intelligence and physical health. In C. Stough, D.H. Saklofske, & J.D.A. Parker (Eds.), *The Springer series on human exceptionality. Assessing emotional intelligence: Theory, research, and applications* (pp. 191–218). New York: Springer.

Kiecolt-Glaser, J. K., McGuire, L., Robles, T. F., & Glaser, R. (2002). Psychoneuroimmunology: Psychological influences on immune function and health. *Journal of Consulting and Clinical Psychology, 70*(3), 537–547.

Kirmayer, L. J., & Taillefer, S. (1997). Somatoform disorders. In S. M. Turner & M. Hersen (Eds.), *Adult psychopathology and diagnosis* (3rd ed., pp. 333–383). New York: Wiley.

Kleinstäuber, M., Witthöft, M., & Hiller, W. (2011). Efficacy of short-term psychotherapy for multiple medically unexplained physical symptoms: A meta-analysis. *Clinical Psychology Review, 31*(1), 146–160.

Kolk, A. M. M., Hanewald, G. J. F. P., Schagen, S., & Gijsbers van Wijk, C. M. T. (2002). Predicting medically unexplained physical symptoms and health care utilization: A symptom-perception approach. *Journal of Psychosomatic Research, 52*(1), 35–44.

Kolk, A. M., Hanewald, G., Schagen, S., & Van Wijk, C. M. T. (2003). A symptom perception approach to common physical symptoms. *Social Science & Medicine, 57*, 2343–2354.

Kroenke, K. (2003). Patients presenting with somatic complaints: Epidemiology, psychiatric comorbidity and management. *International Journal of Methods in Psychiatric Research, 12*(1), 34–43.

Kleinstäuber, M., Gottschalk, J., Berking, M., Rau, J. & Rief, W. (2016). Enriching Cognitive Behavior Therapy with Emotion Regulation Training for Patients with Multiple Medically Unexplained Symptoms (ENCERT): Design and implementation of a multicenter, randomized, active-controlled trial. *Contemporary Clinical Trials, 47*, 54–63.

Landgrebe, M., Barta, W., Rosengarth, K., Frick, U., Hauser, S., Langguth, B., … Eichhammer, P. (2008). Neuronal correlates of symptom formation in functional somatic syndromes: A fMRI study. *Neuroimage, 41*(4), 1336–1344.

Larsen, R. J. (1992). Neuroticism and selective encoding and recall of symptoms: Evidence from a combined concurrent-retrospective study. *Journal of Personality and Social Psychology, 62*, 480–488.

Leventhal, E. A., Hansell, S., Diefenbach, M., Leventhal, H., & Glass, D. C. (1996). Negative affect and self-report of physical symptoms: Two longitudinal studies of older adults. *Health Psychology, 15*, 193–199.

Lieberman, M. D., Eisenberger, N. I., Crockett, M. J., Tom, S. M., Pfeifer, J. H., & Way, B. M. (2007). Putting feelings into words: Affect labeling disrupts amygdala activity in response to affective stimuli. *Psychological Science, 18*(5), 421–428.

Marsland, A. L., Walsh, C., Lockwood, K., & John-Henderson, N. A. (2017). The effects of acute psychological stress on circulating and stimulated inflammatory markers: A systematic review and meta-analysis. *Brain, Behavior, and Immunity, 64*, 208–219.

Mattila, A. K., Kronholm, E., Jula, A., Salminen, J. K., Koivisto, A. M., Mielonen, R. L., & Joukamaa, M. (2008). Alexithymia and somatization in general population. *Psychosomatic Medicine, 70*(6), 716–722.

Meagher, M. W., Arnau, R. C., & Rhudy, J. L. (2001). Pain and emotion: Effects of affective picture modulation. *Psychosomatic Medicine, 63*(1), 79–90.

Meerman, E. E., Verkuil, B., & Brosschot, J. F. (2011). Decreasing pain tolerance outside of awareness. *Journal of Psychosomatic Research, 70*(3), 250–257.

Montoro, C. I., Reyes del Paso, G. A., & Duschek, S. (2016). Alexithymia in fibromyalgia syndrome. *Personality and Individual Differences, 102*, 170–179.

Montoya, P., Sitges, C., García-Herrera, M., Izquierdo, R., Truyols, M., Blay, N., & Collado, D. (2005). Abnormal affective modulation of somatosensory brain processing among patients with fibromyalgia. *Psychosomatic Medicine, 67*, 957–963.

Mor, N., & Winquist, J. (2002). Self-focused attention and negative affect: A meta-analysis. *Psychological Bulletin, 128*(4), 638–662.

Mussgay, L., Klinkenberg, N., & Ruddel, H. (1999). Heart beat perception in patients with depressive, somatoform, and personality disorders. *Journal of Psychophysiology, 13*, 27–36.

Orenius, T. I., Raij, T. T., Nuortimo, A., Näätänen, P., Lipsanen, J., & Karlsson, H. (2017). The interaction of emotion and pain in the insula and secondary somatosensory cortex. *Neuroscience, 349*, 185–194.

Palfai, T. P., & Salovey, P. (1992). The influence of affect on self-focused attention: Conceptual and methodological issues. *Consciousness and Cognition, 1*(3), 306–339.

Pedrosa Gil, F., Ridout, N., Kessler, H., Neuffer, M., Schoechlin, C., Traue, H.C. & Nickel, M. (2009). Facial emotion recognition and alexithymia in adults with somatoform disorders, *Depression and Anxiety, 26* (1), E26–E33.

Pennebaker, J. W. (1982). *The psychology of physical symptoms*. New York: Springer.

Pennebaker, J. W. (1997). Writing about emotional experiences as a therapeutic process. *Psychological Science, 8*(3), 162–166.

Phillips, M. L., Gregory, L. J., Cullen, S., Cohen, S., Ng, V., Andrew, C., ... Aziz, Q. (2003). The effect of negative emotional context on neural and behavioural responses to oesophageal stimulation. *Brain, 126*, 669–684.

Pourtois, G., Schettino, A., & Vuilleumier, P. (2013). Brain mechanisms for emotional influences on perception and attention: What is magic and what is not. *Biological Psychology, 92*(3), 492–512.

Rafienia, P., Azadfallah, P., Fathi-Ashtiani, A., & Rasoulzadeh-Tabatabaiei, K. (2008). The role of extraversion, neuroticism and positive and negative mood in emotional information processing. *Personality and Individual Differences, 44*(2), 392–402.

Reid, S., Whooley, D., Crayford, T., & Hotopf, M. (2001). Medically unexplained symptoms—GPs' attitudes towards their cause and management. *Family Practice, 18*(5), 519–523.

Reiner, K., Tibi, L., & Lipsitz, J. D. (2013). Do mindfulness-based interventions reduce pain intensity? A critical review of the literature. *Pain Medicine, 14*(2), 230–242.

Rhudy, J. L., DelVentura, J. L., Terry, E. L., Bartley, E. J., Olech, E., Palit, S., & Kerr, K. L. (2013). Emotional modulation of pain and spinal nociception in fibromyalgia. *Pain, 154*(7), 1045–1056.

Rhudy, J. L., Williams, A. E., McCabe, K. M., Russell, J. L., & Maynard, L. J. (2008). Emotional control of nociceptive reactions (ECON): Do affective valence and arousal play a role? *Pain, 136*, 250–261.

Rief, W., & Barsky, A. J. (2005). Psychobiological perspectives on somatoform disorders. *Psychoneuroendocrinology, 30*, 996–1002.

Rief, W., Hessel, A., & Braehler, E. (2001). Somatization symptoms and hypochondriacal features in the general population. *Psychosomatic Medicine, 63*(4), 595–602.

Rief, W., & Martin, A. (2014). How to use the new DSM-5 somatic symptom disorder diagnosis in research and practice: A critical evaluation and a proposal for modifications. *Annual Review of Clinical Psychology, 10*, 339–367.

Rietveld, S., Everaerd, W., & Van Beest, I. (2000). Excessive breathlessness through emotional imagery in asthma. *Behaviour Research and Therapy, 38*(10), 1005–1014.

Rietveld, S., & van Beest, I. (2007). Rollercoaster asthma: When positive emotional stress interferes with dyspnea perception. *Behaviour Research and Therapy, 45*(5), 977–987.

Ring, A., Dowrick, C. F., Humphris, G. M., Davies, J., & Salmon, P. (2005). The somatising effect of clinical consultation: What patients and doctors say and do not say when patients present medically unexplained physical symptoms. *Social Science & Medicine, 61*(7), 1505–1515.

Rosmalen, J. G., Neeleman, J., Gans, R. O., & de Jonge, P. (2007). The association between neuroticism and self-reported common somatic symptoms in a population cohort. *Journal of Psychosomatic Research, 62*(3), 305–311.

Rusting, C. L. (1998). Personality, mood, and cognitive processing of emotional information: Three conceptual frameworks. *Psychological Bulletin, 124*(2), 165–196.
Rusting, C. L., & DeHart, T. (2000). Retrieving positive memories to regulate negative mood: Consequences for mood-congruent memory. *Journal of Personality and Social Psychology, 78*(4), 737–752.
Salovey, P., O'Leary, A., Stretton, M. S., Fishkin, S. A., & Drake, C. A. (1991). Influence of mood on judgments about health and illness. In J. P. Forgas (Ed.), *Emotion and social judgment* (pp. 241–262). Oxford: Pergamon.
Salovey, P., Stroud, L. R., Woolery, A., & Epel, E. S. (2002). Perceived emotional intelligence, stress reactivity, and symptom reports: Further explorations using the trait meta-mood scale. *Psychology and Health, 17*(5), 611–627.
Schaefer, M., Egloff, B., & Witthöft, M. (2012). Is interoceptive awareness really altered in somatoform disorders? Testing competing theories with two paradigms of heartbeat perception. *Journal of Abnormal Psychology, 121*, 719–724.
Schwarz, J., Rief, W., Radkovsky, A., Berking, M., & Kleinstäuber, M. (2017). Negative affect as mediator between emotion regulation and medically unexplained symptoms. *Journal of Psychosomatic Research, 101*, 114–121.
Segerstrom, S. C., & Miller, G. E. (2004). Psychological stress and the human immune system: A meta-analytic study of 30 years of inquiry. *Psychological Bulletin, 130*(4), 601–630.
Sharpe, M. (2002). Medically unexplained symptoms and syndromes. *Clinical Medicine, 2*(6), 501–504.
Sibelli, A., Chalder, T., Everitt, H., Workman, P., Windgassen, S., & Moss-Morris, R. (2016). A systematic review with meta-analysis of the role of anxiety and depression in irritable bowel syndrome onset. *Psychological Medicine, 46*(15), 3065–3080.
Simon, G. E., VonKorff, M., Piccinelli, M., Fullerton, C., & Ormel, J. (1999). An international study of the relation between somatic symptoms and depression. *New England Journal of Medicine, 341*(18), 1329–1335.
Singer, J. A., & Salovey, P. (1988). Mood and memory: Evaluating the network theory of affect. *Clinical Psychology Review, 8*(2), 211–251.
Skelton, J. A., Loveland, J. E., & Yeagley, J. L. (1996). Recalling symptom episodes affects reports of immediately-experienced symptoms: Inducing symptom suggestibility. *Psychology and Health, 11*(2), 183–201.
Skelton, J. A., & Strohmetz, D. B. (1990). Priming symptom reports with health-related cognitive activity. *Personality and Social Psychology Bulletin, 16*(3), 449–464.
Stegen, K., Van Diest, I., Van de Woestijne, K. P., & Van den Bergh, O. (2001). Do persons with negative affect have an attentional bias to bodily sensations? *Cognition & Emotion, 15*(6), 813–829.
Steinbrecher, N., Koerber, S., Frieser, D., & Hiller, W. (2011). The prevalence of medically unexplained symptoms in primary care. *Psychosomatics, 52*(3), 263–271.
Suls, J., & Howren, M. B. (2012). Understanding the physical-symptom experience the distinctive contributions of anxiety and depression. *Current Directions in Psychological Science, 21*(2), 129–134.
Tak, L. M., Cleare, A. J., Ormel, J., Manoharan, A., Kok, I. C., Wessely, S., & Rosmalen, J. G. (2011). Meta-analysis and meta-regression of hypothalamic-pituitary-adrenal axis activity in functional somatic disorders. *Biological Psychology, 87*(2), 183–194.
Tillisch, K., Mayer, E. A., & Labus, J. S. (2011). Quantitative meta-analysis identifies brain regions activated during rectal distension in irritable bowel syndrome. *Gastroenterology, 140*(1), 91–100.
Toft, T., Fink, P. E. R., Oernboel, E. V. A., Christensen, K. A. J., Frostholm, L., & Olesen, F. (2005). Mental disorders in primary care: Prevalence and co-morbidity among disorders. Results from the functional illness in primary care (FIP) study. *Psychological Medicine, 35*(8), 1175–1184.
van Diest, I., De Peuter, S., Eertmans, A., Bogaerts, K., Victoir, A., & Van den Bergh, O. (2005). Negative affectivity and enhanced symptom reports: Differentiating between symptoms in men and women. *Social Science & Medicine, 61*(8), 1835–1845.

van Middendorp, H., Lumley, M. A., Houtveen, J. H., Jacobs, J. W., Bijlsma, J. W., & Geenen, R. (2013). The impact of emotion-related autonomic nervous system responsiveness on pain sensitivity in female patients with fibromyalgia. *Psychosomatic Medicine, 75*(8), 765–773.

van Middendorp, H., Lumley, M. A., Jacobs, J. W. G., van Doornen, L. J. P., Bijlsma, J. W. J., & Geenen, R. (2008). Emotions and emotional approach and avoidance strategies in fibromyalgia. *Journal of Psychosomatic Research, 64*, 159–167.

Van den Bergh, O., Stegen, K., & Van de Woestijne, K. P. (1998). Memory effects on symptom reporting in a respiratory learning paradigm. *Health Psychology, 17*(3), 241–248.

Van Den Houte, M., Bogaerts, K., Van Diest, I., De Bie, J., Persoons, P., Van Oudenhove, L., & Van den Bergh, O. (2017). Inducing somatic symptoms in functional syndrome patients: Effects of manipulating state negative affect. *Psychosomatic Medicine, 79*(9), 1000–1007. https://doi.org/10.1097/PSY.0000000000000527

Van Middendorp, H., Lumley, M. A., Moerbeek, M., Jacobs, J. W., Bijlsma, J. W., & Geenen, R. (2010). Effects of anger and anger regulation styles on pain in daily life of women with fibromyalgia: A diary study. *European Journal of Pain, 14*(2), 176–182.

Villemure, C., & Bushnell, M. C. (2009). Mood influences supraspinal pain processing separately from attention. *The Journal of Neuroscience, 29*(3), 705–715.

Villemure, C., Slotnick, B. M., & Bushnell, M. C. (2003). Effects of odors on pain perception: Deciphering the roles of emotion and attention. *Pain, 106*(1), 101–108.

Von Leupoldt, A., Mertz, C., Kegat, S., Burmester, S., & Dahme, B. (2006). The impact of emotions on the sensory and affective dimension of perceived dyspnea. *Psychophysiology, 43*, 382–386.

Walentynowicz, M., Van Diest, I., Raes, F., & Van den Bergh, O. (2017). Ways of encoding somatic information and their effects on retrospective symptom reporting. *British Journal of Health Psychology, 22*(2), 362–378.

Waller, E., & Scheidt, C. E. (2004). Somatoform disorders as disorders of affect regulation: A study comparing the TAS-20 with non-self-report measures of alexithymia. *Journal of Psychosomatic Research, 57*(3), 239–247.

Watson, D., & Clark, L. A. (1984). Negative affectivity: The disposition to experience aversive emotional states. *Psychological Bulletin, 96*, 465–490.

Watson, D., & Pennebaker, J. W. (1989). Health complaints, stress, and distress: Exploring the central role of negative affectivity. *Psychological Review, 96*(2), 234–254.

Wessely, S., Nimnuan, C., & Sharpe, M. (1999). Functional somatic syndromes: One or many? *Lancet, 354*, 936–939.

Wiech, K., & Tracey, I. (2009). The influence of negative emotions on pain: Behavioral effects and neural mechanisms. *Neuroimage, 47*(3), 987–994.

Williams, P. G., & Wiebe, D. J. (2000). Individual differences in self-assessed health: Neuroticism, gender, and physical symptom reports. *Personality and Individual Differences, 28*, 823–835.

Winkielman, P., Knutson, B., Paulus, M., & Trujillo, J. L. (2007). Affective influence on judgments and decisions: Moving towards core mechanisms. *Review of General Psychology, 11*(2), 179–192.

Williams, P. G., Wasserman, M. S., & Lotto, A. J. (2003). Individual differences in self-assessed health: An information-processing investigation of health and illness cognition. *Health Psychology, 22*(1), 3–11.

Zaki, J., Davis, J. I., & Ochsner, K. N. (2012). Overlapping activity in anterior insula during interoception and emotional experience. *Neuroimage, 62*(1), 493–499.

Chapter 5
Alexithymia as a Core Trait in Psychosomatic and Other Psychological Disorders

Georgia Panayiotou

Alexithymia is a term derived from the psychoanalytic tradition (Krystal, 1988) and used to describe the difficulties observed in psychosomatic patients when reporting on their emotions during clinical interviews (Sifneos, 1973). The term is derived from the Greek language and literally means the absence of words for emotions. Its composite "thymos" is the Greek word for affect, as used by the ancient philosopher Plato, who claimed that "victory over the self represents our first and greatest victory." Underlying this statement is an early proclamation of the significance of emotion regulation, which is considered as a central deficit in alexithymia.

Given the evolutionary significance of emotions for survival-related action (Lang, 1993), deficits in the ability to process, regulate, understand, or express them represent serious challenges for well-being and physical and mental health. According to contemporary theories, emotions are essential sources of information about the self and predispositions for actions that are required for survival (Lang, 1979). Deficiencies or aberrations related to the emotion system are present in most categories of psychological disorders, which further attests to the significance of the ability to appropriately process and respond to emotional information for mental health. Given the role of emotions in psychopathology, it is to no surprise that alexithymia, with emotional dysfunctions at its center, has been linked to a multitude of psychological and physical health problems in the large body of literature that has examined this construct over the last five decades (e.g., Bankier, Aigner, & Bach, 2001). It has been linked to a wide range of problems including depression, somatization/medically unexplained symptoms, chronic/somatoform pain, health anxiety, irritable bowel syndrome, autism, substance use, eating disorders, anxiety disorders, and gastrointestinal problems, among others (Foran & O'Leary, 2012; Marchesi, Fontò, Balista, Cimmino, & Maggini, 2005; Taylor & Bagby, 2004).

G. Panayiotou (✉)
Department of Psychology and Center for Applied Neuroscience, University of Cyprus, Nicosia, Cyprus
e-mail: georgiap@ucy.ac.cy

C. Charis, G. Panayiotou (eds.), *Somatoform and Other Psychosomatic Disorders*,
https://doi.org/10.1007/978-3-319-89360-0_5

Through associations between poor emotion regulation, sustained stress responses, and aberrant production of glucocorticoids and catecholamines, the immune response may become deficient, and the cardiovascular system may incur wear and tear leading also to physical disease processes (Fredrikson & Matthews, 1990; McEwen, 2008). Because of the strong link between alexithymia and almost any disorder examined to date, it has been described by some as a general, transdiagnostic risk factor for mental and physical health (Kojima et al., 2012). Understanding what goes wrong with emotions in alexithymia has significant implications, as it may provide insights regarding the role of emotion in psychopathology and health. Developing interventions for alexithymia may also be a way to prevent the psychological and physical disorders that have been linked to this construct.

Based on an extensive literature, alexithymia appears to involve both emotion processing and emotion regulation difficulties (Connelly & Denney, 2007; Herbert, Herbert, & Pollatos, 2011). However, in order to understand alexithymic deficits, some deliberation on how normal emotions are understood by contemporary researchers is required. According to dominant and well-supported theories, like Lang's bioinformational theory (Lang, 1979), emotional information is stored in associative networks in memory, which contain semantic information about emotional events (subjective experience, memories, descriptions, ratings of emotion stimuli, etc.), physiological reactions associated with the specific emotion (e.g., autonomic arousal, reflex activation), and corresponding actions (behavioral repertoires, facial expressions, communication of emotion and defensive actions). Activating one part of the system, for example, by recalling an emotional situation in memory, or imagining the emotional scene, typically starts to activate the other components of the network, including associated physiology and action preparation.

Emotional information tends to vary along two primary dimensions, based on factor analytic findings on emotion adjectives and ratings of emotional materials across cultures. These orthogonal dimensions are *valence* (how positive or negative an emotion is) and *arousal* (how intense the emotion is), whereas a third dimension, *dominance* (how much in control one feels in the emotional situation), is positively related to valence (Mehrabian & Russell, 1974; Panayiotou, 2008). Emotions are first perceived at an automatic or preconscious level, and many of the associated responses, physiological and behavioral, begin to appear at this stage, even before the emotional experience becomes labeled and subjectively recognized as an emotion (Russell, 2003). Once the emotion becomes conscious, attempts to regulate it come into play including attempts to maintain it, increase it, or decrease it (Gross, 1998). Notably, less conscious, implicit, or automatic emotion regulation efforts may also take place as soon as an emotional stimulus becomes encountered (e.g., attention deployment, expressive suppression), during anticipatory stages of processing (e.g., vigilance), or even at earlier stages of planning one's actions with regard to the emotional event (e.g., behavioral avoidance). Thus, although valence and arousal systems are primarily responsible for our emotional experience and associated action preparation, functions related to the executive control system, including inhibitory systems in the medial prefrontal cortex, help to maintain adaptation and self-regulation in the face of hedonic stimuli (Thayer & Lane, 2007).

With regard to alexithymia, empirical evidence has provided indications of malfunction across all emotion response systems, subjective, physiological, and behavioral, and across all stages of emotion processing including initial perception, response, and regulation (Luminet, Rimé, Bagby, & Taylor, 2004; Pollatos & Gramann, 2011). Although there are some indications that alexithymic deficits pertain mostly to the arousal dimension of emotion (Peasley-Miklus, Panayiotou, & Vrana, 2016; Roedema & Simons, 1999), this remains to be further determined. Results regarding all aspects of alexithymic emotional difficulties are to a large degree mixed, partly due to the diverse experimental paradigms used and the selection criteria for alexithymic participants, leading to the need for more research in order to clarify the nature of alexithymia and its role in physical and mental health.

In most contemporary theories, alexithymia is considered as a personality trait found on a continuum in the general population (Mikolajczak & Luminet, 2006). Its central characteristics involve difficulty describing emotions verbally, difficulty identifying emotions in self and others, and an externally oriented, concrete thinking style. It is highly correlated with self-reported physical symptoms and illness perception, and this is believed to be due to a tendency of alexithymic individuals to confuse emotions, and particularly their associated physiology, with physical symptoms (Taylor & Bagby, 2004). In fact, alexithymic individuals seem to lack the ability to represent symbolically the meaning of somatic experiences, including the physiological component of emotions, a characteristic which has been termed "blindfeel" (Lane, Ahern, Schwartz, & Kaszniak, 1997). That is, in spite of potentially normal physiological reactivity to emotional events, the alexithymic individual has been thought to fail in having the corresponding subjective experience and realization that the physical sensations represent an emotion. Emotion-related difficulties are not the only ones apparent in alexithymia, however. The trait has also been related to limited fantasy, dreaming, and imagery ability, while aberrations in self-awareness seem to form another cornerstone of the construct (Taylor, Ryan, & Bagby, 1985). All of these aspects need to be kept in mind in order to better understand the role of alexithymia in mental and physical health and its potential association with somatization and health anxiety symptoms.

Epidemiologically, alexithymia is found at all social levels but in higher prevalence rates among middle-aged, low-educated men, which suggests that it is in part environmentally determined (Kauhanen, Kaplan, Julkunen, Wilson, & Salonen, 1993). Although generally considered as a personality trait, it has also been found to be acquired after psychological trauma and at times following brain injury and lesions to particular emotion-related regions in the brain.

Case Example:

A 45-year-old woman presents for psychological therapy because "something is wrong and her husband asked her to seek help." She has lost 20 pounds over the last 6 months and has increased need for sleep and experienced fatigue. She has been almost unable to engage in any housework and barely makes it to her work. The patient denies feeling depressed or sad; however she appears nervous and agitated. The main disturbing experience she describes is a feeling of "tension" and sensations of "uneasiness" in her chest. When asked for details, she is unable to describe this further or connect it to any specific concerns or feelings of anxiety, but it seems to occur when she is traveling to work and may be running late. When prompted for other potential symptoms of panic attacks, she does not report any, and she is not aware of any specific worries that may be troubling her. Her symptoms started after a conflict between her family and a contractor over a house they are building. She believes the contractor cheated them and used inferior materials in the house. She plans to sue the contractor for compensation. When asked for details about how she feels about this situation, she is unable to report any specific feelings. She insists that the reason she is preoccupied with the situation is that what the contractor did is "wrong." She believes he should honor his agreements and be considerate of the damage to others.

This case example highlights many of the essential features of alexithymia. This patient, like many alexithymic individuals, lacks self-awareness, especially of her emotions. She has difficulties labeling and reporting on her emotional experience, and although she is aware of the physical arousal associated with emotions, she interprets this as a worrisome physical or illness-related symptom. Her focus and approach to resolving her difficulties are externally oriented, while her thinking of the situation is concrete and lacks insight into her situation and behavior. She also may be experiencing difficulty empathizing with the other individuals involved in her current problems.

Research Findings from Our Laboratory

What follows is a summary of recent research findings from our laboratory, the "Clinical Psychology and Psychophysiology Lab" at the University of Cyprus, that may contribute to the understanding of the distinguishing mechanisms in alexithymia and its role in psychological and somatic/medically unexplained symptoms.

The aim of our research into alexithymia is to further understand this construct and its implications for psychopathology and to additionally inform emotion theory in general on how dysfunctions in emotional processes are conducive to the etiology and maintenance of psychological disorders. With regard to alexithymia, our specific aims are to examine what the specific emotion deficits are, that is, which specific emotional mechanisms appear to malfunction and at which stage of emotion processing and regulation these difficulties mostly appear. We additionally aim to find how these deficits are related to emotional, physical, and somatoform disorders and to consider whether they are malleable to change, through the use of experimental interventions that can inform treatments for alexithymia and prevention programs for other emotion disorders in the future.

In our studies, we have used the dominant, validated assessment tool in the literature for the measurement of alexithymia, the Toronto Alexithymia Scale-20 (TAS-20, Parker,

Taylor, & Bagby, 2003). Although other instruments exist and have attracted the interest of researchers, the TAS-20 remains the "gold standard" through which alexithymia is typically identified. It relies upon internationally accepted cutoff scores, where total scores of 60 or above designate the existence of alexithymia, whereas scores below 51 mark its absence. However, as alexithymia is considered a trait found on a continuum in the general population, TAS-20 scores have also been used as a continuous dimension. The tool yields three factors which describe the primary deficits associated with the construct, difficulty identifying feelings (DIF), difficulty describing feelings (DDF), and externally oriented thinking (EOT). Although all factors are important aspects of the alexithymia construct, there is substantial evidence in the literature that they may show differential correlations with other behaviors and characteristics, including mental health.

In order to examine physiological and subjective reactivity to emotions, we typically use the emotional tone-cued imagery paradigm, which has been used extensively by emotion researchers in the past (Vrana & Lang, 1990; Panayiotou, Brown, & Vrana, 2007; Panayiotou, Witvliet, Robinson, & Vrana, 2011). Mental imagery of emotional events is believed to activate all aspects of the mnemonic network, including physiology and action preparation, initiating corresponding efferent response systems. Imagery is based on standardized scripts that participants memorize and recall on the basis of tone cues and have to imagine for a few seconds as if they are actually participating in the situation, based on standard instructions. Scripts are normed on large samples in terms of the valence and arousal they evoke, and materials used in our studies are based on widely used sets of imagery materials (van Oyen Witvliet & Vrana, 1995) normed in the local population (Panayiotou, 2008). Examples of imagery scenes meant to evoke Joy and Fear are presented below.

FEAR: *A strange man is following me through a bad part of town; sweat pours down my face as I listen to his footsteps coming closer.*

JOY: *I jump up with excitement as my husband drives up the road with my Christmas present, a brand new car!*

To assess reactivity to emotions, we measure physiological reactions and subjective ratings to each scene imagined. We typically collect measures of autonomic reactivity including heart rate (HR), skin conductance (SC), behavioral measures, including facial expressions through facial EMG at the corrugator and zygomatic muscles (frown and smile respectively), and the startle reflex as a measure of defensive preparation, the amplitude of which is an excellent index of negative valence and especially the emotion of fear.

In two recently published studies (Constantinou, Panayiotou, & Theodorou, 2014; Peasley-Miklus et al., 2016), we addressed the question if alexithymia is related to physiological hypo-arousal compared to controls in relation to normal or exaggerated subjective responses, or if alexithymia, in accordance to the "blindfeel" hypothesis, involves hyper-arousal (increased or typical physiological reactivity) in relation to decreased subjective response and awareness of emotion. In the literature, findings are mixed with support for both hypotheses, perhaps due to the multiple paradigms and measures of emotional reactivity used (Connelly & Denney, 2007;

Eastabrook, Lanteigne, & Hollenstein, 2013; Stone & Nielson, 2001). Prior findings also do not provide conclusive evidence as to whether alexithymic participants have difficulties processing the valence or the arousal dimensions of emotions, which the present studies can more clearly address through the inclusion of both arousal (HR, SC, self-report) and valence measures (facial EMG, startle reflex, self-report). However, a recent systematic review of the literature by our team is beginning to converge onto the idea that (a) alexithymic individuals tend to show hyporeactivity on multiple indices of autonomic arousal and that (b) their deficits are primarily arousal based (Panayiotou, Panteli, & Vlemincx, in press). Testing these hypotheses in our own samples was the primary aim of the first two studies reviewed below with college student samples, in Cyprus and the USA, respectively.

Emotion processing and regulation in alexithymia In the Peasley-Miklus et al. (2016) study, we found no significant differences between alexithymia and control groups in valence ratings (i.e., how pleasant or unpleasant this scene was) or facial expressions (EMG) at the corrugator or zygomatic facial muscles, suggesting no valence processing dysfunction when participants were asked to imagine standardized scenes involving fear, joy, or neutral situations. Findings were in accord with other evidence (Roedema & Simons, 1999; see Vanman, Dawson, & Brennan, 1998, for an exception), which showed that alexithymic difficulties are mostly arousal and not valence based. In fact, in our study, high-alexithymic participants showed better differentiation by rating neutral and joy scenes as more distinct in valence than control participants.

Instead, our findings suggested an arousal-based deficit during emotional imagery. As alexithymia scores increased, there was less differentiation between neutral and arousing emotional imagery (joy and fear) in heart rate increase from baseline. This finding is consistent with a hypo-arousal view of alexithymia, with decreased autonomic mobilization during emotions, across valences. Importantly, this effect was specific to emotional imagery; the study had also included non-emotional, "action" imagery (e.g., sports scenes); no HR deficits in arousal were identified for that type of imagery in alexithymia.

In the Constantinou et al. (2014) study, we found evidence also consistent with hyporeactivity in alexithymia but, in this case, mostly with regards to the startle reflex, an index of defensive mobilization. Alexithymic participants compared to controls showed significantly slower startle latencies and marginally smaller startle reflex amplitudes than controls especially during fear imagery, when the response is expected to be most potentiated. It was notable that the effect was strongest for latency than for amplitude, as startle reflex latency is considered to be more sensitive to arousal than valence aspects of emotion. A finding worth noting across both studies is a tendency for high-alexithymic participants to be over-aroused rather than under-aroused during conditions when a more relaxed state might have been appropriate: In the Peasley-Miklus et al. study, increased TAS-20 scores were associated with increased heart rate to neutral emotional imagery, while in the Constantinou et al. study, alexithymic participants had larger startle reflex amplitudes than controls during resting baseline.

Furthermore, across both studies, evidence is presented consistent with the idea of poor symbolic representation of bodily experiences in alexithymia, which may partly explain its association with somatoform symptoms, where patients appear to misreport emotional experiences as signs of illness (Eastabrook et al., 2013; Papciak, Feuerstein, & Spiegel, 1985). Specifically, Peasley-Miklus et al. (2016) found evidence of decoupling (disassociation) among emotion systems in the sense that as alexithymia increased, there was less HR increase in high arousal emotional imagery, whereas as alexithymia decreased, the HR response increased in tandem with the arousal ratings of emotional scenes. Similarly, Constantinou et al. (2014) found significantly smaller within-subject correlations between subjective ratings of arousal and both heart rate and skin conductance level in high-alexithymic participants, in accordance with substantial previous evidence of decoupling between self-report and physiological response systems in alexithymia (e.g., Martin & Pihl, 1986).

These findings provide information, which helps to reconcile previous evidence and is consistent with the overall conclusions of the Panayiotou et al. (in press) review, specifically that the tendency of alexithymic individuals is toward hyporeactivity in autonomic and reflexive action preparation during emotions, that the deficits seem to pertain mostly to the arousal system, and that they are specific to emotional arousal rather than arousal in general.

But why do these individuals respond with decreased physiological activation to emotional situations? The mechanism of action remains obscure, while the effect is reminiscent of the "affective blunting" observed in other clinical populations, including those with some anxiety disorders like generalized anxiety disorder (Borkovec & Roemer, 1995), post-traumatic stress disorder (McTeague et al., 2010), or comorbid anxiety with depression (McTeague & Lang, 2012). These populations are characterized by general "nonspecific" negative affect and significant subjective distress co-occurring with decreased physiological reactions, especially to their own idiographic fearful conditions. This effect has been explained as the outcome of severity, chronicity of the condition, and comorbidity with depression and negative affectivity, which are marked by behavioral immobilization, as indexed by the blunting of autonomic and behavioral/reflexive responses (McTeague & Lang, 2012; Panayiotou, Karekla, Georgiou, Constantinou, & Paraskeva-Siamata, 2017). The picture painted by ours and other studies for alexithymia is similar to this, with the modification that subjective experience of arousal may also be dampened in some cases, although evidence from the majority of alexithymic decoupling studies points to the idea that dampened reactivity is mostly in terms of physiology (Panayiotou et al., in press). Given the high associations between alexithymia and depression in the literature, it may be important for future studies to delineate if physiological under-reactivity still remains a characteristic of this condition when the effect of depression is controlled for, something that has not been done in many existing studies.

Findings like this are consistent with conceptualizations of alexithymia as an emotion regulation disorder, which emphasize the possibility that the emotion dysfunctions presented by this population are a result of the reliance on emotion regulation or defense mechanisms involving repression, suppression, and denial

(Swart, Kortekaas, & Aleman, 2009). The question surfaces then, whether the hyporeactivity of alexithymic individuals represents an innate inability to process emotional aspects or is a learned defense or regulation mechanism reinforced by its ability to protect the individual from the awareness of unwanted experiences. Although this issue remains open to investigation, some preliminary findings from our lab suggest that poor emotion regulation ability, probably due to failed learning of appropriate regulation strategies, may be responsible. We repeatedly find associations between alexithymia and avoidant coping, especially avoidance of unwanted experiences (Panayiotou et al., 2015). Some recent unpublished data from an experiment involving a letter search task while emotional distractors were presented on some trials suggested that alexithymic individuals indeed perceived and were affected by the emotional qualities of distractors, even though they may have effortfully attempted to prevent such emotional influences (Panayiotou, Theodorou, Vrana & Konstantinou, under review).

A second important issue that arises from our findings is that alexithymic deficits seem centered to the arousal system, which raises questions as to why alexithymic individuals are able to process appropriately the valence aspect of emotion, irrespective of their deficits. One potential explanation might be that due to their externally oriented thinking, they focus their attention on external cues (in the case of our experiments the imagery scripts they were given to memorize) to decipher what they "should" feel rather than relying in interoceptive cues in order to report what they actually feel (Peasley-Miklus et al., 2016). That is, they are able to remain relatively accurate in their reports and behavior (facial EMG) not because they know what they feel but because they figure out what they should be feeling using external sources of information, especially in the context of a structured experimental session. To the contrary, in the case of unstructured clinical interviews, offering few cues as to how one should feel, alexithymic patients may present with a difficulty in reporting on their emotions, which had led to the initial conceptualization of alexithymia as a problem in the verbal reporting of affect.

Can alexithymic emotion processing deficits be remediated The next topic that we addressed in our research is whether alexithymia deficits are malleable to change. Few attempts exist in the literature to directly treat alexithymia, and alexithymic patients are well known as being difficult to treat, due to their limited insight and ability to describe their emotional experiences (Joyce, Nordhagen, Ogrodniczuk, Stovel, & Bjorge, 2015). One previous study found that training in anger expression among alexithymic individuals was an effective intervention for headache sufferers (Lumley, 2004), while another study found that traditional CBT for affective disorders, not specifically targeted for alexithymia, was associated with a posttreatment decrease in alexithymia scores (Panayiotou et al., 2015). We mostly applied experimental manipulations in the lab, based on the premise that to the degree that hypo-arousal is a learned coping mechanism, alexithymic individuals should be able to show improvement in their reactivity following appropriate guidance or training in how to process and regulate emotions. Hence, another question that was addressed in the Constantinou et al. (2014) study was whether guidance in how to process emotional situations more effectively could have an impact on alexithymic emotional responses, in an initial attempt to identify modes of potential interventions to remedy the impact of this trait.

In that study, participants were asked to imagine the situations in two different ways, either in a shallow or in a deep manner. During shallow processing, they had to pay attention to the various descriptive elements in the imagery scene, so that they could recall them when asked. During deep processing, they had to imagine the situation while paying attention to how they felt, their reactions, thoughts, and sensations, as if they had to describe them to an actor in order to accurately impersonate them. The study provided initial evidence that deep emotion processing somewhat decreased the hypo-arousal phenomenon in alexithymic participants. They demonstrated faster startle reflex latencies during deep processing compared to shallow and higher HR response during deep fear imagery. However deep processing was associated with some unexpected "side effects." High-alexithymic participants reported less dominance during deep processing of fear compared to shallow processing and less subjective arousal in that same condition with simultaneous greater reported arousal during deep processing of neutral imagery. Currently, studies are underway both in our lab and others, evaluating interventions, like mindfulness, as a way to help alexithymic individuals to process emotion more deeply and effectively.

Summing up these findings, they seem to suggest that alexithymic individuals can be taught different ways to process emotion, which may address some of their emotional deficits. Specifically, guidance in deeper processing may help increase their somatic reactivity, which in turn may help them become more aware of physical sensations as emotional experiences and combat their interoceptive inaccuracy (Herbert et al., 2011) by decreasing decoupling between different emotion systems. The mechanism behind this change may involve the increased focus on the self and its experiences that was the result of the deepening instructions provided. Though not an intervention itself, these experimental results may provide some preliminary clues on elements that might comprise future intervention programs designed specifically for alexithymia.

But what does the unexpected decreased reporting of arousal at higher levels of physiological reactivity (due to deepening) mean? Although still a preliminary finding in need of further replication, it may provide a hint regarding the mechanism behind alexithymic decoupling. In accord with previous reports that alexithymia can result from trauma and may entail defense mechanism that decrease self-awareness (suppression, avoidance; Bilotta, Giacomantonio, Leone, Mancini, & Coriale, 2015; Laloyaux, Fantini, Lemaire, Luminet, & Larøi, 2015; Venta, Sharp, & Hart, 2012), these findings may indicate a "shutting down" or blunting of emotions, when external or internal cues suggest that the emotion will be intense or overwhelming. In this direction, it is of interest that both studies found increased subjective reports of arousal among alexithymic individuals during neutral emotional situations, perhaps perceived as the least threatening. Based on these findings, the next set of questions that arise pertain to the ability of alexithymic individuals to regulate emotions in ways that are compatible with mental health and the association between their observed emotion processing and regulation difficulties with health and psychological symptoms.

Alexithymia and emotion regulation Although it is generally accepted that poor emotion regulation is a hallmark of alexithymia, this assertion has been supported mostly by self-report studies. More recently, some brain imaging studies have provided supportive evidence of decreased activation in emotion regulation areas in alexithymia (Mériau et al., 2006). Evidence already exists that alexithymia is specifically related to "maladaptive" regulation and coping strategies including suppression and low reappraisal so that in fact alexithymic individuals use these strategies more "efficiently." Additional evidence suggests that alexithymic individuals also rely on avoidant coping, especially experiential avoidance (Venta et al., 2012), an effortful attempt to not come into contact with unwanted internal experiences (Hayes, Wilson, Gifford, Follette, & Strosahl, 1996). In order to examine emotion regulation in alexithymia, we analyzed data that were collected in the context of the same study reported in Constantinou et al. (2014). Specifically, we used two indices of emotion regulation typically neglected in the alexithymia literature, heart rate variability (HRV) at baseline, as a measure of trait emotion regulation ability, and recovery/habituation of physiological responses as an index of emotion downregulation. In normally functioning individuals, the rhythm of the heart shows variability as the organism adjusts to the changing environmental demands, while a "locked," inflexible autonomic response (low HRV) has been associated with poor physical and psychological health (Beauchaine & Thayer, 2015; Thayer, Åhs, Fredrikson, Sollers, & Wager, 2012) and delayed recovery from stressors (Weber et al., 2010). To the contrary, individuals with greater emotion regulation ability have higher resting HRV (Thayer & Lane, 2007). Similarly, normally functioning individuals habituate to repeated or prolonged presentation of stimuli (stressors), a sign of adjustment and self-regulation.

In this study (Panayiotou & Constantinou, 2017), we compared the startle reflex amplitude of alexithymic and control participants over time that is during an initial baseline, during the imagery exposure (first exposure) to fear scenes, and during a second exposure to the same scenes. As reported above, participants had to imagine the same scene with either deep or shallow processing instruction during first exposure only. At reexposure, they were allowed to imagine the scene as they normally would without further instruction. HRV was assessed during an initial 2-min baseline prior to the start of the experiment.

During shallow processing, alexithymic participants demonstrated marginally lower startle reflex amplitudes at exposure than controls. During deep processing, their responses were larger relative to shallow processing of fear, but this was true across all phases, including baseline and reexposure, demonstrating the impact of deep processing instructions to combat hyporeactivity. However, among alexithymic participants, there was no apparent increase in startle amplitude during exposure and no apparent habituation during reexposure, demonstrating poor adjustment to the changing demands of the context, suggesting poor emotion regulation abilities and autonomic inflexibity.

To further examine this question, group differences in baseline HRV were examined, along with the ability of HRV to predict startle reflex responses in both groups. We found a trend for lower HRV in alexithymia, especially of high-frequency domain measures, which indicate parasympathetic control of the heart, and significant correlations between the same indices and the difficulty identifying feelings aspect of the TAS-20. Using linear regression, we also found that the model where HRV indices were set to predict startle reflex amplitude during different phases of the experiment was significant for alexithymics but not controls. Startle amplitude habituation during re-exposure to fear imagery was predicted by increased parasympathetic control (time domain components, high-frequency component) and decreased sympathetic control (low-frequency/high-frequency ratio). These effects were only true during deep processing when emotion engagement was expected to be at its greatest.

According to the above findings, in addition to emotion processing difficulties (low reactivity), alexithymic individuals show poor emotion regulation ability demonstrated as lower tonic HRV and poor habituation of defensive activation to fear imagery, which indicates poorer adjustment to the varying demands of the environment. Decreased parasympathetic control of the heart was a predictor of this adjustment difficulty. These findings lead to the hypothesis that low emotion regulation ability may form the link between alexithymia and psychopathology. For example, it has been previously suggested that low baseline HRV, especially among anxious individuals, means difficulty in processing "safety signals." The question arises as to whether alexithymic individuals share this tendency, which may make them particularly cautious to engage in intense negative affective situations. In the context of the literature linking alexithymia to traumatic experiences, the experience of unpleasant or traumatic uncontrollable events may explain their poor processing of safety signals (Melzig, Weike, Hamm, & Thayer, 2009). The inability to more adaptively regulate emotions may additionally explain their tendency for blunting and experiential avoidance (as well as low ratings of dominance during deeply processed arousing affect found in Constantinou et al. (2014), as emotional situations may appear overwhelming; see Fig. 5.1).

Associations between alexithymia and psychopathology In the context of further understanding the association between poor emotion regulation in alexithymia and psychological pathology, a series of additional studies were conducted using a correlational approach of questionnaire self-report data. In one study, using a college sample in Cyprus and a clinical sample of mixed affective disorder presentations in the USA (Panayiotou et al., 2015), we assessed the association between TAS-20 indices and psychosomatic and depression symptoms using the psychological health questionnaire (Kroenke, Spitzer, & Williams, 2002) and Beck Depression Inventory II (Beck, Steer, & Brown, 1996), respectively, and examined a putative mechanism for this association, namely, experiential avoidance, the

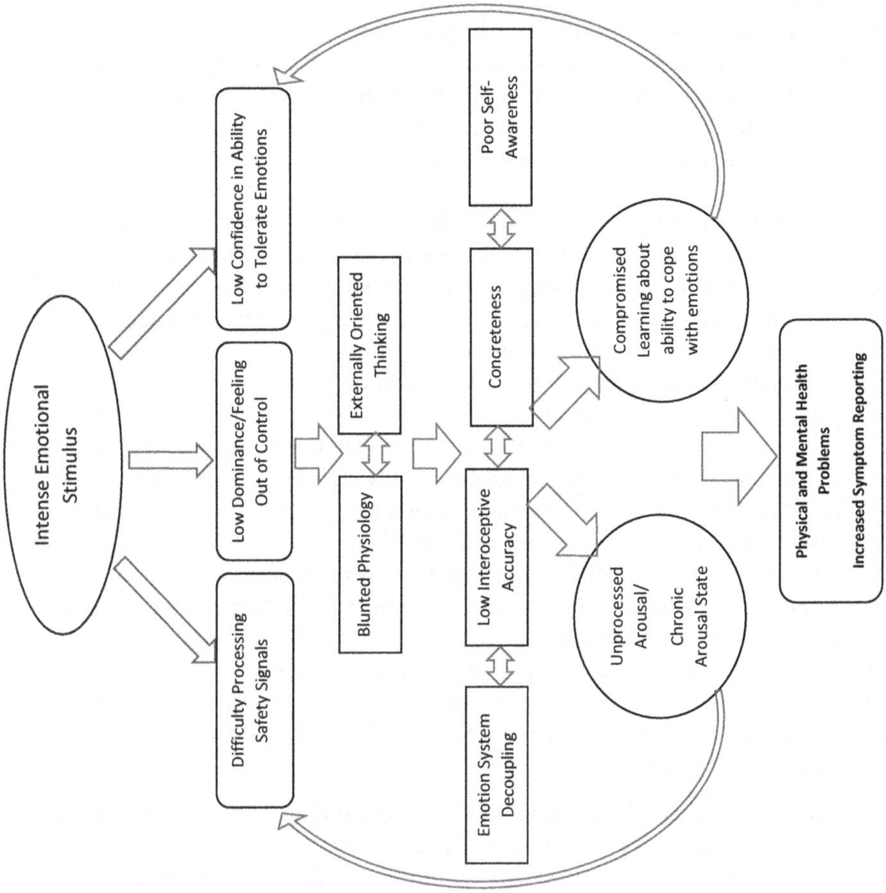

Fig. 5.1 Diagrammatic depiction of a conceptual model describing emotion processing difficulties in Alexithymia

emotion regulation strategy focused on trying not to come into contact with unwanted experiences.

Strong associations were observed between TAS-20 factors and experiential avoidance and also between TAS-20 and psychosomatic symptoms in the college sample. Notably, the externally oriented thinking (EOT) factor of TAS-20 showed the smallest/nonsignificant associations with both symptoms and experiential avoidance. In the clinical sample, TAS-20 was similarly strongly associated with both depression symptoms and experiential avoidance, with EOT not being significantly associated with symptoms. In both samples, we found that experiential avoidance mediated the association between alexithymia and psychological symptoms. This finding provides evidence in support of the hypothesis that this type of (poor) emotion regulation strategy, focused on attempts to decrease awareness of emotions, may be a viable hypothetical mechanism linking alexithymia to psychological disorders.

Similar results were obtained in another study conducted with a college sample (Panayiotou, Leonidou, Constantinou, and Michaelides, 2018), which also found alexithymia to be associated with psychological symptoms, specifically of social anxiety, and this association to be mediated by experiential avoidance. The finding that the EOT factor is the least strongly related to both symptoms and reports of experiential avoidance was also replicated. This study additionally showed a negative association between all aspects of TAS-20, especially EOT and private self-consciousness, an aspect of self-awareness measured by the Self-Consciousness Scale (Fenigstein, Scheier, & Buss, 1975). This finding was expected on the basis of previous assertions that alexithymia involves low awareness of self and emotions and that it entails concrete and externally oriented thinking. Notably, however, in unpublished data from the same study, a negative association was observed between self-reflectiveness, a negative variant of self-awareness involving self-scrutiny and criticism (Panayiotou & Kokkinos, 2006) and EOT, which was apparently linked to low self-awareness of all types, including positive self-knowledge. Given that associations between many other emotional disorders and experiential avoidance have been found consistently in the past, what is unique about alexithymia may be its characteristic low self-awareness and externally oriented thinking. Thus, not only do individuals high in alexithymia engage in avoidance, much like other individuals with anxiety and affective symptoms, but they seem to have little awareness both of their distress (demonstrated by the low correlation between EOT and all types of symptoms assessed) and their attempt to avoid it (shown in low associations between EOT and experiential avoidance, when at the same time the other aspects of alexithymia show strong correlations with this type of emotion regulation strategy). Externally oriented thinking and low self-awareness probably increase the risk for psychological symptoms in alexithymia because of reduced self-knowledge that could activate self-regulation and coping, but at the same time, they may serve a protective function against distress (Davydov, Luminet, & Zech, 2013), at least in the short run.

In upublished data (available upon request), we also examined the association between alexithymia and emotion regulation strategies as measured by the Cognitive

Emotion Regulation Questionnaire short form (Garnefski & Kraaij, 2006) and the Emotion Regulation Questionnaire (Gross & John, 2003). All aspects of alexithymia were found to be positively related to suppression and negatively to reappraisal, in support of previous findings showing a link between alexithymia and poor emotion regulation strategies. Notably, EOT was negatively correlated to all types of emotion regulation strategies requiring mental processing (e.g., reappraisal, positive reframing, rumination), reflecting the externally focused tendencies of alexithymic individuals. To the contrary, the other facets of alexithymia, difficulty identifying feelings and difficulty describing feelings, were positively related to maladaptive types of emotion regulation, typically found in samples with emotional disorders as well, such as self-blame, other blame, and catastrophizing. Based on these findings, EOT may play a protective role against distress. Figure 5.1 depicts a theoretical model of alexithymia and its relation to emotion processing and regulation difficulties.

Concluding Comments

The summary of the literature and findings from our own lab presented above leads to some preliminary conclusions and raises a number of questions for further study in alexithymia and its role in psychopathology, including somatoform illness and medically unexplained symptoms. First, additional replication using standardized experimental designs is needed to draw definitive conclusions that alexithymia involves hyporeactivity of the physiological response system during the processing of emotions, paired with normal self-report of distress. Current evidence points to that direction, and the alexithymic emotion response profile looks remarkably similar to that of patients with emotional disorders who show physiological blunting in intense affective situations but may report high levels of negative affect. This picture results in the relatively consistent finding of a decoupling in alexithymic individuals between emotion response systems, which may be associated with their tendency to confuse physical sensations with signs of illness. What may be a distinguishing feature of alexithymia in relation to other emotional disorders is the externally oriented thinking and low self-awareness, which may play a protective role against distress by directing the focus of attention away from emotional symptoms and experiences and even away from efforts to regulate these emotions, which apparently include strategies like suppression and avoidance. In fact, in all of our studies, a very notable strong correlate of alexithymia was experiential avoidance, which is believed to be an effortful attempt to decrease awareness of unwanted experiences. This is different from anxiety and emotional disorders, which typically entail painful self-awareness, self-focused attention, and rumination.

Although research into effective interventions for alexithymia is still in its infancy, there is preliminary evidence that traditional cognitive behavior therapy may be effective (Panayiotou et al., 2015) and that interventions focused on increasing awareness of ones' own emotions while decreasing the use of avoidance for coping may be important for alexithymia. Given the pathogenic role of avoidance in all anxiety and psychosomatic disorders (Leonidou, Panayiotou, Bati, & Karekla, 2016; Panayiotou, Karekla, & Panayiotou, 2014), decreasing this tendency may serve to reduce the role of alexithymia as a general risk factor for psychopathology. Additionally, alexithymic individuals seem to respond well to interventions involving deepening of emotional experience, though this will need further study regarding its long-term effectiveness, while training in stress/emotion tolerance and acceptance may need to happen simultaneously to combat avoidance tendencies. Mindfulness training may be an important skill in this direction, which has not been applied to alexithymia previously. Given the major role of externally oriented thinking in alexithymia, interventions that focus on the retraining of attention to focus on internal rather than external stimuli may also be promising, such as attention bias modification training (Hakamata et al., 2010), as this has been applied to the treatment of anxiety disorders.

Lessons learned from existing alexithymia research is that replication is required to reconcile conflicting findings and that designs that take into account multiple emotion response systems, different dimensions of emotion, and the timeline of affective responses, from initial processing to regulation, may be valuable to deepen our understanding of alexithymia as a trait that represents a risk factor for many psychological and physical conditions.

References

Bankier, B., Aigner, M., & Bach, M. (2001). Alexithymia in DSM-IV disorder: Comparative evaluation of somatoform disorder, panic disorder, obsessive-compulsive disorder, and depression. *Psychosomatics, 42*, 235–240.

Beauchaine, T. P., & Thayer, J. F. (2015). Heart rate variability as a transdiagnostic biomarker of psychopathology. *International Journal of Psychophysiology, 98*, 338–350.

Beck, A. T., Steer, R. A., & Brown, G. K. (1996). *Manual for the Beck depression inventory-II*. San Antonio, TX: Psychological Corporation.

Bilotta, E., Giacomantonio, M., Leone, L., Mancini, F., & Coriale, G. (2015). Being alexithymic: Necessity or convenience. Negative emotionality× avoidant coping interactions and alexithymia. *Psychology and Psychotherapy: Theory, Research and Practice, 89*, 261–275.

Borkovec, T. D., & Roemer, L. (1995). Perceived functions of worry among generalized anxiety disorder subjects: Distraction from more emotionally distressing topics? *Journal of Behavior Therapy and Experimental Psychiatry, 26*, 25–30.

Connelly, M., & Denney, D. R. (2007). Regulation of emotions during experimental stress in alexithymia. *Journal of Psychosomatic Research, 62*, 649–656.

Constantinou, E., Panayiotou, G., & Theodorou, M. (2014). Emotion processing deficits in alexithymia and response to a depth of processing intervention. *Biological Psychology, 103*, 212–222.

Davydov, D. M., Luminet, O., & Zech, E. (2013). An externally oriented style of thinking as a moderator of responses to affective films in women. *International Journal of Psychophysiology, 87*, 152–164.

Eastabrook, J. M., Lanteigne, D. M., & Hollenstein, T. (2013). Decoupling between physiological, self-reported, and expressed emotional responses in alexithymia. *Personality and Individual Differences, 55*(8), 978–982. https://doi.org/10.1016/j.paid.2013.08.001

Fenigstein, A., Scheier, M. F., & Buss, A. H. (1975). Public and private self-consciousness: Assessment and theory. *Journal of Consulting and Clinical Psychology, 43*(4), 522–527. https://doi.org/10.1037/h0076760
Foran, H. M., & O'Leary, K. D. (2012). The role of relationships in understanding the alexithymia-depression link. *European Journal of Personality, 27*, 470–480. https://doi.org/10.1002/per.1887
Fredrikson, M., & Matthews, K. A. (1990). Cardiovascular responses to behavioral stress and hypertension: A meta-analytic review. *Annals of Behavioral Medicine, 12*(1), 30–39.
Garnefski, N., & Kraaij, V. (2006). Cognitive emotion regulation questionnaire—Development of a short 18-item version (CERQ-short). *Personality and Individual Differences, 41*(6), 1045–1053. https://doi.org/10.1016/j.paid.2006.04.010
Gross, J. J. (1998). Antecedent- and response-focused emotion regulation: Divergent consequences for experience, expression, and physiology. *Journal of Personality and Social Psychology, 74*(1), 224–237. https://doi.org/10.1037/0022-3514.74.1.224
Gross, J. J., & John, O. P. (2003). Individual differences in two emotion regulation processes: Implications for affect, relationships, and well-being. *Journal of Personality and Social Psychology, 85*(2), 348–362. https://doi.org/10.1037/0022-3514.85.2.348
Hakamata, Y., Lissek, S., Bar-Haim, Y., Britton, J. C., Fox, N. A., Leibenluft, E., … Pine, D. S. (2010). Attention bias modification treatment: A meta-analysis toward the establishment of novel treatment for anxiety. *Biological Psychiatry, 68*, 982–990.
Hayes, S. C., Wilson, K. G., Gifford, E. V., Follette, V. M., & Strosahl, K. (1996). Experiential avoidance and behavioral disorders: A functional dimensional approach to diagnosis and treatment. *Journal of Consulting and Clinical Psychology, 64*(6), 1152–1168. https://doi.org/10.1037/0022-006X.64.6.1152
Herbert, B. M., Herbert, C., & Pollatos, O. (2011). On the relationship between interoceptive awareness and alexithymia: Is interoceptive awareness related to emotional awareness? *Journal of Personality, 79*, 1149–1175.
Joyce, A. S., Nordhagen, A., Ogrodniczuk, J. S., Stovel, L. E., & Bjorge, A. (2015). Partial hospitalization treatment of the alexithymic patient: A case study. *Journal of Clinical Psychology, 71*, 167–177.
Kauhanen, J., Kaplan, G. A., Julkunen, J., Wilson, T. W., & Salonen, J. T. (1993). Social factors in alexithymia. *Comprehensive Psychiatry, 34*, 330–335.
Kojima, M., Taylor, G., Bagby, R., Parker, J., Sifneos, P., Fassino, S., … Arakawa, H. (2012). Alexithymia as a prognostic risk factor for health problems: A brief review of epidemiological studies. *BioPsychoSocial Medicine, 6*(1), 21. https://doi.org/10.1186/1751-0759-6-21
Kroenke, K., Spitzer, R. L., & Williams, J. B. (2002). The PHQ-15: Validity of a new measure for evaluating the severity of somatic symptoms. *Psychosomatic Medicine, 64*, 258–266.
Krystal, J. H. (1988). Assessing alexithymia. In H. Krystal (Ed.), *Integration and self-healing: Affect, trauma, alexithymia* (pp. 286–310). Hillsdale, NJ: Analytic Press.
Laloyaux, J., Fantini, C., Lemaire, M., Luminet, O., & Larøi, F. (2015). Evidence of contrasting patterns for suppression and reappraisal emotion regulation strategies in alexithymia. *The Journal of Nervous and Mental Disease, 203*, 709–717.
Lane, R. D., Ahern, G. L., Schwartz, G. E., & Kaszniak, A. W. (1997). Is alexithymia the emotional equivalent of blindsight? *Biological Psychiatry, 42*, 834–844.
Lang, P. J. (1979). A bio-informational theory of emotional imagery. *Psychophysiology, 16*, 495–512.
Lang, P. J. (1993). The network model of emotion: Motivational connections. In R. S. Wyer & T. K. Srull (Eds.), *Advances in social cognition* (Vol. 6). Hillsdale, NJ: Lawrence Erlbaum.
Leonidou, C., Panayiotou, G., Bati, A., & Karekla, M. (2016). Coping with psychosomatic symptoms: The buffering role of psychological flexibility and impact on quality of life. *Journal of Health Psychology*, 1359105316666657.
Luminet, O., Rimé, B., Bagby, R. M., & Taylor, G. (2004). A multimodal investigation of emotional responding in alexithymia. *Cognition and Emotion, 18*, 741–766.

Lumley, M. A. (2004). Alexithymia, emotional disclosure, and health: A program of research. *Journal of Personality, 72*(6), 1271–1300.

Marchesi, C., Fontò, S., Balista, C., Cimmino, C., & Maggini, C. (2005). Relationship between alexithymia and panic disorder: A longitudinal study to answer an open question. *Psychotherapy and Psychosomatics, 74*(1), 56–60. https://doi.org/10.1159/000082028

Martin, J. B., & Pihl, R. O. (1986). Influence of alexithymic characteristics on physiological and subjective stress responses in normal individuals. *Psychotherapy and Psychosomatics, 45*, 66–77.

McEwen, B. S. (2008). Central effects of stress hormones in health and disease: Understanding the protective and damaging effects of stress and stress mediators. *European Journal of Pharmacology, 583*, 174–185.

McTeague, L. M., & Lang, P. J. (2012). The anxiety spectrum and the reflex physiology of defense: From circumscribed fear to broad distress. *Depression and Anxiety, 29*(4), 264–281.

McTeague, L. M., Lang, P. J., Laplante, M. C., Cuthbert, B. N., Shumen, J. R., & Bradley, M. M. (2010). Aversive imagery in posttraumatic stress disorder: Trauma recurrence, comorbidity, and physiological reactivity. *Biological Psychiatry, 67*(4), 346–356.

Mehrabian, A., & Russell, J. A. (1974). *An approach to experimental psychology*. Cambridge, MA: MIT Press.

Melzig, C. A., Weike, A. I., Hamm, A. O., & Thayer, J. F. (2009). Individual differences in fear-potentiated startle as a function of resting heart rate variability: Implications for panic disorder. *International Journal of Psychophysiology, 71*, 109–117.

Mériau, K., Wartenburger, I., Kazzer, P., Prehn, K., Lammers, C. H., Van der Meer, E., … Heekeren, H. R. (2006). A neural network reflecting individual differences in cognitive processing of emotions during perceptual decision making. *NeuroImage, 33*, 1016–1027.

Mikolajczak, M., & Luminet, O. (2006). Is alexithymia affected by situational stress or is it a stable trait related to emotion regulation? *Personality and Individual Differences, 40*, 1399–1408.

Panayiotou, G. (2008). Emotional dimensions reflected in ratings of affective scripts. *Personality and Individual Differences, 44*, 1795–1806.

Panayiotou, G., Brown, R., & Vrana, S. R. (2007). Emotional dimensions as determinants of self-focused attention. *Cognition and Emotion, 21*, 982–998.

Panayiotou, G., & Constantinou, E. (2017). Emotion dysregulation in alexithymia: Startle reactivity to fearful affective imagery and its relation to heart rate variability. *Psychophysiology, 54*, 1323–1334.

Panayiotou, G., Karekla, M., Georgiou, D., Constantinou, E., & Paraskeva-Siamata, M. (2017). Psychophysiological and self-reported reactivity associated with social anxiety and public speaking fear symptoms: Effects of fear versus distress. *Psychiatry Research, 255*, 278–286.

Panayiotou, G., Karekla, M., & Panayiotou, M. (2014). Direct and indirect predictors of social anxiety: The role of anxiety sensitivity, behavioral inhibition, experiential avoidance and self-consciousness. *Comprehensive Psychiatry, 55*, 1875–1882.

Panayiotou, G., & Kokkinos, C. M. (2006). Self-consciousness and psychological distress: A study using the Greek SCS. *Personality and Individual Differences, 41*, 83–93.

Panayiotou, G., Leonidou, C., Constantinou, E., & Michaelides, M. P. (2018). Self-Awareness in alexithymia and associations with social anxiety. *Current Psychology*, 1–10.

Panayiotou, G., Leonidou, C., Constantinou, E., Hart, J., Rinehart, K. L., Sy, J. T., & Björgvinsson, T. (2015). Do alexithymic individuals avoid their feelings? Experiential avoidance mediates the association between alexithymia, psychosomatic, and depressive symptoms in a community and a clinical sample. *Comprehensive Psychiatry, 56*, 206–216.

Panayiotou, G., Panteli, M., & Vlemincx, E. (in press). Processing emotions in alexithymia: A systematic review of physiological markers.

Panayiotou, G., Witvliet, C. O., Robinson, J. D., & Vrana, S. R. (2011). A startling absence of emotion effects: Active attention to the startle probe as a motor task cue appears to eliminate modulation of the startle reflex by valence and arousal. *Biological Psychology, 87*, 226–233.

Panayiotou, G., Theodorou, M., Konstantinou, N., & Vrana, S. (under review). I can take my eyes off of you! Processing emotional faces under different perceptual load conditions and the effects of alexithymia and heart rate variability

Papciak, A. S., Feuerstein, M., & Spiegel, J. A. (1985). Stress reactivity in alexithymia: Decoupling of physiological and cognitive responses. *Journal of Human Stress, 11*, 135–142.

Parker, J. D., Taylor, G. J., & Bagby, R. M. (2003). The 20-Item Toronto Alexithymia Scale: III. Reliability and factorial validity in a community population. *Journal of Psychosomatic Research, 55*, 269–275.

Peasley-Miklus, C. E., Panayiotou, G., & Vrana, S. R. (2016). Alexithymia predicts arousal-based processing deficits and discordance between emotion response systems during emotional imagery. *Emotion, 16*, 164–174.

Pollatos, O., & Gramann, K. (2011). Electrophysiological evidence of early processing deficits in alexithymia. *Biological Psychology, 87*, 113–121.

Roedema, T. M., & Simons, R. F. (1999). Emotion-processing deficit in alexithymia. *Psychophysiology, 36*, 379–387.

Russell, J. A. (2003). Core affect and the psychological construction of emotion. *Psychological Review, 110*, 145–172.

Sifneos, P. E. (1973). The prevalence of 'alexithymic' characteristics in psychosomatic patients. *Psychotherapy and Psychosomatics, 22*, 255–262.

Stone, L. A., & Nielson, K. A. (2001). Intact physiological response to arousal with impaired emotional recognition in alexithymia. *Psychotherapy and Psychosomatics, 70*, 92–102.

Swart, M., Kortekaas, R., & Aleman, A. (2009). Dealing with feelings: Characterization of trait alexithymia on emotion regulation strategies and cognitive-emotional processing. *PLoS One, 4*, e5751.

Taylor, G. J., & Bagby, R. M. (2004). New trends in alexithymia research. *Psychotherapy and Psychosomatics, 73*(2), 68–77. https://doi.org/10.1159/000075537

Taylor, G. J., Ryan, D., & Bagby, R. M. (1985). Toward the development of a new self-report alexithymia scale. *Psychotherapy and Psychosomatics, 44*, 191–199.

Thayer, J. F., Åhs, F., Fredrikson, M., Sollers, J. J., & Wager, T. D. (2012). A meta-analysis of heart rate variability and neuroimaging studies: Implications for heart rate variability as a marker of stress and health. *Neuroscience & Biobehavioral Reviews, 36*, 747–756.

Thayer, J. F., & Lane, R. D. (2007). The role of vagal function in the risk for cardiovascular disease and mortality. *Biological Psychology, 74*, 224–242.

Van Oyen Witvliet, C., & Vrana, S. R. (1995). Psychophysiological responses as indices of affective dimensions. *Psychophysiology, 32*, 436–443.

Vanman, E. J., Dawson, M. E., & Brennan, P. A. (1998). Affective reactions in the blink of an eye: Individual differences in subjective experience and psychological responses to emotional stimuli. *Personality & Social Psychology Bulletin, 24*, 994–1005.

Venta, A., Sharp, C., & Hart, J. (2012). The relation between anxiety disorder and experiential avoidance in inpatient adolescents. *Psychological Assessment, 24*(1), 240–248. https://doi.org/10.1037/a0025362

Vrana, S. R., & Lang, P. J. (1990). Fear imagery and the startle-probe index. *Journal of Abnormal Psychology, 99*, 181–189.

Weber, C. S., Thayer, J. F., Rudat, M., Wirtz, P. H., Zimmermann-Viehoff, F., Thomas, A., ... & Deter, H. C. (2010). Low vagal tone is associated with impaired post stress recovery of cardiovascular, endocrine, and immune markers. *European Journal of Applied Physiology, 109*, 201–211.

Chapter 6
Trauma and Its Consequences for the Body and Mind

Werner Bohleber

Introduction

For a long time, research on trauma was more or less a blank page in the theoretical and clinical psychoanalytical discourse. Although psychoanalysis had begun as a theory of trauma, and although Freud would return time and again to trauma (particularly during the First World War), and despite the looming barbarism of National Socialism, psychoanalysis, as a whole, it had not attributed the significance it ought to have to political and social violence. While the psychic consequences of both world wars compelled one to focus on traumatization, interest therein paled and was extinguished altogether a short time thereafter. Given the multiple catastrophes and extreme experiences that people were exposed to and suffered from during the twentieth century, trauma ultimately became the signature mark of the entire century. Considerable time was to elapse; however, before psychoanalysis, psychiatry and other human sciences took up this theme and made it a central theme of research. Only after the Vietnam War, once the diagnosis of PTSD became part of psychiatric nomenclature in 1980, did comprehensive research on traumatization get under way. In psychoanalysis, it was, above all, the survivors of the Holocaust who enforced a renewed and sustained pursuit of the theory and treatment of trauma. They confronted psychoanalysts with the effects of extreme experience, which were hitherto unknown. Through the feminist movement in the 1980s, a public debate was initiated on the subject of sexual abuse and its consequences, which then brought about a renewed pursuit thereof within psychoanalysis. Taken as a whole, and in recent decades, trauma has experienced a huge boost in attention, so much so that in everyday communication, the concept has assumed an almost banal character. Today, trauma research is anchored in many disciplines, beginning with psychiatry through to literary studies.

W. Bohleber (✉)
Private Practice, Frankfurt am Main, Germany

C. Charis, G. Panayiotou (eds.), *Somatoform and Other Psychosomatic Disorders*,
https://doi.org/10.1007/978-3-319-89360-0_6

That, for a considerable period of time, psychoanalysis experienced difficulties with the theoretical and clinical understanding of trauma, is a circumstance that goes back to its theoretical preferences. The field of psychoanalysis was the inner world of the human being—the unconscious and unconscious fantasies. For many analysts, the adequate integration of external reality seemed like an intrusion on psychic reality and the meaning of the unconscious. As a consequence, the research and adequate treatment of traumatization lagged considerably behind. This is owing to the fact that trauma is not only the consequence of a shaking to the core of the psyche's structure but also that the ego/self is abruptly overwhelmed and reacts with helplessness, fear of death, and annihilation anxiety: The psychic processing mechanisms become paralysed, and only emergency reactions are possible. This experience of massive psychic overwhelming then results in permanent change to the psyche's organization. Naturally, not every traumatic situation impacts upon everyone in the same way; predisposing factors also play a role. The normal functioning of psychic organization is, however, suspended. While the traumatic event and the experience thereof are registered, they are not psychically integrated by way of the associative formation of meaning. The attempt at integration is only subsequently set in motion, where the ego/self—challenged by repetition compulsion—attempts to process the consequences and to integrate the trauma into its patterns of experience.

This description of traumatic processes remains relatively cursory serving only to emphasize the psychically unbearable weight, the "too much" which characterizes external reality in the case of traumatization. Detailed consideration reveals, however, that the situation is more complex. The reason for addressing the topic here is to elucidate why, for a considerable period of time, analysts have had such great difficulties when it comes to appropriately conceptualizing traumatic phenomena.

The Concept of Posttraumatic Stress Disorder (PTSD)

Before describing the psychoanalytic models, I want to present the definition and description of PTSD. This conception of trauma is used mainly in psychiatry and in trauma research.

PTSD is characterized by the presence of three distinct, but co-occurring, symptom clusters:

- *Re-experiencing symptoms* describe spontaneous, often insuppressible intrusions of the traumatic memory in the form of images or nightmares that are accompanied by intense physiological distress.
- *Avoidance symptoms* involve restricting thoughts and distancing oneself from reminders of the traumatic event, as well as more generalized emotional and social withdrawal.

- *Hyperarousal symptoms* reflect more overt physiological manifestations, such as insomnia, irritability, impaired concentration, hypervigilance, and increased startle responses.

These symptoms must be severe enough to impair social, occupational, or interpersonal function and co-occur for at least 1 month. The impairment from PTSD is amplified by poor coping strategies, substance abuse, co-occurring mood and anxiety disorders, lack of social support, and the accelerated development of stress-related medical conditions (Yehuda & LeDoux, 2007).

It is important to understand that PTSD as a full syndrome does not begin on the day of trauma. The disorder that occurs immediately after exposure to a trauma is a prolonged response of the exposure but not PTSD. It has become apparent that PTSD is more complex than a simple extension of the traumatic stress response (for the following see McFarlane, Yehuda, & Clark, 2002).

1. PTSD develops only in a proportion of individuals who are exposed to traumatic events, whereas in most people the acute stress response symptom has a dramatic decline occurring by 3 months after the traumatic event.
2. In some individuals, PTSD symptoms appear to first emerge months, years, or even decades after exposure to a traumatic event. In others, there may be a lifelong pattern of oscillation between active PTSD and remitted symptoms.
3. There is a greater prevalence of PTSD following exposure to interpersonal violence as compared with accidents. Interpersonal violence provides an increased "dosage" of trauma.
4. It is now widely appreciated that most individuals who experience a traumatic event will immediately experience some intrusive and distressing recollections of the event. However, only a subgroup of these individuals develops symptoms of avoidance, hyperarousal, and intrusive memories. It has been suggested that the intrusive and distressing recollections, rather than the direct experience of the traumatic event, actually drive the biological and psychological dimensions of PTSD. Thus, the traumatic event, although necessary for the induction of PTSD, is not a sufficient explanation for the emergence of the syndrome.
5. Intrusive thoughts and recollections of the traumatic event have a central position in understanding and trying to explain the symptoms of PTSD.

McFarlane et al. (2002) suggest that an individual's cognitive and affective adaptability is actually impaired by the dominance of internal memories.

This last point is an important conclusion. I will come back to these problems of traumatic internal memories and the pathological consequences of enduring intrusions, but I will first present the psychoanalytic models of trauma. As you will see, psychoanalysis has a much broader understanding of trauma than the concept of PTSD.

The Phenomenology of Trauma and the Difficulties to Define It Psychoanalytically

Trauma involves a concept linking an external event or, more generally, influences from the external world to their specific consequences for internal psychic realities. Both the complexity and ambiguity of the psychoanalytical concept of trauma turn on this dual referentiality and specific intermeshing of the external and the internal. Laplanche (1976) characterizes trauma as a form of "outside-inside" formed like a "thorn in the flesh". One such metaphor affiliated to this thorn in the flesh is that of the "foreign body", which plays a substantial role in trauma theory when characterizing an externally intrusive factor of which it is impossible to psychically process and integrate in a habitual manner.

Trauma is not an unambiguously defined concept. In the mid-1980s, Joseph Sandler carried out a project in collaboration with staff at the Sigmund Freud Institute in Frankfurt (Sandler, Dreher, & Drews, 1991). Ten leading psychoanalysts each presented three cases of traumatized patients. They were subsequently interviewed on their conception of trauma and its treatment. The aim was to identify those dimensions in the meaning of the trauma relevant to practice. The following core dimensions were singled out:

- The external event
- The subjective experience of such an event
- The short- and long-term outcomes of such a traumatic experience

It became conspicuously evident that many psychoanalysts applied the term imprecisely in its relation to the event, to the direct experience, and to an entire series of consequences. The external event alone would frequently be defined as trauma, whereas clinical material showed that the actual traumatic outcome was bound to the *subjective perception* of the situation. A further result was that attached to the concept of the trauma was an unavoidable, though influenceable after-effect. A pathogenic agent, more than a mere memory, remained.

Henry Krystal (1988) pointed out that what is often characterized as psychic trauma in literature on the subject is actually just a trauma-like situation which does not expand into a traumatic situation. For him, the central factor is the *experienced* helplessness. It is not the traumatic situation itself that triggers this helplessness but its subjective evaluation. The accuracy of this is initially irrelevant for the mental reaction. If the danger is regarded as unavoidable, the helplessness changes into an inner sense of giving up on oneself, of surrender. The affective state shifts from hyperalert and hyperactive response (anxiety), to one of blocking emotions and progressive inhibition (p. 143). For Krystal, this experience of having the defence function, as well as the expressive function of anxiety overwhelmed and its attendant inhibition, is the actual trauma.

Arnold Cooper (1986) defined trauma by referring to Freud's psychoeconomic model: "a psychic trauma is any psychological event which abruptly overwhelms the ego's capacity to provide a minimal sense of safety and integrative intactness, resulting in overwhelming anxiety or helplessness, or the threat of it, and producing an enduring change in the psychic organization" (p. 44). A major factor in this definition is the sudden, disruptive, uncontrollable aspect of the traumatic event and the experience of a "too much" that renders one helpless. The prototype of this definition is the shock trauma.

There are, however, other kinds of traumatization which proceed differently and for which this definition appears inadequate: sexual abuse, extreme emotional neglect, separation trauma, attachment trauma, and cumulative trauma, among others. In the definition of such traumas, focus is no longer placed on the stimulus barrier—as was still the case with Freud—which is broken through by way of disproportionately large quantities of excitation, too great to be mastered; rather, its position as protective shield is now adopted from the network of signifiers (Kirshner, 1994) regulating our life more preconsciously than consciously. Without this net, the safety and self-evidence in many aspects of our daily lives would be shattered. This situation involves what Erikson called basic trust. The decisive factor is no longer the suddenness of the traumatic irruption, but that due to its unexpected nature, the traumatic occurrence can no longer be absorbed by existing meaning structures. They are broken through like a texture, resulting in the loss of trust in the shared, symbolically mediated world by which we are preconsciously connected. The trauma sufferer's trust in his world and in his objects shatters. It can never be fully re-established.

Looking at these different kinds of trauma, it isn't surprising that we can find different models of trauma in psychoanalysis.

Psychoanalytic Models of the Trauma

How do psychoanalysts describe the psychic reality of traumatic experiences today? For a psychoanalyst, it is not enough to study the affective-cognitive storage of traumatic memories; the aim is rather to also comprehend the horror, the pain, the abandonment, the fear of death, and the annihilation which shattered the psychic equilibrium and which then form the inner core of the traumatic experience. Before pursing this in greater detail, I would like first to give a brief presentation of two of the main models of trauma which we find in psychoanalytic theory. They also form the basis for the further discussion. The first is based on Freud's psychoeconomic model, and the second on Ferenczi's object relations psychological approach.

Sigmund Freud's Psychoeconomic Model of Trauma In *Beyond the Pleasure Principle* (1920), Freud developed a model of trauma from a psychoeconomic point of view. In the moment of traumatization, the excessive quantum of excitation cannot be psychically bound and overwhelms the ego, breaking through the protective shield. The force of the surging quantities of excitation is too great to be mastered. In order to accomplish the task of psychic binding, the psychic apparatus regresses to more primitive modes of response. Freud introduces the concept of the repetition compulsion in order to describe the special nature of this experience beyond the dynamics of the pleasure-unpleasure principle. Through the repetition compulsion, the traumatic experience is actualized in the hope of thereby psychically binding the excitation and setting the pleasure principle back in motion, as well as its associated forms of psychic response.

In *Inhibitions, Symptoms and Anxiety* (1926), Freud connected the psychoeconomic view of trauma with his theory of anxiety. He draws on the concept of automatic anxiety that he developed for the actual neuroses. The excessive quantity of excitation in the traumatic situation gives rise to a massive anxiety. It floods the ego, which is defenceless against this onslaught, and renders it absolutely helpless. Automatic anxiety has an indefinite quality and lacks an object. In a first attempt at mastery, the ego attempts to convert the automatic anxiety into signal anxiety, which makes it possible for the absolute helplessness to be transformed into an expectation. The ego thereby develops an inner activity and repeats the traumatic experience "actively in a weakened version, in the hope of being able itself to direct its course" (1926, p. 167). The situation of external dangers is thereby internalized and acquires significance for the ego. The anxiety is symbolized and no longer remains indefinite and objectless. The traumatic experience thus acquires a hermeneutic structure and becomes possible to overcome.

In *Inhibitions, Symptoms and Anxiety*, Freud repeatedly described the helplessness experienced by the ego as the consequence of an object loss. This form of complete loss of internal protective objects constitutes the foundation of the second model of trauma.

The Model of Trauma in Object Relations Theory With the development of object-relations theories, quantitative considerations concerning an intolerable mass of excitation that floods the ego were rejected. The paradigm for the model is no longer an isolated experience with a shock impact—such as an accident—but the object relationship itself. Ferenczi anticipated many insights of later research into trauma. Michael Balint (1969) was the first to follow him in this respect. He emphasized that the traumatogenic quality of a situation depends on whether an intensive relationship has developed between the child and the object. The object relationship itself thus acquires a traumatic quality. As later studies (Steele, 1994) confirmed, it is not primarily the child's injuries from physical force that produce a traumatic disorder; rather, the most intensely pathogenic element is mistreatment or abuse by the person whose protection and care is actually needed. This viewpoint broadens the understanding of psychic reality in a traumatic situation. The greater the trauma, the more severe the damage to the internal object relationship, and the more severe the breakdown in the protective, stabilizing internal communication between self- and object-representations. This gives rise to isolated fragments of traumatic experience that are encapsulated and cut off from the internal communication.

The object relations theory approach to trauma theory was further developed by research into the severe traumatization that was suffered during the Holocaust. A key psychic consequence of such experiences is the breakdown of the empathic process. The communicative inner dyad between the self and its good internal objects breaks down, resulting in absolute internal isolation and the most intense desolation. The internal good object becomes silent as an empathic mediator between self and environment and the trust in the continual presence of good objects and the expectation of human empathy are destroyed (Cohen, 1985; Kirshner, 1994; Laub & Podell, 1995). This conception gives us a better understanding of the experiential core of severe traumatization. It consists of a domain of experience that is almost incommunicable: a catastrophic isolation and an inner abandonment that not only paralyses the self and its possibilities of action, but also annihilates it, while at the same time, accompanied by mortal fear, hatred, shame, and despair.

Attachment research has also developed, in a similar way, a conception of an inner traumatic core which is almost incommunicable. An attachment trauma is generated by neglecting the child in the sense of leaving the child psychologically alone in the midst of emotional distress. Allen described this point with extreme simplicity: "the essence of traumatic experience is being afraid and alone" (Allen, 2013, 164). Being alone means that there is no one to help regulate the intense emotional distress. The traumatic experience is conceptualized as an unmentalized inner core of experience.

The conceptions in object relations theory represent a major advance in the understanding of trauma. We nevertheless require both the psychoeconomic models and the models based on object relations theory in order to comprehensively cover the psychic processes of traumatization. Kindly allow me to recapitulate how the different conceptualizations of trauma have described the intrusion of an excessive reality and its effect on the psychic organization. The psychoeconomic models centre on the violence and abruptness of the intrusion of an overwhelming outside reality into the psychic organization. Metaphorically speaking, the psychic texture cannot absorb or bind the stimuli because of their excessiveness of excitation. Other concepts used in this context are "automatic objectless anxiety", "pure trauma", and an "absolute helplessness of the ego". The object relational models however centre on the destruction of the empathic protective shield which is formed by the internalized primary objects, a destruction with absolute inner loneliness and the most extreme hopelessness as a consequence thereof. Other concepts used in this context are a quasi-autistic incommunicable region, an "unmentalized foreign body", a "rupture of the network of signifiers" (Kirshner, 1994), and a "black hole" (Kinston & Cohen, 1986).

Seeing both models together then, the object relational group of concepts are better suited to explain the psychic phenomena of loss of trust in the continuous presence of good objects and the loss of trust in the shared symbolically mediated world by which we are preconsciously connected. They are also better suited to explain the traumatic breakdown of the very construction process by which we generate meanings. However, and for the explanation of the direct traumatizing force, which is a massive surplus, a "too much" that ruptures the psychic structure, we also need the psychoeconomic models. After this review of psychoanalytic concepts of trauma, I would now like to turn our attention to some clinical problems in the treatment of traumatized patients.

Traumatic Memories

The excessive arousal in a traumatic situation significantly alters the processes of encoding and storing, thereby disrupting or prohibiting the subsequent consolidation of a memory. The integrative function of memory is overwhelmed and shuts down, as the self and its functions collapse, surrendering to the situation by numbing physical and emotional pain (Krystal, 1988). Consequently, this leads to the emergence of a dissociated self-state, as a result of the fact that the traumatic experience and the resulting memories have become encapsulated. Metaphorically, this had long been characterized as a "foreign body" within the psychic matrix. This means that it cannot connect or exchange with the associative tissue of the psyche. The dissociation and encapsulation of the traumatic experience could be so strong that it gives rise to an amnesia which can extend itself retrograde. One example is:

A 35-year-old man, Mr. M., comes for analytic treatment because of severe depressive states. He is afraid that he will no longer be able to practice his profession as a social worker and provide for his family and might instead have to kill himself someday. The anamnesis reveals that his father killed himself by jumping off a high-rise building when the patient was 8. After his father's death, Mr. M. developed obsessive-compulsive behaviour and other symptoms. Growing up with one other sibling, a sister who is 2 years older, he describes how he became the mother's darling and had very good grades in school. His identity problem began to appear during adolescence. He did not really know who he actually was. During his university studies and in the first years of his professional life he was an active and very friendly colleague during the day. His mood changed in the evenings, however, and he often sat home alone, severely depressed, drinking a great deal of alcohol. When he was 25, his sister killed herself. During treatment a central memory came back to him with increasing clarity but without affect: the scene in which the family learns that the father has killed himself. A neighbour came into the house, and the patient saw from a distance how after he began talking to the mother, she suddenly broke into tears. He also started crying without really understanding what had happened. The mother told him not the truth but a lie that the father died of a heart attack. The dissociation of this traumatic memory developed its own dynamic and attracted more and more of his whole life before the age of 8 which remains split off and the memories of that time were not accessible to consciousness anymore. He has photographs and letters from that time and has also asked among his relatives and learned that his father tried to kill himself several times before. In the long psychoanalytic treatment it wasn't possible to dissolve this extended amnesia of his childhood, only small memories were retrieved.

In most cases, however, this dissociative encapsulation is not a complete isolation but rather a matter of *degree* in the limitations it places on possible connections between thoughts. Seen in terms of neurobiology, Siegel (2006) considers an unprocessed trauma to be an interrupted cortical consolidation process, whereby the memory of the traumatic events cannot be transferred into permanent, explicit memory. Regarding these problems of processing of traumatic memories, the area of hippocampus plays a major role in integrating cortical functioning and in the mediation of the storage of memories in the cortical system. Many neuroscientific studies have demonstrated smaller hippocampal volumes in PTSD. But today—as Yehuda and LeDoux (2007) have shown—prospective longitudinal studies have failed to show change in hippocampal volume over time in persons followed in the acute aftermath of trauma and longitudinally. Because of that reason, the smaller hippocampal volume is seen by some investigators as representing a pre-existing marker of vulnerability to PTSD. For these persons it is more difficult to contextualize and reinterpret the experience of trauma in a way that can facilitate recovery. Other studies showed that in PTSD there is a decreased activation of Broca's area in the left hemisphere and increased activation in a number of right hemisphere regions. These findings suggest that, in PTSD subjects, trauma-related material is processed less in the language domain and more in the limbic structures involved in the affective representation of the memory (McFarlane et al., 2002).

Psychoanalysis conceptualized this restricted contextualization and integration of traumatic memories in a different way. Traumatic memories unfold their own dynamics. They can irrupt suddenly into consciousness when this encapsulated self-state is activated. However, and this is important, these intrusions or flashbacks are not photographically accurate replicas of the traumatic experiences. Often they are mixtures of real memory images with visualized anxieties, in which the worst fears can express themselves (Schacter, 1996). But it is true that the isolated encapsulated traumatic material cannot be brought into a free exchange with other parts of the associative network of the mind. Depending on the severity of the trauma, this exchange is obstructed, yet not completely excluded from the associative stream of psychic material, or from any transformation of the material.

What we discover again and again in therapeutic work with traumatized persons are certain typical psychic transformations in traumatic memories.

1. The traumatic experience confronts the ego with a "fait accompli" (Furst, 1978). The ego's reactions are too late in coming. They do not come in response to an impending danger, but only after the event, and once the ego has been passively subjected to the shock of trauma. The collapse of the self in the traumatic situation can cause long pre-existing, threatening, and repressed fantasies to break into consciousness. Internal archaic convictions can then present themselves as having become true, just as central, frightening images can also become almost insolubly fused with the experience of the traumatic situation.
2. The paralysed psychic activity of the traumatized self freezes the mental sense of time, producing an internal, temporal standstill. Posttraumatic states are often described as the kind of sensation that a part of the self has been left behind, more or less remaining the same (i.e. as when it was so left behind) because it can no longer be exposed to life. It is also described in terms of "standing aside" or as a "darkened existence". Others simply say that their inner clock stopped at the moment of traumatization.
3. Another type of transformation can occur after the traumatic event. This is because the trauma suffered tends to be revived and to repeat itself in flashbacks,

in nightmares, and through symptoms. The repetition has the character of something intrusive and not comprehended, but at the same time, it is also the ego's attempt to master the incomprehensible. The traumatized person attempts to tame and attenuate the pure trauma, in that he seeks to integrate it into a comprehensible causal processing system. One typical form of subsequent processing following the traumatic experience prompts some victims of trauma to attempt escaping from this ensuing sense of passivity—of being completely at another's mercy—by blaming themselves for what happened in order to create the semblance of activity induced by themselves. This consequently gives rise to guilt feelings, split-off convictions, and screen memories.

These are but a few examples which I mention here in order to illustrate what is meant by the psychic transformation of traumatic memories. If we accept this process as a fact, then, in therapy, it will not suffice to simply make the encapsulated, dissociated memory of the trauma accessible again and to then integrate it into memory. The situation is rather more complex, and I would now like to describe the main issues in this regard.

Some Problems in the Psychoanalytic Treatment of Traumatized Patients

Reconstruction and Historicization of the Trauma Discovering the reality of the trauma and its associated affects—namely, its historicization, however fragmentary or approximate—is the first step or prerequisite for elucidating and comprehending its secondary revision and transformation by unconscious phantasies and meanings which, for example, are filled by feelings of guilt and punitive impulses. Fantasy and traumatic reality are thereby disentangled, and the ego acquires an alleviating context of understanding. Historicization also involves recognizing the traumatic fact and understanding the individual experience together with the emerging long-term consequences. When such a reconstructive interpretation succeeds, patients often speak of astonishing improvements in their condition. The sensation of psychic integration they report indicates that self-organization is at work restructuring itself. In addition, the previously encapsulated traumatic part can now become more associatively interconnected. Similarly, the past can be more clearly distinguished from the present. This does not primarily involve a cognitive differentiation, however, but an altered affective regulation.

By way of example, we would like to outline a central reconstructive intervention in the treatment of Mrs. A (Bohleber, 2010). As a 5-year-old child, she was hospitalized and diagnosed with diabetes, type I. During this hospitalization she developed dissociative states. Prior to an upcoming laser treatment of her retina, the patient experienced panic attacks and began to dissociate again—a typical response whenever she had to visit an ophthalmologist. During the session, she described, for the first time, the details of the traumatic events surrounding the operation on her crossing eye at the age of 3 1/2. After the operation, she was tied down because she had attempted to tear off the bandage and get out of bed. She still remembered how she had hovered up to the ceiling and looked down upon herself. She was not in her body with her feelings. My spontaneous remark with respect to this peritraumatic dissociation was "That was when you left your body and when the break within you occurred". She later recalled that it had felt as if a shock or a charge of adrenaline had shot through her the moment I made the remark. The reconstruction of this trauma, which had now become possible, caused an affective restructuring and a stronger mental integration. Her internal agitation and chronic hyperarousal began to disappear. She no longer had to exert such strong control over herself. The dissociative inner splitting into different persons disappeared, and she now felt more or less like one person. She noted that a split had been eliminated deep within her. Moreover, she was suddenly able to see things in sharper focus. The imminent laser operation then transpired without any major intrusion of anxiety, and the same held for all subsequent visits to the doctor. It was as if a clamp had been loosened, she said. She no longer felt all bound up with anxiety as had previously been the case.

However, a reconstructive interpretation of the traumatic reality remains insufficient without the interpretation of the secondary transformation of meaning. One must recognize what has been suffered, to articulate screen memories and split-off convictions and to understand and interpret these in connection with the traumatic events. This is not to say, however, that all aspects of experience can be verbalized. Dissociated contents are organized at various levels of psychic representation. Further, a number of gaps must be bridged by constructions, for example, based on somatic symptoms, repetitive dreams, or external hints from others. In a reconstructive, that is, verbal formulation of the traumatic event that had overwhelmed the patient, the self-state dissociated through the trauma can be reconnected to non-dissociated mental material. The narrative emerging from this reconstruction both articulates and furthers an ongoing process of mental integration.

One central aspect of the interpretation and narration of traumatic experience is that it be tied to an awareness that something *real* has, in fact, occurred—no matter how fragmentary its reconstruction might have been. This knowledge can provide patients with a sense of truth and security which they can then use for understanding their traumatic transformations of the self, object relationships, and affects, instead of simply processing them in terms of guilt. What is at issue here is the reconstruction of the historical truth of the traumatic experience. Hence, merely constructing a meaningful narrative for integrating the dissociated mental material misses the mark.

The Irreparable Break of Basic Trust and the Need to Control Relationships Psychoanalysts often underestimate consequences of traumatization. I would like to emphasize here just one such consequence. Traumas generate an irreversible break in the trust in a predictable and secure environment. The break no longer heals. We cannot treat a traumatized person in the same way one does a neurotic patient with whom it may be sufficient to actualize conflict scenarios and structures as well as their defences in transference and to work them through. In the case of traumatized persons, by contrast, the traumatic intrusion of the external world causing the inner catastrophe creates an entirely different situation. The core traumatic experience is the destruction of the sense of basic trust or, as described by Krystal (1988): "having experienced its own mortality and helplessness, no living creature is quite the same again. The reconstruction of one's feeling of security, or even faith, is never again complete. It is as if the encounter had provided a black background upon which the rest of one's life will be painted" (p. 158). Naturally, the severity of the trauma is also relevant here. But neither do lighter forms of traumatization remediate the problem—the feeling of being abandoned by the protecting powers of the parents or that fate is overwhelming. Many of our patients who have endured massive traumatization in early childhood expressed a feeling that they feel like someone who has fallen out of the world. Or they articulate a childlike feeling of being absolutely lost in the world. As a means of defence, one patient hyperactively sought to prove that he has a place in the world and is not insignificant. The trauma has to do with an existential, deeply anchored sense of the meaningfulness of life which has been destroyed. Here, the meaning itself is put into question. We remain blind to these aspects of a destroyed sense of basic trust if we only interpret it from the perspective of the defences so as to once again restore it.

Restoring the Paralysed Agency of the Traumatized Self All analysts who work with traumatized patients are familiar with the problem of how memories of the trauma, as triggered by specific stimuli, break into consciousness and paralyse the ego. Here, Freud (1939) talks of repetition compulsion by which he meant an "attempt at cure" (p. 77). The ego attempts to attribute meaning to the occurrence, to incorporate it into a comprehensible causal system of action so as to thereby regain its ability to act and inner activity. As we have gathered from trauma research (Shalev, 1996), repetition compulsion—the longer these intrusions appear—increasingly loses its healing function. The intrusions chronify themselves and are experienced as a pure sense of being overwhelmed to which the ego is passively subject. In this respect, intrusions represent something of a double-edged sword: while they can advance mental integration and the discovery of meaning, they also threaten with disruption and the sense of being overwhelmed. In the latter case, recurring intrusions can have a re-traumatizing effect, once again rendering the individual passive and leaving him helplessly at the mercy of the event. The ego loses its sense of agency; it feels numbed, petrified, or frozen. As part of the intrusion, an altered state of consciousness begins to set in. Some refer to this as a "not-me self-state". In many cases, this weakness of the ego is yet further enhanced through attacks by the super-ego, which apportions blame to the ego for the renewed traumatic intrusion. In such situations, often the only choice a weakened ego has is a phobic attitude by means of which the traumatized individual attempts to interrupt and avoid all associative connections to the core traumatic experience.

How a traumatically weakened and numbed ego can regain its agency represents a complex issue in treatment. It is of central importance because the regaining of agency can change the helplessness repeatedly actualized by recurrent intrusions.

Based on his clinical experience, Krystal (1988) has ascertained that any type of activity during the traumatic situation reduces the severity of the aftereffects (p. 232). We consider the regaining of the ego's agency to be one of the central factors of a therapeutic change in the treatment of traumatized patients.

An increase of agency can be the result of the therapeutic work, which very generally brings with it a strengthening of the ego. Here, reconstructive interpretations occupy a special function. They are an aid to dissolving the false connections the patient makes in explaining the trauma. This relieves the ego from charges of guilt for the occurrence and can bring with it a sense of self-expansion. The ego is no longer completely, passively subject to repetition compulsion along with its intrusions but achieves a sense of distance. It understands what happens to him in a new way. In this manner, the ego regains a certain degree of activity and is no longer passively exposed to the whole issue. As a rule, however, achieving such a change cannot result from a single reconstructive interpretation. Each recurrent intrusion requires renewed interpretation of the traumatic experience and the suffering entailed by the loss of one's own agency.

References

Allen, J. (2013). *Mentalizing in the development and treatment of attachment trauma*. London: Karnac.

Balint, M. (1969). Trauma and object relationship. *The International Journal of Psycho-Analysis, 50*, 429–436.

Bohleber, W. (2010). *Destructiveness, intersubjectivity, and trauma. The identity crisis of modern psychoanalysis*. London: Karnac.

Cohen, J. (1985). Trauma and repression. *Psychoanalytic Inquiry, 5*, 163–189.

Cooper, A. (1986). Toward a limited definition of psychic trauma. In A. Rothstein (Ed.), *The reconstruction of trauma. Its significance in clinical work* (pp. 41–56). Madison, CT: International Universities Press.

Freud, S. (1920). Beyond the pleasure principle. *Standard Edition, 18*, 7–64.

Freud, S. (1926). Inhibitions, symptoms and anxiety. *Standard Edition, 20*, 77–174.

Freud, S. (1939). Moses and monotheism. *Standard Edition, 23*, 7–137.

Furst, S. (1978). The stimulus barrier and the pathogenicity of trauma. *International Journal of Psycho-Analysis, 59*, 345–352.

Kinston, W., & Cohen, J. (1986). Primal repression: Clinical and theoretical aspects. *International Journal of Psycho-Analysis, 67*, 337–355.

Kirshner, L. A. (1994). Trauma, the good object and the symbolic: A theoretical integration. *International Journal of Psycho-Analysis, 75*, 235–242.

Krystal, H. (1988). *Integration and self-healing. Affect, trauma, alexithymia*. Hillsdale: Analytic Press.

Laplanche, J. (1976). *Life and death in psychoanalysis*. Baltimore, MD: John Hopkins University Press.

Laub, D., & Podell, D. (1995). Art and trauma. *International Journal of Psycho-Analysis, 76*, 991–1005.

McFarlane, A. C., Yehuda, R., & Clark, C. R. (2002). Biologic models of traumatic memories and post-traumatic stress disorder: The role of neural networks. *Psychiatric Clinics of North America, 25*, 253–270.

Sandler, J., Dreher, A. U., & Drews, S. (1991). An approach to conceptual research in psychoanalysis illustrated by a consideration of psychic trauma. *International Review of Psycho-Analysis, 18*, 133–142.

Schacter, D. (1996). *Searching for memory. The brain, the mind, and the past*. New York: Basic Books.

Shalev, A. Y. (1996). Stress versus traumatic stress. From acute homeostatic reactions to chronic psychopathology. In B. van der Kolk, A. Mc Farlane, & L. Weisaeth (Eds.), *Traumatic stress. The effects of overwhelming experience on mind, body and society* (pp. 77–101). New York, NY: Guilford Press.

Steele, B. F. (1994). Psychoanalysis and the maltreatment of children. *Journal of the American Psychoanalytic Association, 42*, 1001–1025.

Siegel, D. (2006). Entwicklungspsychologische, interpersonelle und neurobiologische Dimensionen des Gedächtnisses. Ein Überblick. In H. Welzer, & H. Markowitsch (Hg.), Warum Menschen sich erinnern können. Fortschritte in der interdisziplinären Gedächtnisforschung (pp. 19–49). Stuttgart: Klett-Cotta.

Yehuda, R., & LeDoux, J. (2007). Response variation following trauma: A translational neuroscience approach to understanding PTSD. *Neuron, 56*, 19–32.

Chapter 7
Embodiment: A New Key to the Unconscious?

Marianne Leuzinger-Bohleber

Introduction

The short- and long-term consequence of severe traumatizations and their transmission to the next generation is a topic which has been in the focus of clinical and extraclinical research of the Sigmund Freud Institute for years. To mention just one example: one of the unexpected results of the LAC depression study[1] has been that more than 80% of the chronic depressed patients of our study had undergone severe, cumulative traumatizations during their childhood. Various forms of traumatizations also have been frequently observed in the many different projects on early prevention as well as in the current projects with refugees in the outdoor service for refugees and the pilot project "STEP BY STEP" supporting refugees in the first reception institution "Michaelisdorf" in Darmstadt. In all these projects, we can observe the complex interconnections and interactions of inner and outside factors determinating the consequences of traumatizations in the individuals as well as in the German society (see, e.g. Leuzinger-Bohleber, 2014a).

Man-made disasters destroy the lives of the traumatized individuals and cast their shadows onto the second and third generation. They also determine the atmosphere of the traumatized societies in complex, hidden and painful ways. Only artists, e.g. Boualem Sansal (2011), in his novel *The Village of the German*, are capable to communicate these complex unconscious interconnections in their narratives in

[1] LAC study (**La**ngzeitbehandlungen **c**hronisch Depressiver): a randomized controlled study comparing the outcomes of long-term psychoanalytical and cognitive behavioural psychotherapies with chronic depressed patients (see www. Sigmund-freud-institut.de)

This paper will be published in another version in German in a book on trauma, edited by Heinz Weiss.

M. Leuzinger-Bohleber (✉)
Sigmund Freud Institut, Frankfurt am Main, Germany
e-mail: Leuzinger-Bohleber@sigmund-freud-institut.de

C. Charis, G. Panayiotou (eds.), *Somatoform and Other Psychosomatic Disorders*,
https://doi.org/10.1007/978-3-319-89360-0_7

a precise and "true" way. Hans Schiller, who was highly involved in the development of cyclone B and in other crimes of the SS during the Holocaust, went underground in the small village in Deb in Algeria. He succeeds to become a highly recognized leader, Scheich Hassan. He sends his two adolescent sons to Paris. The older son Rachel becomes an internationally successful businessman. The younger one, Malrich, a jobless adolescent, lives in the Banlieus and experiences the Islamistic radicalization due to the Mafia structures of the fundamentalistic Islamists in his "city", a part of the Banlieus. Islamistic terrorists kill both parents in a very brutal way. The older son discovers some secret documents of the father concerning his involvements in the Nazi regime. He begins to investigate the past of his father and follows his traces through Europe: from Frankfurt, Hamburg, Uelzen, Auschwitz, via Turkey, Libya to Cairo. Finally he commits suicide in order to atone from the sins of his father by gas in his garage in Paris.

In the centre of the novel, testifying the transgenerational guilt is the famous poem by Primo Levy:

IS THIS A MAN

In your warm houses,
Who return at evening to find
Hot food and friendly faces:

Consider whether this is a man,
Who labours in the mud
Who knows no peace
Who fights for a crust of bread
Who dies at a yes or a no.
Consider whether this is a woman,
Without hair or name
With no more strength to remember
Eyes empty and womb cold
As a frog in winter.

Consider that this has been:
I commend these words to you.
Engrave them on your hearts
When you are in your house, when you walk on your way,
When you go to bed, when you rise.
Repeat them to your children.
Or may your house crumble,
Disease render you powerless,
Your offspring avert their faces from you.
(Primo Levy)

Rachel adds the following paragraph:

The children do not know;
They live, they play, they love.
And when what has happened reaches them;
The dramas inherited from the parents
They are confronted with foreign questions,
of icy silence,
of nameless shadows.

My house has broken down and the pain
presses me down;
And I do not know why.
My father has not told me anything.

Boualem Sansal: The Village of the German, p. 69/70 (Merlin Verlag)

Indeed, as we know from numerous psychoanalytical studies, the burden of denied, split-off traumatic experiences, connected with man-made disasters, may cause that the houses of children in the second generation of persecutors and bystanders are breaking down.

This has been the case with Mrs. M. as I will discuss in this paper.

In order to discuss how the unrepresented, transgenerational traces of trauma have been discovered in the transference, I will refer to the concept of embodiment, a concept which is not yet known very well in psychoanalysis. In a second step, I will use this concept for illustrating my clinical experiences that it proves to be indispensable for a process of transformation in psychoanalysis to approach the "historical truth" of trauma in the transference.

My clinical experiences are based, e.g. on a third analysis with a patient who had suffered from a serious poliomyelitis during her fifth year of life. She was grateful for her two former long psychoanalyses because they had proven to be very helpful for her. However, one of the most painful symptoms, her "psychotic breakdowns", had not changed and thus had been such a burden that her husband planned to get divorced. In our psychoanalyses we found out that her "psychotic breakdowns" had nothing to do with a psychotic state of the mind but were determined by "embodied memories" of the totally unexpected, extremely painful onset of her polio. Only after Mrs. M. had understood these memories in detail and was able to work them through in transference she was able to "overcome this madness". "How much pain and despair would have been saved to myself, my husband and my children if I – and my analysts – would have had the courage to look at all this much earlier..." she said (Leuzinger-Bohleber, 2008).

Therefore I hope to initiate a discussion in this issue.

"Embodied" Countertransference Reactions: Keys to the Nonrepresented Trauma?

Freud wrote in 1914 in *Remembering, Repeating and Working-through*:

> "Above all, the patient will *begin* his treatment with a repetition of this kind... What interests us most of all is naturally the relation of this compulsion to repeat to the transference and to resistance... The greater the resistance, the more extensively will acting out (repetition) replace remembering." (Freud, 1914, p. 150)

Generations of psychoanalysts since Freud have concerned themselves with the way in which repetition in transference can be rendered a healing process of remembering. This primarily involves symbolically represented and repressed memories or relationship patterns. However, theory and clinical psychoanalysis has focused for quite some time on psychic material present in the analytical relationship in other ways. Levine, Reed, and Scarfone entitled their anthology *Unrepresented States and the Construction of Meaning* (2013, in honour of André Green) and focus on the question of the search for meaning in the unrepresented from a contemporary perspective. With his broadly received concept of "dead mother", Green (2007) described the early identification with an absent mother leading to a withdrawal cathexis and thus to a disappearance of the inner representation which, in the transference relationship, can be perceived by the analyst as an empty, negative hallucination of the object, "a representation of the absence of representation" (Green, 1999, p. 196, quoted from Reed, 2013, p. 39). Reed (2013, p. 29ff.) points out that this negative hallucination of the object leads to an emptiness rather than a representation of the lost object—an empty mirror—which, with these patients, is always there but which is frequently observed in the analysand's extreme reactions to separation from the analyst.

Green is concerned with the process of de-objectification, namely, the obliteration of representation. Other psychoanalysts, by contrast, focused on the psychic material of patients, which had only insufficiently, if at all, gone through the processes of symbolization. Dominique Scarfone (2013) presented a conceptual integration of different forms of psychic representation and their various psychoanalytic conceptualizations. He compared Pierce's sign theory to Freud's conception of primary and secondary processes; Lacan's theory of the real, the imaginary and the symbolic; Wilfred Bion's beta- and alpha elements; Jean Laplanche's infantile sexual theories and their decoding in analytic discourse; and Pierra Aulangier's concept of the primary, such as "primary violence", which entered the stage ("mis-en-scène") and that could ultimately open up the discourse on secondary processes: a brilliant example of contemporary concept research.

Here, I pursue another path by drawing on several studies in the field of basic research, more specifically, embodied cognitive science and the cognitive neurosciences, so as to show that these disciplines offer first explanations for this clinically important phenomenon, such as the analyst's spontaneous inspiration, which represents an initial central step to understanding hitherto unrepresented psychic material and which is capable of making psychoanalytic processing accessible. Hence, this should provide new perspectives on familiar concepts, such as "scenic understanding" (Argelander, Lorenzer), "hearing with the third ear" (Reik), "cracking up" (Bollas) or the "now moments" by the Boston Change Process Study Group. Furthermore, aspects of current discourse on intersubjective psychoanalysis and on enactment are touched on, as well as further understanding of countertransference around the bodily sensations of the analyst (cf. also Scharff, 2010). Reference to works on musicality, dynamically emotional syntax and performance of the analytic relationship is plausible (cf., among others, Buchholz & Gödde, 2013; Dantlgraber, 2008; Leikert, 2013).

In the following, I draw on a clinical example from a first interview as starting point so as to show how these more recent interdisciplinary conceptualizations of recollection and memory prove fruitful.

Enactment and Countertransference Reactions in an Assessment Interview: A Clinical Example

Hardly had I opened the door before Ms. M. stormed in across the threshold. She clasped my hand feverishly, pressing it between hers in a peculiar and sexually stimulating manner while stepping up very close to me, thus encroaching on my normal sense of distance: "Well, hi there …I'm so glad to have the opportunity of speaking with you…" I immediately noted a forceful, negatively emotional reaction combined with an aversive physical response: what an overwhelming woman! I find this too much. "She's really coming too close for comfort… Why did I propose an appointment? Will I ever be able to send her away? Evidently, she is very needy…"

After enquiring about the location of the toilet, she made her way in leaving the door wide open, which I found thoroughly strange.

Only once having seated herself in the chair opposite me did I first notice her pretty, girlish face as it clearly endeavoured to maintain a permanent smile, and her beautiful female form, which she apparently sought to conceal beneath loose-fitting jeans and a frayed, plain pullover. Though in her mid-forties, her mannerisms are rather characteristic of a 60 year-old. She had previously informed me over the telephone that her family doctor had recommended she seek out psychotherapeutic help. She is ill and suffering from burn-out syndrome with attendant heavy depression: "I can't go on any longer – I haven't been able to sleep at night for weeks, can barely eat, am unable to work – and I am scarcely able to tolerate the teenagers who I supervise in my work as social worker. I repeatedly break down in tears in front of them".

Characteristic for her in the interview situation is that she begins by enquiring into *my* frame of mind—whether it is alright for her to come at this late hour in the evening, whether I am too tired to listen to her after such a tiring day at work, etc. Only after having explicitly confirmed that I am not exhausted but would like to learn more about her is she then able to begin her narrative. "I have no idea what happened to me – I have always functioned very well. Nothing works now…" When enquiring about the context of her "collapse" she explained that her boyfriend, with whom she has been in a relationship over some years, had just announced his plans to move to another city. And further, that the daily confrontations between her 14 year-old daughter and her mother are increasing. "But these things are just trifling matters – my boyfriend does not really mean that much to me anyway, and quarrels with an adolescent are anyway more than normal. I have no idea why I have now fallen into such a deep hole… things no longer seem to make any sense. I'm now completely out of energy…"

In the following section, I would like to start out from this initial scene before moving on to show how Ms. M.'s bizarre physical behaviour contains the key to early traumatic experiences, embodied memories and the significance of which we were only able to understand together in transference, thanks to the very detailed observations during the third year of psychoanalysis:

In the following theoretical part of my paper, I would like to show that the concept of "embodiment" has proven helpful for recognizing indicators for earlier traumatization in the transference and, as outlined above, combine these with images, metaphors and language.

Finding the Body in the Mind: An Old Problem and a Revolutionary Concept

What are "embodied memories"?

Marcel Proust has described the fundamental ideas of embodiment and decides before the embodied revolution:

> Many years had elapsed during which nothing of Combray, save what was comprised in the theatre and the drama of my going to be there, had any existence for me, when one day in winter, as I came home, my mother, seeing that I was cold, offered me some tea, a thing I did not ordinarily take. I declined at first and, then, for no particular reason, change my mind. She sent out for one of those short, plump little cakes called "petites madeleines", which look as though they had been moulded in the fluted scallop of a pilgrim's shell. And soon, mechanically, weary after a dull day with the prospect of a depressing morrow, I raised to my lips a spoonful of the tea in which I had soaked a morsel of the cake. No sooner had the warm liquid, and the crumbs with it, touched my plate than a shudder ran through my whole body, and I stopped, intent upon the extraordinary changes that were to take place. An exquisite pleasure had invaded my sense, but individual, detached, with no suggestion of its origin. And at once the vicissitudes of life had become indifferent to me, its disasters innocuous, its brevity illusory—this new sensation having had on me the effect which love has of filling me with a precious essence, or rather this essence was not in me, it was myself. I had ceased nor to feel mediocre, accidental, mortal. Whence would it have come to me, this all-powerful joy? I was conscious that it was connected with the taste of tea and cake, but that it infinitely transcended those savours, could not, indeed, be of the same nature as theirs. Whence did it come? What did it signify? How could I seize upon and define it? […] I drink a second mouthful, in which I find nothing more than in the first, a third, which gives me rather less than the second. It is time to stop; the potion is losing is magic. It is plain that the object of my quest, the truth, lies not in the cup but in myself. The tea has called up in me, but does not itself understand, and can only repeat indefinitely with a gradual loss of strength, the same testimony; which I, too, cannot interpret, though I hope at least to be able to call upon the tea for it again and to find it there presently, intact and at my disposal, for my final enlightenment. I put down my cup and examine my own mind. It is for it to discover the truth. But how? What an abyss of uncertainty whenever the mind feels that some part of it has strayed beyond its own borders; when it the seeker, is at once the dark region through which it must go seeking, where all its equipment will avail it nothing. Seek? More than that: create. "It is the face with something which does not so far exist, to which it alone can give reality and substance, which it alone can bring into the light of day. **[...]** *And suddenly the memory returns. The taste was that of the little crumb of madeleine which on Sunday mornings at Combray (because on those mornings I did not go out before church-time), when I went to say good day to her in her bedroom, my aunt Léonie used to give me, dipping it first in her own cup of real or of lime-flower tea.*" (Marcel Proust, Remembrance of Things Past, [transl. C.K. Scott Moncrieff] 1922, p. 61ff.; accentuation by the author.)

With respect to the impressiveness of its force and precision, Marcel Proust's description of "embodied memories" remains unsurpassed: the struggle in deciphering unexpected and, thus, initially incomprehensible bodily sensations in a specific, present situation of interaction: in the body—by way of analogous sensomotoric coordination—at lightning speed and initially unconscious memories of an earlier situation are constructed with analogous bodily sensations: "No sooner had the warm liquid, and the crumbs with it, touched my pallet than a shudder ran through my whole body, and I stopped, intent upon the extraordinary changes that were to take place. An exquisite pleasure had invaded my sense, but individual, detached, with no suggestion of its origin. [...]" The memory is there immediately, but, as Proust indicates, it must first be present in images and language "and then, at once, the memory was there" (Proust, 1978, p. 61ff.).

In spite of Marcel Proust and other poets who described memories with comparable degrees of lucidity, psychoanalysis would still need till the close of the twentieth century before finally conceptualizing these relevant processes as embodied memories. In the psychoanalytic model of representation and in the computer metaphor derived from "classic cognitive science", memory and recollection were for a long time understood as processes whereby (statically) retained knowledge was transformed from long-term memory to short-time memory and called up into a current problem-solving situation. We still find comparable thinking in some textbooks in clinical psychology. Aristotle's famous example comparing memory to a wax tablet into which experiences etch themselves appears to live on. This (erroneous) idea of memory has also entered popular language usage: "we call up saved knowledge" or "we search for forgotten names in memory" (much like the search for an object in a wardrobe).

Researchers of the embodied cognitive science developed alternative and more suitable conceptualizations of memory and human problem-solving by taking up knowledge and inspirations from the so-called life sciences, biology, genetics, developmental research and the modern neurosciences.

Embodiment: A New Perspective from Basic Sciences on the "Mind-Body Problem"

Memory as a function of the whole organism The distinction between the new, biologically inspired and "classical" models of memory becomes very clear in a diagram published by Gerald Edelman in 1992 (cf. also Leuzinger-Bohleber & Pfeifer, 1998, S. 897ff.). In the case of traditional models of memory—analogous to information processing in computers—one assumes a precise storage of knowledge, which is static and unchanging, and thus making transference to new problem-solving possible.

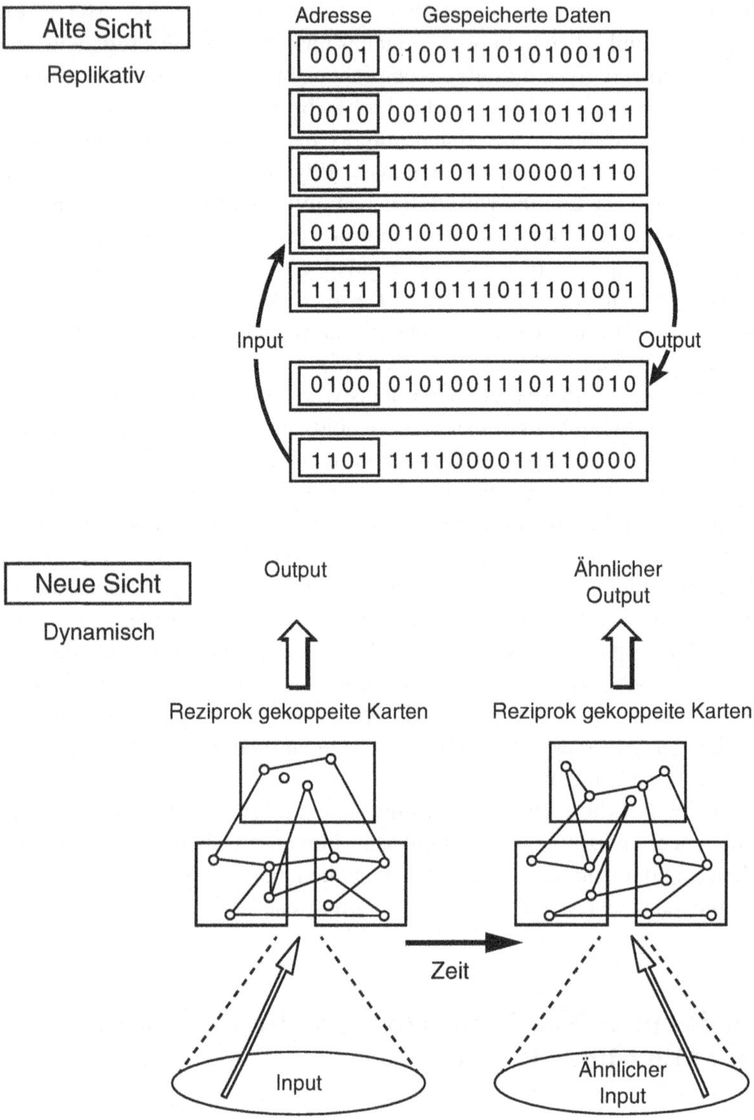

Illustration 3 A comparison of "Classic" and "Embodied" memories according to Gerald Edelman

By contrast, "knowledge storing" in the dynamic models of embodied cognitive science, though less exact, precisely through this quality enables optimum generalization and adaptation to a new situation. In the process, so-called neuronal maps are produced through the functional circulation of the organism's constant interaction with its environment.

> "These consist of several 10000s of neurons, which work functionally in one direction. Thus, each system of perception has, e.g. the visual apparatus, the sensuous surface of the skin, etc. and a multiplicity of maps which are stimulated by qualitatively different impressions: colour, touch, direction, warmth, etc. These maps are connected to one another by parallel and reciprocal fibres, which guarantee the renewed and repeated entry, flow and exchange of signals. If one map is selected by way of the stimulation of groups of neurons, then a stimulation of the maps to which it is connected simultaneously results. Due to the reciprocal connections ('reentry'), the nerve impulses are returned, whereby the reinforcement or attenuation of synapsis in the neuronal groups occurs in the synapses of each map: the connections of the maps themselves undergo modification. Through this, new selective qualities emerge, in other words, 'automatic' re-categorizations of current stimuli from different sense channels" (Leuzinger-Bohleber & Pfeifer, 1998, p. 898f.).

Through such "sensomotoric coordination", which is connected with permanent re-categorizations, the organism ensures a sustained ability to orient itself in the environment, namely, to connect current experience with previous experience whereby, due to the new situation, previous re-categorizations are adapted by way of the retained stimuli.

Hence, due to the above outlined radical conceptual rethinking in embodied cognitive science, memory is understood as a function of the total organism and the product of complex, invariably "embodied", dynamic re-categorizing and interactive processes (cf. among others, Leuzinger-Bohleber & Pfeifer, 2013a).

Gerald Edelman's (1987) book *Neural Darwinism*, António Damásio's (1994) *Descartes' Error*, Lakoff and Johnson's (1999) *Philosophy in the Flesh. The Embodied Mind and Its Challenge to Western Thought* and Rolf Pfeifer and Josh Bongard's (2007) *How the body shapes the way we think* are probably the most well-known examples which show that the Cartesian dualism between the mind and body must be revised in favour of a radically new perception of an "embodiment" of the psyche in the body.

> "There exists no Kantian radically autonomous person, with absolute freedom and a transcendent reason, that correctly dictates what is and isn't moral. Reason, arising from the body, doesn't transcend the body. What universal aspects of reason there are arise from communalities of our bodies and brain and the environments we inhabit. The existence of these universals does not imply that reason transcends the body. Moreover, since conceptual systems vary significantly, reason is not entirely universal. [...] Since reason is shaped by the body, it is not radically free, because the possible human conceptual systems and the possible forms of reason are limited." (Lakoff & Johnson, 1999, p. 5)

Interaction with the Environment Changes the Organism: A New View to the Nature-Nurture Problem

As indicated in the above, from the viewpoint of embodied cognitive science, psychic processes are constituted only through the subject's adaptive, re-categorizing interaction with the environment, in which memory is actively constructed. One further postulate is that the organism finds itself in ongoing transformation. I would also like to give an example of this from epigenetics, a highly interesting research field for psychoanalysis, which, thanks to recent technical advances in molecular genetics, has brought forth a wealth of interesting studies. Furthermore, proven genetic vulnerabilities do not represent the victim's destiny but first make their appearance where previous, weighty environmental or relationship experiences play a role. Thus, those studies, among others, by Caspi et al. (2003) and Hauser (2008) that were capable of verifying genetic vulnerability by way of the so-called moderated 5—HHT allele of the serotonin transporter gene were given considerable attention. This proved that people with this genotype only then suffer from depression when subjected to ongoing weighty life circumstances or earlier traumas, such as child abuse. Kaufman et al. (2006) and Goldberg (2009) were also able to show that a responsive, empathetic motherly behaviour in the first months of life represents a protective factor, whereby the risk of becoming ill from depression is also reduced in cases of proven vulnerability (cf. also Suomi, 2011).

These studies on epigenetics confirm the basic psychoanalytic thesis of an ongoing and determining interaction between genetics and environment, between biology and social experience, especially in early and earliest childhood. The developmental perspectives of embodied cognitive science differentiate these general theses, among others, by empirically showing that the organism's interaction with the environment, as one has imagined for considerable time, is not regulated exclusively by a "genetic programme" but by an ongoing dynamic and "embodied" interaction between subject and environment, namely, from the outset.

To summarize just some of the theses concerning embodiment and trauma:

1. Learning, problem-solving and memory are thus no longer functions of a "saving in the brain" but invariably the product of complex, self-regulated, sensomotoric coordination.
2. Psychic processes, such as "unconscious memories" or affects and fantasies evoked in a certain situation, are "constructed" between subject and environment in the here and now of a current interaction: consequently, thinking, feeling and action thus arise only interactively; the subject cannot learn in an insular quasi-autistic capsule and further develop itself: it requires interaction with the environment.
3. The concept of "embodiment" is thus radically "historical", as psychic processes in the present always take place as the product of sensomotoric coordinations analogous to those in the subject's idiosyncratic past: the past inevitably impacts the present and future, that is, for the most part, unconsciously.
4. In that each new experience further develops sensomotoric coordinations, earlier experiences are permanently rewritten. Hence, the "historic truth" can never be reconstructed "one to one" on the basis of specific behaviour in the present. Put more bluntly: this is the subjective part of all psychic experience. And yet, in the sensomotoric coordinations, past real experiences are retained "objectively" ("embodied") and can be measured, in principle, with the aid of neurobiological methods. For this reason, psychic experience such as memory always receives a "subjective" as well as an "objective" side (the social history of the individual

has a constitutional influence even on the hardware of the brain; researchers use the term "social brain").

If an individual experiences a trauma, the capability of continuous adaptation to new situations may completely break down or at least becomes very limited. Therefore the "inadequate, embodied" reactions in a current situation (e.g. in the transference) may offer some keys for the original traumatic situation.

Embodiment: A New Insight into Early Developmental Processes and "Early Parenting"

The following table in Gerald Edelman's book *Neural Darwinism* illustrates the above-mentioned central thesis of "embodied cognitive science", namely, that neuronal networks are in a permanent state of dynamic development. Environmental experiences in the uterus lead to a developmental selection as early as the embryonic stage and thus to the formation of the primary repertoires. Environmental influence, namely, of social relations, is increased in the first year of life: experience selection leads to the formation of secondary repertoires. All these processes correspond to the principles of a neuronal Darwinism: successful, used connections between the nerve cells are strengthened—those which are not used atrophy and wither away (for a more detailed discussion, cf. Leuzinger-Bohleber & Pfeifer, 1998, p. 897ff.).

What is important is the reciprocal coupling of maps based on sensomotoric coordinates. Embodiment, therefore, means that social experience finds sustained expression through sensomotoric coordinates and literally enters the hardware of the body and brain. Hence, leading neuroscientists refer to the "social brain". However, they must also always add that this "social brain" cannot be considered in isolation but as part of a "social body", a position which supports the "intersubjective turn in psychoanalysis" (cf. for further detail see also Gallese, 2009, 2013a, 2013b; Knox, 2009; Fuchs, Sattel, & Henningsen, 2010).

Thus, "embodied" means far more than simply "non-verbal" or based in the body: memory arises through a coupling of sensoric and motoric processes, which reciprocally influence one another without central regulation. This coupling is implemented biologically by way of neuronal maps embedded in the organisms' sensomotoric system. Thus, Clancey, for example, defines (1994) memory as the possibility of coordinating neurological processes and to thus categorize sensoric and motoric processes such as these occurred in comparable earlier situations.

This central thesis of embodied cognitive science was further supported by Makaken through the discovery of mirror neurons by Giacomo Rizzolatti and his

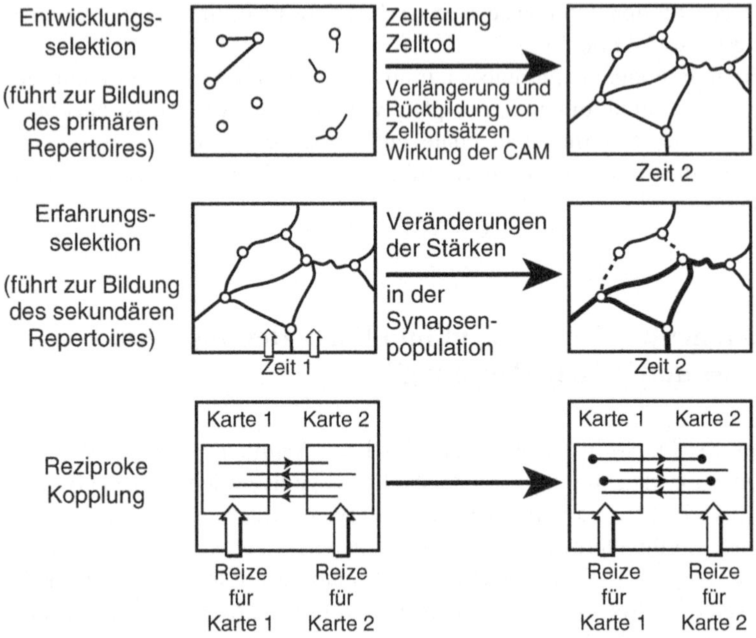

Fig. 3 Principles of neuronal Darwinism in the development of neuronal networks (on the definition of maps, cf. legend illustration 3)

colleagues (1992). Their findings have meanwhile been verified for human infants by way of numerous experiments. These studies increase awareness of the fact that the infant is influenced by way of earlier identification process with its first relationship persons (with the aid of mirror neurons) long prior to developing consciousness and language. These earliest identifications are reflected in the sensomotoric coordinations (maps etc.), which influence later interactions. Gallese (2013a, 2013b) also discussed the significance of mirror neurons for early embodied interaction processes in the intersubjective consideration of emotional, social and therapeutic exchange, among others, when he wrote:

> "The discovery of the actions responsible for the mirror neuron mechanism led to the hypothesis that the mirror neurons most probably constitute the mere tip of a huge, hitherto undiscovered iceberg, which is concealed in the sphere of emotional and physical sensibilities (Gallese, 2013a, 2013b; Goldman & Gallese, 2000). This hypothesis is also supported by empirical findings… Taken as a whole, these results suggest that one important aspect of intersubjectivity when observing the expression of important aspects of external emotions and sensations may be understood as re-utilisation of the same circuit which constitutes the foundation of our own emotional and sensory experiences … One supported the thesis that a common functional mechanism, namely, 'embodied simulation' (ES), is capable of coherently and neuro-biologically explaining the multiplicity of intersubjective phenomena". (Gallese, 2013b, p. 95ff.) (italics M.L.-B.)

The many studies that have meanwhile been carried out on the infant's processes of early, prelinguistic identification with primary attachment figures correspond to the psychoanalytic view that the early object relationships express themselves in the basic melody of the psyche. Now well known, the so-called Still Face Experiment (Tronick, 2003) provides impressive empirical evidence about the degree to which the infant's psychic sensitivities are dependent on a resonant, affective and consistent interaction with its mother. A mother is requested following a "customary" affective resonant game sequence with its 1-year-old baby to show no mimic reactions, a "still face". The baby reacts immediately and attempts with all means at its disposal to regain her "normal" behavioural interaction. When unable to achieve this, the infant reacts in a visibly irritated manner and turns away before beginning to cry bitterly.

Hence, there emerges a close connection between embodiment and early development: as "embodied memories" the early experiences of interaction determine subsequent development and the spontaneous (not cognitive) expectations and unconscious interpretations of new interaction situations. Psychoanalytic knowledge as to just how decisive and definitive are the first relationship experiences during the initial weeks and months over the long term—determined as these are by extreme vulnerability and enormous plasticity—are given fascinating empirical support by way of interdisciplinary research on "embodiment" and early parenthood. As is well known, Freud had already claimed that originally the ego was a bodily one.

To mention just one example: early interaction of depressive mothers with their infants has been well researched empirically and clinically (cf., among others, Stern, 2010/1985; Beebe & Lachmann, 2004; Feldman, 2012; Rutherford, Goldberg, Luvten, Bridgett, & Mayes, 2013). Due to its depression, sensitivity and emotional resonance for the infant's individual needs are severely restricted or even break down to a large extent. How infants of depressive mothers have no choice other than to identify with their "dead mothers" in order to establish a proximity to their primary objects is described impressively by Daniel Stern. One of the four possible coping strategies he outlines that strongly influence the emerging personality is the development of a "false self" (cf. also Leuzinger-Bohleber, 2012). As I will discuss in a moment, this has been the case with Mrs. M.

As all these studies show, the early, "embodied" experiences of interaction with primary objects are deposited in a formative manner. Because in these earliest interactions with the primary objects the sensomotor coordinations are built, these experiences intensively unconsciously determine later feelings, thoughts and actions. These unconscious sources of mental functioning can hardly be overestimated. To use a metaphor: in the earliest relationships, the "body of sound" of the psychic "Stradivari" is constructed, which is brought into music in later human interactions.

Naturally, this does not mean that only the earliest relationship experiences express themselves as "embodied memories", although these, as already indicated, determine the psychic basic melody, or—to use spatial terminology—the basic orientation of the sensomotoric coordinations taken up by further development.

Later experiences also enter into the body in the form of a continuous development process. Of decisive importance here are, above all, traumatic experiences which, due to their extreme, psychic non-processable quality, metaphorically speaking bring previous sensomotoric coordinations to the point of collapse at any age, thus affecting the same for psychic self-regulation, creativity and integrative problem-solving. To cite one of Edelman's metaphors: in later analogous relationship situations, unconscious memories of traumatic object relations trigger "storms" in the body and the brain, which render mature psychic functioning impossible and repeat the traumatic experience time and again (as in the case of Ms. M.).

A Deeper Understanding of Clinical Processes of Transformation in Psychoanalysis: The Decoding of the Unrepresented by Way of Embodied Memories in Transference or "How Do Thoughts of the Unrepresented Emerge"?

As mentioned in the introduction, the question as to how it is possible to not only sense that which remains unrepresented in the analytic situation, but to also articulate it in visualizations, images and language, and thereby transfer unconscious repetition in a transforming therapeutic memory process, has remained largely unclear in contemporary psychoanalytic literature. Here, as is well known, the analyst's associations, and spontaneous thoughts, provide a first key to understanding the meaning of that which, hitherto, has remained entirely misunderstood and which is then operative in the transference. In analytic literature, this spontaneous knowledge and these spontaneous insights and thoughts are frequently rewritten metaphorically as "turning points" in the treatment, the "meeting of the minds", the communication of unconscious to unconscious, the "now moments", etc. And yet, as far as I am aware, no plausible explanations have been given, to date, for the occurrence of these important thoughts. This is precisely what the knowledge of embodied cognitive science as summarized in this paper offers: as outlined in the above, categories form in the interaction between the subject and his environment (in "system environment interactions") and are always based on sensomotoric coordination, namely, are "automatic" and are not centrally regulated but self-regulative. The human brain and the human psyche find themselves in a perpetual process of re-categorizing experience: without spontaneously self-forming (unconscious) "categories of understanding", all orientation in a new situation is missing; the organism could not survive in the present and would not be able to orient itself in the present; there would be no adaptive reactions; no processes of problem-solving; no spontaneous memories that play out, which could be fruitful for the current situation; and no learning (cf. the above-mentioned experiment by Pfeifer and Bogart). The same holds for the analytic relationship.

As explained in the above, the mirror neuron system enables the analyst to identify with the analysand's current sensomotoric coordinations (the unconscious memory processes) while at the same time bringing this to bear in his own countertransference, namely, in his own body. Through this, analogous sensomotoric coordinations in current interaction are activated, as they are in the analysand. These processes bring forth categories—automatically, spontaneously and unconsciously—which, thanks to the processes of identification, are connected with the analysand's unconsciously running memory processes from earlier, important relationship experiences. In the case of traumatized patients, it is above all memories of psychically unbearable flooding experiences, of extreme powerlessness, and of doubt, pain, panic and the fear of death. Through the identification processes in his spontaneously self-forming categories, the analyst re-categorizes these reactions—as conditioned by traumatic experiences, namely, unconscious "understanding". However, the extreme qualities of the traumatic experiences also lead to spontaneous defence and initially hinder the process of becoming conscious. Consequently, at first contact, namely, at the first interview, he predominantly registers a combination of immediate sensomotorically categorized perceptions and his own defence processes, as illustrated by the example of Ms. M. "woman! I find this all too much. She's really getting under my skin … Why did I offer her an appointment? These (conscious) thoughts clearly contained both the perception of an overpowering quality of the patient's psychic reality as caused by a trauma as well as my own defence movements.

The first, unconscious perception of the specific traumatic experiences of the analysand did not involve a singular occurrence but rather a complex process that repeats itself continually. On the one hand, by way of the identification with the many variations of occurring sensomotoric coordinations, it requires a constantly repeating enactment in the transference so as to ultimately be able to re-categorize the traumatization suffered in one's own embodied countertransference. On the other hand, it is inevitable that the analyst processes his defence against a possible flooding through the patient's traumatic material (unconsciously) so as to become conscious of the unconsciously formed categories about the traumatizations suffered by the patient. As clinical-psychoanalytical experiences have shown in various ways—especially with severely traumatized patients—a direct revival of the traumatic experience in the transfer of both parties is only then possible if a supporting, retaining and containing analytical relationship has developed.

In the language of cognitive science: in the therapeutic interaction (new), sensomotoric coordinations develop, which build successively on carrying capacity, of being understood through a new, psychoanalytic object. As is well known, among the most sustained experiences of severe traumatizations is the complete breakdown of trust in a helping object. Connected to this are the unconscious convictions and fantasies to which the person affected attributes self-guilt for the traumatic experience. Thus, initially unconsciously, traumatic patients will continually repeat this "inner truth" in transference and only due to alternative forms of relationships begin to limit their validity. In other words, the sensomotoric coordinations, analogous to the traumatic experiences of relationships, cannot be deleted; they are repeated time and again in the analytic relationship—and yet alternative sensomotoric coordinations (namely, metaphorically speaking, alternative neuronal paths) connected with categories, such as "security", "reliability", "understanding" and "survival", can be successively built up. The "old" re-categorization processes based on traumatic relationship experiences run disconnected and parallel to the new re-categorization processes forming in the psychoanalytic relationship. Only once the "new" re-categorization has finally led to the more or less stable categories, such as "trust", "security", etc., do the two paths of sensomotoric coordinations (the maps) become connected to one another. Now the analyst is in a position to access the hitherto unconscious category "trauma" by way of an accurate, specific idea (e.g., sexual abuse) and thereby open up a first door for a psychoanalytic processing of the traumatization. I will briefly illustrate these complex processes by way of the clinical example:

Only in the third year of psychoanalysis did the meaning reveal itself in the above scenes in the first interview. The intrusive behaviour outlined in the above was repeated in several variations in the analytic treatment (e.g., Ms. M. repeatedly used our private WC, opened the doors to our private rooms, got into my car to turn off the light, etc.). One day before the analysis session to be described below, Ms. M.'s intrusive behaviour once again irritated me considerably. She appeared, unannounced, at my lectures in a public institution and seated herself in the first row. When listening to Ms. M. for 10 min in the subsequent session in silence while she explained to me that her uncle had told her shortly before his death how, on each occasion, she would impatiently wait for him in front of his studio, it suddenly occurred to me that this could involve a case of sexual abuse perpetrated by the uncle. A: "Could it be that what you remember of your impatience and the visits to your uncle was your initiative, indeed, that you actively sought his closeness, because it was too painful to think that your uncle had abused the longing you felt for your father and had thus transgressed the boundaries of intimacy?" M: "Naturally, we shared mutual affections – but I enjoyed this. When he touched my breast, I finally felt like an attractive young woman …", said Ms. M. to my great surprise.

The subject disappeared from the sessions for considerable time, but then brutally sexualized scenes increasingly began to emerge in her dreams, which I once again sought to address: "You were already adolescent when you began visiting your uncle, and can probably remember the experience of the time. You told me some time ago that affections had been exchanged between you and your uncle. Could it be that you are reluctant to think about any further details which occurred between you, because it could be too shameful to talk about your memories?" Ms. M. reacted vehemently to this question. She went to the toilet and vomited.

In subsequent sessions she was able to relate her memories of the coitus experiences with her uncle that were marked by violence. Nausea, disgust and aversion appeared: the acting out of the overwhelming, traumatic experiences gave way to successive memory and verbalization.

Ms. M. blamed herself for these events: "I was so in need of affection. No wonder that my uncle responded to this…"

Only gradually was she able to admit that this really was a case of abuse that had a major impact on her adolescence and her sexuality as a woman "When visiting my uncle as a thirteen-year-old, I would always storm into the studio and take the initiative in our sexual adventures: I was the one who sought emancipation, to be unconventional, and not him. I found this interesting…".

Only then did I understand that the indicated scenes in the first interview contained unconscious "embodied memories" of her traumatic experiences with her uncle: I was also, quite literally, overrun and overwhelmed by her in the first interview, and she "got under my skin". However, at that time it was not yet possible to decode these unconscious memories in the enactment of Ms. M., only once I had got to know the analysand much better and had often directly experienced the intrusive encroachments in the transfer relationship to me while simultaneously building a supporting psychoanalytic relationship to her—something which allowed for great empathy to the desperate, traumatized child in Ms. M.—did a decisive thought occur to me.

Again, expressed in the language of embodied cognitive science: only once I had—unconsciously—repeatedly experienced the characteristic sensomotoric coordinations of Ms. M. in the psychoanalytic sessions, and adopted them through identifications in my "embodied" countertransference reactions, and only once new categories of a sustainable psychoanalytic relationship had developed, did it then become possible to connect the hitherto disconnected paths of memory with one another. Much like in Proust's "Madeleine scene", ultimately this connection all of a sudden gave rise to the thought (the category) of "sexual abuse" due to my own (unconscious) sensomotoric coordinations. Naturally, unconsciously, it was linked to the "embodied memories" mediated by the repeated sensomotoric coordinations.

With this I had evidently hit the mark. As then became evident, Ms. M. had been sexually abused by her uncle from the age of 13–20. And yet, only through the ongoing psychoanalytic relationship was it possible for her to admit, by way of new memories of brutal scenes, that this was really a matter of sexual assault and had nothing to do with an "emancipated" "happy" affair which she had initiated. Only through the secure psychoanalytic relationship did it become possible to admit the painful insight as to how destructive these experiences had been for her; they had been a major contribution to her inability to allow herself a constant, affectionate and at the same time passionate love relationship but must instead, among others, remain content with the boyfriend mentioned above, a married man, and to live a very limited sexual life over which she has tight control.

My thought made it possible for the first time to articulate in language that which had hitherto remained unrepresented and to thereby initiate a process of working through in the transference relationship. The scope of the present volume limits a more detailed discussion, though mention must be made of the fact that—as the concept of embodied memories postulates—Ms. M.'s traumatic experiences were repeatedly overwritten. Thus, in the fourth year of psychoanalysis, dreams led to a further unexpected discovery: along with her adolescent experience of abuse, Ms. M. enacted other unconscious "embodied memories" of a brutal rape of her mother by Russian soldiers during the Second World War, to which she bore witness as a 3-year-old; furthermore, these were traumatic memories which unconsciously prompted her during late adolescence to engage in dangerous sexual adventures that had led to seven abortions within the space of 10 years. The unconscious feelings of guilt which this triggered determined, among others, her depressive state, as later revealed itself in psychoanalysis.

These "embodied memories" were ultimately closely connected to the traumatic experience of separation in her mother's severe postpartum depression during Ms. M.'s first year of life, which were, incidentally, also contained in the initial scene: the way in which Ms. M. pressed my hand between her two own hands, not only had a sexually stimulating character, but we also understood it as an attempt to, quite literally, hold on to me and not let me go. "Will I ever be able to send her away? She seems so needy…" were my categories of understanding which spontaneously formed at the time and which—in retrospect—were already perceived as early separation trauma but which—also due to my own above-mentioned defence reactions—could not be decoded in detail.

Summary

Psychoanalytic literature is rich with creative metaphors of the unrepresented and the unconscious which open up the understanding and, as are expressed in enactment, that transform the patient's split traumatic memory into painful, though healing, processes of remembering. In this chapter I discussed how concepts of basic research and studies in the field of so-called embodied cognitive science and cognitive neurosciences offer first explanations for the spontaneous, "theory-free" appearance of innovative, creative thoughts in analysts. They constitute the first decisive step for grasping that which has hitherto been unrepresented in images and language.

With reference to techniques of treatment, it becomes evident that the consideration of the new memory theories based on biology influences psychoanalytic attitudes to the extent that they sensitize one to one's own, subtle (embodied) bodily responses. In the case of fault-prone attempts to decode unconscious elements in the enactments of the analysand, for the analyst, the couch setting has proven a great help, since it eases the processes of identification with the sensomotoric coordinations of the analysand, as well as the direction of one's own antenna to the most subtle embodied countertransference reactions. In a face-to-face setting, the subtle resonance mirror processes are continually overlayered by current sensomotoric coordinations and thus complicate the perception of dissociated, split psychic realities (cf. also Bender, 2014).

Finally, psychoanalytic research in recent years has also experienced that both exclusive work with transference and an exclusive (mostly intellectual) reconstruction of the analysand's (traumatic) life history do not lead to a sustained therapeutic change. Above all, psychoanalyses with severe traumatic patients require both the reflection of a horizontal as well as vertical dimension of psychic processes (cf.

Buchholz & Gödde, 2013). On the one hand, psychic processes invariably play out in the subject's current interaction situation with his environment (or his persons of reference) and are thus invariably "horizontal", "intersubjective" and determined by the present, which means in the transference relationship with the analyst. On the other hand, current experiences are invariably determined by sensomotoric coordinations, which have formed in the subject's idiosyncratic (biographic) past. The distinctive history of the individual is, thus, "embodied" because the sensomotoric coordinations emerged in the earliest relationship experiences and, as outlined, continually (causally) determine the later, current, psychic processes in relationships.

This conceptualization has far-reaching clinical consequences (cf. also Bohleber, 2012; Leuzinger-Bohleber, 2008; Bohleber & Leuzinger-Bohleber, 2016). In psychoanalyses with severely traumatized analysands, it has proven indispensable for approaching the distinctive life and trauma history, the "historical reality of the trauma", even when it is never possible to discover the historical truth of the trauma in a one-to-one sense. While life historical events—in the sense of resentment—are time and again rewritten and adapted to the current present, the "historical truth" nevertheless remains in essence. Thus, the successive analytical process of understanding in "embodied memories" and their working through in the analytic relationship allow especially traumatized patients to better psychically integrate the dissociative states, the fragmentations of the self and the inner objects. Thus, as in the case of Ms. M., the analysand gained a healing access to her own, distinctive trauma and life history.

Bibliography

Bauer, J. (2006). *Kleine Zelle, große Gefühle—Wie Spiegelneurone funktionieren*. SWR2. Retrieved January 8, 2006, from www.swr.de/swr2/programm/sendungen/wissen/swr2-wissen-aula-kleinezellen-grossegefuehle/-/id=660374/did=1639788/nid=660374/81ikf0/index.html.

Beebe, B., & Lachmann, F. M. (2004 [2002]). *Säuglingsforschung und die Psychotherapie Erwachsener. Wie interaktive Prozesse entstehen und zu Veränderungen führen*. Übers. H. Haase. Stuttgart: Klett-Cotta.

Bender, T. (2014). *Triebschicksal, Körper-Ich und Realitätssinn: Anmerkungen zur Wiederentdeckung des Körperlichen*. Vortrag, DPV-Frühjahrstagung, 28–31 May 2014, Freiburg im Breisgau.

Bloom, K. (2006). *The embodied self: Movement and psychoanalysis*. London: Karnac.

Bohleber, W. (2010). *Destructiveness, intersubjectivity, and trauma: The identity crisis of modern psychoanalysis*. London: Karnac.

Bohleber, W. (2012). *Was Psychoanalyse heute leistet. Identität und Intersubjektivität, Trauma und Therapie, Gewalt und Gesellschaft*. Stuttgart: Klett-Cotta.

Bohleber, W., & Leuzinger-Bohleber, M. (2016). The special problem of interpretation in the treatment of traumatized patients. *Psychoanalytic Inquiry, 36*, 60–76.

Buchholz, M. B., & Gödde, G. (2013). Balance, Rhythmus, Resonanz: Auf dem Weg zu einer Komplementarität zwischen "vertikaler" und "resonanter" Dimension des Unbewussten. *Psyche, 67*, 844–880.

Caspi, A., Sugden, K., Moffitt, T. E., Taylor, A., Craig, I. W., Harrington, H. L., ... Poulton, R. (2003). Influence of life stress on depression: Moderation by a polymorphism in the 5-HTT gene. *Science, 301*, 386–389.

Clancey, W. J. (1994). Situated cognition: How representations are created and given meaning. In: R. Lewis, & P. Mendelsohn (Eds.), *Lessons from learning: working conference, proceedings*, 6–8 Sept 1993, North-Holland, Amsterdam, pp. 231–242.

Corrigall, J., Payne, H., & Wilkinson, H. (Eds.). (2006). *About a body: Working with the embodied mind in psychotherapy*. London, New York: Routledge.

Damasio, A. R. (1997 [1994]). *Descartes' Irrtum. Fühlen, Denken und das menschliche Gehirn*. Übers. H. Kober. München (dtv).

Dantlgraber, J. (2008). "Musikalisches Zuhören". Zugangswege zu den Vorgängen in der unbewussten Kommunikation. *Forum Psychoanalyse, 24*, 161–176.

di Pellegrino, G., Fadiga, L., Gallese, V., & Rizzolatti, G. (1992). Understanding motor events: A neurophysiological study. *Experimental Brain Research, 91*, 176–180.

Edelman, G. M. (1989). *The remembered present: A biological theory of consciousness*. New York: Basic Books.

Edelman, G. M. (1993 [1987]). *Unser Gehirn—ein dynamisches System. Die Theorie des neuronalen Darwinismus und die biologischen Grundlagen der Wahrnehmung*. Übers. F. Griese. München: Piper.

Edelman, G. M. (1995 [1992]). *Göttliche Luft, vernichtendes Feuer. Wie der Geist im Gehirn entsteht. Die revolutionäre Vision des Medizin-Nobelpreisträgers*. Übers. A. Ehlers. München: Piper.

Emde, R. N., & Leuzinger-Bohleber, M. (Eds.) (2014). *Early parenting and prevention of disorder: Psychoanalytic research at interdisciplinary frontiers*. London: Karnac.

Feldman, R. (2012). *The neurobiological basis of intersubjectivity: Oxytocin, brain, and interactive synchrony*. Vortrag, 13. Joseph Sandler Psychoanalytic Research Conference, "Research in Early Parenting and the Prevention of Disorder", Frankfurt/M., 2–4 March 2012.

Freud, S. (1896). L'hérédité et l'étiologie des névroses. *GW 1*, 407–422.

Freud, S. (1899). Über Deckerinnerungen. *GW 1*, 531–554.

Freud, S. (1914). Erinnern, Wiederholen und Durcharbeiten. *GW 10*, 126–136.

Frie, R. (2008). Fundamentally embodied: The experience of psychological agency. *Contemporary Psychoanalysis, 44*, 367–376.

Fuchs, T., Sattel, H. & Henningsen, P. (Hg.) (2010). *The embodied self: Dimensions, coherence and disorders*. Stuttgart: Schattauer.

Gaensbauer, T. J. (2011). Embodied simulation, mirror neurons, and the reenactment of trauma in early childhood. *Neuropsychoanalysis, 13*, 91–107.

Gaensbauer, T. J. (2014). Frühes Trauma und seine Repräsentation über die Lebensspanne vom frühkindlichen Stadium bis zum Beginn des Erwachsenenalters. Eine Falldarstellung. *Psyche, 68*, 997–1029.

Gallese, V. (2009). Mirror neurons, embodied simulation, and the neural basis of social identification. *Psychoanalytic Dialogues, 19*, 519–536.

Gallese, V. (2013a). Mirror neurons, embodied simulation and a second-person approach to mindreading. *Cortex, 49*, 2954–2956.

Gallese, V. (2013b). Den Körper im Gehirn finden. Konzeptuelle Überlegungen zu den Spiegelneuronen. In: M. Leuzinger-Bohleber, R. N. Emde, & R. Pfeifer (Hg.), *Embodiment. Ein innovatives Konzept für Entwicklungsforschung und Psychoanalyse*. Göttingen and Bristol, CT, pp. 75–112.

Goldberg, D. (2009). The interplay between biological and psychological factors in determining vulnerability to mental disorders. *Psychoanalytic Psychotherapy, 23*, 236–247.

Goldman, A., & Gallese, V. (2000). Reply to Schulkin. *Trends in cognitive sciences, 4*(7), 255–256.

Green, A. (1999 [1993]). *The work of the negative*. London: Free Association.

Green, A. (2007). *Resonance of suffering: Countertransference in non-neurotic structures*. London: International Psychoanalytic Association.

Green, S. R. (2010). Embodied female experience through the lens of imagination. *The Journal of Analytical Psychology, 55*, 339–360.

Hagner, M. (2008). *Homo cerebralis: Der Wandel vom Seelenorgan zum Gehirn*. Berlin: Suhrkamp.

Hampe, M. (2003). Pluralism of sciences and the unity of reason. In M. Leuzinger-Bohleber, A. U. Dreher, & J. Canestri (Eds.), *Pluralism or unity? Methods of research in psychoanalysis* (pp. 45–63). London: International Psychoanalytical Association.
Hannabach, C. (2007). Anxious embodiment, disability, and sexuality: A response to Margrit Shildrick. *Studies in Gender and Sexuality, 8*, 253–261.
Hauser, S. T. (2008). The interplay of genes, environments, and psychoanalysis. *Journal of the American Psychoanalytic Association, 56*, 509–514.
Hill, J. (2009). Developmental perspectives on adult depression. *Psychoanalytic Psychotherapy, 23*, 200–212.
Kaufman, J., Yang, B. Z., Douglas-Palumberi, H., Grasso, D., Lipschitz, D., Houshyar, S., ... Gelernter, J. (2006). Brain-derived neurotrophic factor-5-HTTLPR gene interactions and environmental modifiers of depression in children. *Biological Psychiatry, 59*, 673–680.
Knoblauch, S. H. (2007). The perversion of language in the analyst's activity: Navigating the rhythms of embodiment and symbolization. *International Forum of Psychoanalysis, 16*, 38–42.
Knox, J. (2009). Mirror neurons and embodied simulation in the development of archetypes and self-agency. *The Journal of Analytical Psychology, 54*, 307–323.
Lakoff, G., & Johnson, M. (1999). *Philosophy in the flesh: The embodied mind and its challenge to western thought*. New York: Basic Books.
Langan, R. (2007). Embodiment. *American Journal of Psychoanalysis, 67*, 249–259.
Leikert, S. (2013). *Korrespondenzen und Resonanzen. Psychoanalyse und Musik im Dialog*. Frankfurt am Main: Brandes & Apsel.
Leuzinger-Bohleber, M. (2003). Erinnerungen an frühe Traumatisierungen. Einige Beobachtungen aus einer repräsentativen Katamnesestudie. In E. Brainin (Ed.), *Kindsein in stürmischen Zeiten. Reales Trauma und psychische Bewältigung* (pp. 68–101). Wien: Picus.
Leuzinger-Bohleber, M. (2008). Biographical truths and their clinical consequences: Understanding 'embodied memories' in a third psychoanalysis with a traumatized patient recovered from serve poliomyelitis. *International Journal of Psychoanalysis, 89*, 1165–1187.
Leuzinger-Bohleber, M. (2010). *Psychoanalyse als "Wissenschaft des Unbewussten" im ersten Jahrhundert der IPA*. Internationale Psychoanalyse—Nachrichtenmagazin der IPV 18 (Sonderausg.), pp. 24–26.
Leuzinger-Bohleber, M. (2012): The 'Medea fantasy': An unconscious determinant of psychogenic sterility. In: Mariott, P. (ed.), *The maternal lineage. Identification, desire, and transgenerational issues* (pp. 169–204). London/New York: Routledge.
Leuzinger-Bohleber, M. (2014a). Working with severely traumatized, chronically depressed analysands. *The International Journal of Psycho-Analysis, 96*(3), 611–636.
Leuzinger-Bohleber, M. (2014b). Den Körper in der Seele entdecken-Embodiment und die Annäherung an das Nicht-Repräsentierte. *Psyche, 68*, 922–950.
Leuzinger-Bohleber, M. (2015). *Finding the body in the mind—Embodied memories, trauma, and depression, International Psychoanalytical Association*. London: Karnac.
Leuzinger-Bohleber, M., Emde, R. N., & Pfeifer, R. (2013). *Embodiment. Ein innovatives Konzept für Entwicklungsforschung und Psychoanalyse*. Göttingen: Vandenhoeck & Ruprecht.
Leuzinger-Bohleber, M., & Pfeifer, R. (1998). Erinnern in der Übertragung—Vergangenheit in der Gegenwart? Psychoanalyse und Embodied Cognitive Science: ein interdisziplinärer Dialog zum Gedächtnis. *Psyche, 52*, 884–918.
Leuzinger-Bohleber, M., & Pfeifer, R. (2002). Remembering a depressive primary object: Memory in the dialogue between psychoanalysis and cognitive science. *The International Journal of Psycho-Analysis, 83*, 3–33.
Leuzinger-Bohleber, M., & Pfeifer, R. (2013a). Embodiment: Den Körper in der Seele entdecken—Ein altes Problem und ein revolutionäres Konzept. In M. Leuzinger-Bohleber, R. N. Emde, & R. Pfeifer (Eds.), *Embodiment—ein innovatives Konzept für Entwicklungsforschung und Psychoanalyse* (pp. 14–38). Göttingen: Vandenhoeck & Ruprecht.
Leuzinger-Bohleber, M., & Pfeifer, R. (2013b). Psychoanalyse und Embodied Cognitive Science in Zeiten revolutionären Umdenkens. Erinnern, Übertragung, therapeutische Veränderung

und “embodied metaphors”. In M. Leuzinger-Bohleber, R. N. Emde, & R. Pfeifer (Eds.), *Embodiment—ein innovatives Konzept für Entwicklungsforschung und Psychoanalyse* (pp. 39–74). Göttingen: Vandenhoeck & Ruprecht.

Leuzinger-Bohleber, M., Rickmeyer, C., Tahiri, M., Hettich, N., & Fischmann, T. (2016). Special communication. What can psychoanalysis contribute to the current refugee crisis? Preliminary reports from STEP-BY-STEP: A psychoanalytic pilot project for supporting refugees in a “first reception camp” and crisis interventions with traumatized refugees. *International Journal of Psychoanalysis, 97*(4), 1077–1093.

Leuzinger-Bohleber, M., Roth, G., & Buchheim, A. (Eds.). (2008). *Psychoanalyse—Neurobiologie—Trauma*. Stuttgart: Schattauer.

Levine, H. B., Reed, G. S., & Scarfone, D. (2013). *Unrepresented states and the construction of meaning: Clinical and theoretical contributions*. London: Karnac.

Marshall, K. (2009). The embodied self: Thinking psychoanalytically in a time of ‘science’. *The Journal of Analytical Psychology, 54*, 677–696.

Mizen, R. (2009). The embodied mind. *The Journal of Analytical Psychology, 54*, 253–272.

Pfeifer, R., & Bongard, J. (2007). *How the body shapes the way we think: A new view of intelligence*. Cambridge, MA: MIT Press.

Proust. *Auf der Suche nach der verlorenen Zeit. Frankfurter Ausgabe*. Frankfurt: Suhrkamp.

Proust, M. (2004 [1913]). *Auf der Suche nach der verlorenen Zeit. Bd. 1: Unterwegs zu Swann. Übers. E. Rechel-Mertens, rev. von L. Keller*. Frankfurt am Main: Suhrkamp.

Reed, G. (2013). An empty mirror: Reflections on nonrepresentation. In H. B. Levine, G. S. Reed, & D. Scarfone (Eds.), *Unrepresented states and the construction of meaning: Clinical and theoretical contributions* (pp. 18–41). London: Karnac.

Rizzolatti, G., Fadiga, L., Fogassi, L., & Gallese, V. (2002). From mirror neurons to imitation: Facts and speculations. In A. N. Meltzoff & W. Prinz (Eds.), *The imitative mind: Development, evolution, and brain bases* (pp. 247–266). New York: Cambridge University Press.

Rutherford, H. J., Goldberg, B., Luvten, P., Bridgett, D. J., & Mayes, L. C. (2013). Parental reflective functioning is associated with tolerance of infant distress but not general distress: Evidence for a specific relationship using a simulated baby paradigm. *Infant Behavior & Development, 36*, 635–641.

Sansal, B. (2011). *Das Dorf des Deutschen oder das Tagebuch der Brüder Schiller*: Roman. Merlin-Verlag.

Scarfone, D. (2013). A brief introduction to the work of Jean Laplanche. *The International Journal of Psycho-Analysis, 94*, 545–566.

Scharff, J. M. (2010). *Die leibliche Dimension in der Psychoanalyse*. Frankfurt am Main: Brandes & Apsel.

Shapiro, S. A. (2009). A rush to action: Embodiment, the analyst's subjectivity, and the interpersonal experience. *Studies in Gender and Sexuality, 10*, 93–103.

Sletvold, J. (2011). “The reading of emotional expression”: Wilhelm Reich and the history of embodied analysis. *Psychoanalytic Dialogues, 21*, 453–467.

Sletvold, J. (2012). Training analysts to work with unconscious embodied expressions: Theoretical underpinnings and practical guidelines. *Psychoanalytic Dialogues, 22*, 410–429.

Stern, D. N. (2010 [1985]). *Die Lebenserfahrung des Säuglings. Mit einer neuen Einleitung des Autors* (Übers. W. Krege, bearb. v. E. Vorspohl. 10. Aufl.). Stuttgart: Klett-Cotta.

Stone, M. (2006). The analyst's body as tuning fork: Embodied resonance in countertransference. *The Journal of Analytical Psychology, 51*, 109–124.

Suomi, S. (2011). Trauma und Epigenetik. In: M. Leuzinger-Bohleber, & R. Haubl (Eds.), *Psychoanalyse: interdisziplinär—international—intergenerationell. Schriften des Sigmund-Freud-Instituts* (Reihe 2, Bd. 16). Göttingen: Vandenhoeck & Ruprecht, pp. 295–315.

Tronick, E. Z. (2003). Things still to be done on the still-face effect. *Infancy, 4*, 475–482.

Vivona, J. M. (2009). Embodied language in neuroscience and psychoanalysis. *Journal of the American Psychoanalytic Association, 57*, 1327–1360.

Chapter 8
Case Study of a 29-Year-Old Patient with a Panic Disorder, Recurrent Depressive Disorder, Current Episode Moderate, IBS, Posttraumatic Stress Disorder (ICD-10 F 41.0, F 33.1, F 45.32, F 43.1)

Christos Charis

Presenting Problems

On his own initiative and on the recommendation of a psychiatrist who provided him with 5 mg Escitalopram and 25 mg Atosin, Mr. Y presented himself to me 18 months after the sudden death of his mother and told me that he had suffered the first panic attack 4 weeks previously. He was lying in bed on the Sunday night of that week, was not able to sleep and had an unpleasant feeling with stabbing pains in his abdomen. Soon after that, he experienced flashbacks of the traumatic death of his mother (aged 56), who was being unsuccessfully resuscitated for over 1 h in front of his eyes, triggered by pains in his abdomen. (She had been having an ache in her abdomen just a few minutes before; she had become hot, so she had taken off her clothes in front of his eyes, and an abdominal aneurysm until then unknown had led her to death.) He cried and had himself tested in the emergency department, because he believed that he suffered from the same condition as his mother and he would die as well. He experienced diarrhoea. The emergency doctor diagnosed very high blood pressure and gave him something to calm him down. Later, he had several examinations carried out by physicians. All the examinations came up with a diagnosis of nothing apart from irritable bowel syndrome (IBS). Since then he has always had diarrhoea and pain in his abdomen. When he got pain, he faced the image of the death of his mother in front of him, fearing that he would die too because he had the same fatal illness as his mother. He trembled all over. He suffered the second panic attack on the day on which his girlfriend was having an operation. On that evening he was at home alone. He cried, thinking he could not be

To illustrate conversion symptoms I will present a patient suffering from these symptoms in this chapter.

C. Charis (✉)
Dillenburg, Germany

C. Charis, G. Panayiotou (eds.), *Somatoform and Other Psychosomatic Disorders*,
https://doi.org/10.1007/978-3-319-89360-0_8

alone, because if something happened to him, then he would die without help from anybody. That is why he slept at his girlfriend's mother's apartment. He had become withdrawn after the death of his mother and had been studying for his degree course until about 4 am, because he thought he owed his mother a good degree. Nevertheless, he had to repeat the last semester because he did not pass his examinations.

Case History

The patient reported the following:

His father had died of "a heroin overdose" when the patient was 2 years old. Mr. Y had lived with his mother (+28 years, hairdresser, but worked as a cleaning lady) and his two sisters (+8 years, +2 years). As his mother had always wanted "a boy", he had been "her favourite child". His mother had married as early as 17; her first marriage had ended pretty quickly, however, after she had got pregnant. His oldest sister was a product of this marriage. He experienced his mother as being cheerful and happy, "very strong personality, managed independently, dominant, bossy". She "had only lived for her children" and had not remarried after the death of her second husband, but had had several life partners afterwards. She had hated these men. The time spent with his mother and his two sisters had been pleasant. The patient and his sister had looked after one another and had done their homework independently ("we had to take on responsibility at home"). His mother had taught her children values, such as "respect, diligence and self-reliance". Her wish had been for her children to go to university, since she herself had been forbidden to do so. In the spring of 2013, she had died quite suddenly before his eyes. He describes himself as being "a little sensitive, someone who shies away from conflict", cheerful, introvert, "pretty well-adjusted" in puberty and someone who had good grades in grammar school. Following his A levels, he completed his civilian service and then did an Arts degree. After the death of his mother, with whom he had lived, he had "got stuck into university work". ("I thought I owed it to my mother to graduate well.") Her death had resulted in him having to leave their shared flat, since he had lacked the money to pay the rent. He then moved in with his girlfriend (first girlfriend, same age as him), whom he had known from school (she had also done her A levels, but had not studied at university) and with whom he had been friends for 3 years. Sex is not possible since she suffers from a fistula in the genital area. There are some tensions between them, as his girlfriend wants to remain near her mother, whereas, due to occupational reasons, the patient will have to move away. He notes that she had lost her father when she was 12.

Case Formulation

The fact that the patient thinks he is going to die from the same disease as his mother makes it clear how close his relationship to his mother is; he has not managed to overcome the loss of his mother. The cause of the very close relationship to his mother is, among other things, that the patient grew up without a father. Since his mother reproached the dead father for having left her alone with the three children by his early death, she gave the patient an image of his father which did not allow him to relate to a good male role model. As a result he could not distance himself sufficiently from his mother. (In healthy development, the identification with the father enables the male child to become independent of the mother who is taking care of him. The father passes through the older bond of mother and son in the process; we call that in psychoanalysis "triangulation".) Mr. Y's mother, on the other hand, was dominant and spoiled him as her "favourite child". As a message for life, she told him: "Everything is taken care of!" The patient felt secure with her. Even in puberty, adolescents normally seek to become independent of the parents; Mr. Y seemed to be quite passive. Against the background of his symbiotic attachment to the mother, he is afraid of autonomy, that is, confronted with independent life. The moment he sees his mother die in front of his own eyes, he experiences the panicky fear that he has to master life alone and independently! This fear and his grief about the death of his mother can be ousted at first because he has given the role of his mother (that is to say, to give him security) to his girlfriend, with whom he moved in immediately after his mother's death. Thus he suffers, inwardly and consistently, the second panic attack just before his girlfriend undergoes a fistula surgery. ("If something happens, I am completely alone!") Since the patient can make this connection himself, he comes back to the therapy at this point, again in the sense of an inner consistency. I assume that he has also suffered the first panic attack in connection with a fantasized loss of his girlfriend. For example, it may be that 4 weeks previously he first heard of his girlfriend's surgery. His fear of life, which he must lead independently, is expressed by his symptoms (tremors, panic, etc.), that is, he converts his fears of independent (autonomous) life into a physical expression symptom. Psychoanalytically one could speak of a mobilized autonomy-dependency conflict. The pathological syllogism would be: "Since my mother died, I will also die!" Feelings of helplessness are awakened. While he is resting at night and is experiencing irritable physical sensations through the colon, he associates: "Since my mother had pain in the abdomen and died, I will also die because I have an abdominal pain!" Thus he expresses the psychological pain in a ciphered form (conversion) caused by the loss of his mother and his fears by what he experienced as an abdominal pain. That way of thinking points to two facts: First as already mentioned, he identifies strongly with his mother, from whom he has not resolved. In the way he keeps to his mother, he maintains the connection to her, thereby warding off the pain of the loss. (Why is the pain of the patient a conversion and not an affect equivalent? Because Mr. Y identified himself with his mother through the pain. His mother had pain before she died. Through his pain in his abdomen, he symbolically expresses his fantasy of being one with his mother.) Therefore, he fears, "If I have pain in the abdomen, I have the same disease as my mother and I am about to die of that illness!" and he expresses **that fearful fantasy** with diarrhoea (another conversion symptom.) Secondly, he is afraid of death, a fear that he cannot suppress in the light of his concrete life experiences, unlike most people succeed in suppressing it; thirdly, he became conscious of his limited life expectancy by the death of his mother, who died in front his eyes. Since this death was sudden and unexpected, and in the context of his very close attachment to his mother, he could not mourn the loss of this important reference person, but he denied his concern by fleeing into his studies. A further factor plays an important role in the lack of grief processing: in the context of his biography, he has not learned to regulate his emotions ("structural deficit") and to deal with loss reactions ("everything can be managed"). Instead, the affects flood him; he is overwhelmed by them, and the triggering of fear is the result. This is, e.g. recognizing that he had slept or had to sleep at his "mother-in-law's" home on the day of his girlfriend's operation. Mr. Y begins to realize his emotional dependence on important people in his environment, and thus his lack of independence results in his pronounced separation. The only available resort left to him is to cling to strong women.

Therapy

The psychodynamic therapy consisted of 80 sessions split into weekly visits. Mr. Y stopped taking his antidepressants 3 months after therapy began. During the first course of treatment and throughout large stretches of therapy, the patient seeks a comforting and caring father figure in me by describing his anxiety symptoms and thereby laying bare, albeit carefully, his hardship. In this sense, the initial focus of the treatment was stabilizing the patient. That is to say, the patient repetitively addressed his physical symptoms in the context of an increasingly productive therapeutic relationship. Repeatedly, we talked about all the physical examinations the patient had done following the death of his mother, and the patient became cognisant of the fact that he had been thoroughly examined by experienced professionals, and all examinations had been without any pathological diagnostic findings, a circumstance he deemed credible. Furthermore, the patient could comprehend that his abdominal pain resulted from IBS and not from him having the same illness as his mother had had. Moreover, Mr. Y learnt how to effectively distance himself from intrusions by using relaxation exercises (safe exercise, tree exercise). In light of this positive development, Mr. Y is beginning to feel more self-confident. In this sense, he is starting to prepare for the examination forming part of his bachelor thesis, something he had not succeeded in doing before therapy began. Against this background, his "trauma"—the death of his mother before his own eyes—is dealt with as gently as possible. Hence, the focus of therapy is on grief work. (It seemed important to me to win him over to grieving, in order for him to accept the death of his mother and let go of her.) He cries a lot in this phase. He expresses his marked sense of loneliness and his fear of being left alone. Furthermore, he manages to express his rage at having been left alone by his mother. During this stage of therapy, there is a temporary increase of psychosomatic symptoms and anxiety symptoms, after each session, due to him reliving his trauma and being overwhelmed by his emotions. I take up his implicit accusation that he has been left alone. I make him aware of how acutely he felt left alone after the death of his mother and how much he misses his mother. Against this background, he notes that he is slowly beginning to realize that everything has come to an end. In this context, Mr. Y makes the dreams he has had since the death of his mother the subject of discussion. He reports having been chased and attacked by threatening figures. It was better if he said goodbye to everyone, since he was going to die. Or he reports being trapped somewhere, in a dark room, the door being the limit. He understands these dreams as being a manifestation of his fear of death; he reflects on his own mortality (I think the death of his mother has made him aware of his own mortality). In this context, partly as a result of my recommendation, he is reading the book "Staring at the Sun. Overcoming the Terror of Death" I. Yalom. At this stage, he is visiting seminars that focus intensively on death. My interpretation is that by intensively grappling with death, he is seeking to be close to his mother, allowing me to address the patient's grief but also his separation anxiety. He admits in tears that, yes, he misses her a lot! She was taken from him too soon. Through repeated interpretation in this direction, Mr. Y is allowing himself to grieve more and more, which goes hand in hand with the experience of no longer having nightmares. He recalls life with his mother. He remembers many happy moments with her and acknowledges with gratitude that she devoted her life to her children, although living too little herself. However, she regularly complained about her husband, who had passed away too early and left her alone with the children. This was the reason for her not visiting his grave. She now lies in a gravesite separate to that of her husband. Mr. Y notes that he will not sacrifice himself for his children; he would like to live as well. As he reports, this is something he and his girlfriend often talk about. He speaks to her about whether they should marry and have children. Thereafter, the patient has dreams once more—he has married his girlfriend and they have had children. His girlfriend then died leaving him alone with the child. He bypasses my interpretation that he has lost many people close to him, which in turn triggers his fear of once more losing someone close to him, such as his girlfriend; this in turn results in him shying away from marrying her. Moments later, he denies his fear of separation, claiming marriage would make him feel oppressed. In this phase of therapy, Mr. Y is addressing his fear of marriage and of starting a family. During this process, he behaves ambivalently. On the one hand, he unconsciously expresses his disappointment about how difficult life in a family was for him, and in light of this biographic background, he holds on to his pessimistic interpretation of things. On the other hand, he sees me as a nurturing father figure, who models an alternative path in life. We repeatedly have heated discussions centred on this topic. Gradually, more and more tensions in the relationship to his girlfriend are manifesting. She would like to be taken care of. She expects him to put her to bed, she will not tolerate sex, however, due to pain she experiences. She reacts jealously, since the patient is tutoring a younger student in art history and is in contact with the latter. The patient would like to suspend grief work concerning the death of his mother and focus on the problems between him and his girlfriend. I inform Mr. Y that if we act upon his wish, his physical symptoms will persist once therapy has been concluded and tell him that I am uncertain as to whether we can resolve the problems he has with his girlfriend in the short space of time remaining. I therefore suggested that he and his girlfriend should consult a couple therapist; they both, however, refuse to do so. The patient accepts my paternal advice and reflects on his relationship to his mother. Subsequently, he finds himself able to deal with the grief experienced after his mother's death, meaning the pain experienced through her loss becomes more manageable as a result of therapy. His feeling of living in a dream and when he wakes up all will be alright again is slowly dissipating. The stable therapeutic relationship reinforces his progress; Mr. Y sees me as reliable father figure in whom he can confide his negative emotions. Against this background, the patient manages to detach himself from his mother, to a certain extent, even though he was not able to deal with his fear of separation during the course of this therapy. Furthermore, while reflecting on himself, he notices that he is slowly but gradually maturing. He is, for instance, thinking about starting a family, something he had not wanted to do until recently. I narcissistically support the patient in his findings, by clarifying, "you notice your coping a lot better now". Since the tensions between him and his girlfriend are increasing, he is now seriously contemplating separation. Meanwhile, she has surreptitiously started a new relationship, when asked about it, she denies this. (Mr. Y notes that his girlfriend had also had a secret relationship the last time they were going out). Mr. Y, who has become more independent and self-assured during the course of therapy, exposes his girlfriend's relationship and leaves her. He leaves the flat they shared and moves into a small flat in his paternal grandmother's house. (Once more, this highlights that he has, so far, not been able to face his fear of separation.) To a certain extent, he is sad that his relationship ended badly, but he does not get depressed, and his discussed symptoms do not resurface. Soon after, our therapeutic sessions have come to an end. Six months later we meet once more. We note the treatment outcome has remained stable to this day. Mr. Y no longer has any symptoms.

Chapter 9
Psychotherapy Among HIV Patients: A Look at a Psychoimmunological Research Study After 20 Years

Ann Schaefer, Gerhard Paar, Reinholde Kriebel, and Karl-Heinz Stäcker

Abbreviations

AIDS	Acquired immune deficiency syndrome
HAART	Highly active antiretroviral therapy
HIV	Human immunodeficiency virus

Introduction

An HIV infection leads to a progressive immunodeficiency syndrome. Once it penetrates the bloodstream, the HI virus particularly impairs cellular immunity.

The following can be summarised according to Weinel (2017): infection with the human immunodeficiency virus (HIV) is characterised by a persistent viraemia and a long clinical latency period. The transition from the initial infection to the full clinical picture, the last stage of the disease referred to as acquired immunodeficiency syndrome (AIDS), can be of variable length. The infected person is largely without symptoms in the latency period, and the HIV particles are only verifiable in lower concentration in the blood (viral load). The primary transmission occurs through sexual intercourse, primarily anal intercourse as the most important mode of infection. If untreated, the infection leads via the full clinical picture of AIDS to death. Approximately 90% of those affected die from AIDS. If untreated, about 2–4 years elapse between the first AIDS complication and death. The onset of the full clinical picture can usually be prevented or at least delayed with a combination

A. Schaefer (✉)
Köln, Germany

G. Paar · R. Kriebel
Essen, Germany

K.-H. Stäcker
Department of Psychology, University of Essen-Duisburg, Essen, Germany

C. Charis, G. Panayiotou (eds.), *Somatoform and Other Psychosomatic Disorders*,
https://doi.org/10.1007/978-3-319-89360-0_9

of antiretroviral drugs. A complete cure is, however, still not possible. As a result, an HIV infection is equated with a chronic disease.

In the 80s, the HI virus primarily proliferated among homosexual and bisexual men and posed a massive threat. At that time, the average life expectancy after the initial infection was approx. 10 years (Brodt et al., 1986). Even today the affected persons in this group are exposed to the risk of a double stigmatisation. The disclosure of one's own HIV infection can lead to ostracism due to fears of infection and homophobic attitudes in the social environment. It is obvious that with inadequate integration of homosexual identity, coping with the disease and the possibly necessary change of sexual practices (safer sex) are complicated. Those affected remain highly susceptible to blaming themselves or experiencing recriminations.

The psychological working through of an HIV infection is a complex and long-term process in which the successes of medicinal treatment and altered perceptions of society—also in interaction with each other—are adopted. Before 1996 the medicinal treatment consisted of a less effective monotherapy (reverse transcriptase inhibitors) with a rather marginal lifetime extension (approx. 6 months). The new highly potent antiretroviral combination therapy (HAART, highly active antiretroviral therapy with protease inhibitors) has been available since 1996. Whereas the HIV diagnosis was associated with a threat of death and a massive disruption of the narcissistic balance in the pre-HAART era, the prognosis with HIV infection has improved considerably in the subsequent HAART era. The disease progression can be better controlled, and the life-threatening comorbidities in the full clinical picture of AIDS are less severe (Beck, Freudenreich, & Worth, 2010). The life expectancy of HIV-infected homosexual males in Europe is therefore comparable with noninfected individuals. However, this only applies if the diagnosis is made early and the patient is already offered treatment while the immune system is still less weakened. Moreover, the patient has to take the medications on a regular and lifelong basis (Fätkenheuer, 2015). Pre-HAART era and HAART era differ in terms of the scope and content of the threat.

In the pre-HAART era, the Institute of Medical Psychology conducted an interdisciplinary research project[1] with the Clinic for Dermatology at Essen University Hospital from 1990 to 1993. A psychosocial group offer for HIV-positive homosexual and bisexual men was developed and reviewed within the framework of this project. Of particular interest was the evidence of a psychoimmunological efficacy relating to the psychological level through the positive influence of coping with disease as well as on the somatic level with regard to verifiable positive effects for the immune system.

From today's point of view, the study at that time still seems relevant to us under three aspects:

[1]Research project funded by the BMFT (funding code: V-005 90) and MFW (account number:10330140): *"Über das Mitwirken psychosozialer Faktoren am Verlauf einer HIV-Infektion—Eine Studie an homo- und bisexuellen Männern"*.

1. Psychoimmunological studies were met with great interest in the pre-HAART era (Weber, Atanackovic, & Deter, 2015), since lesser interactions of treatment with the immune system occurred in comparison to today. Medicinal treatment started later and was restricted in its efficacy. That is why psychoimmunological associations were easier to illustrate.
2. In the pre-HAART era, the diagnosis of an HIV infection was associated with a threat of death and the prospect of a limited future. From today's point of view, the notification of the diagnosis at that time can be comprehended as a type I trauma. In the HAART era, the threat of death was relativised to an incurable chronic disease with which a person can live with. The meaning of "incurable" underwent a change: a disease "leading to death" became an aspect of "must live with the disease". Our own investigation provides information regarding which coping mechanisms are mobilised among patients under the threat of death and to what extent these are therapeutically capable of being influenced despite the continued existence of the threat of death. The comparison with results of subsequent studies can provide information regarding whether and how the coping mechanisms change under a "mitigated" threat. In the process, one certainly cannot assume a simple depiction of a strong vs. weak threat of narcissistic vulnerability. Particularly due to the threat of death in the pre-HAART era, there was one possibility of coping for the infected person in the development of a "paradox identity" (Weinel, 2017). The experience of one's own existential peculiarity could give meaning and create detachment in light of imminent death, which is omitted as merely a "chronically ill person". The illness becomes "more banal" and also loses its exceptional status in the eyes of the social environment. Nevertheless, under HAART the adaptation to the lifelong burdensome treatment of the infection constitutes a daily challenge for the regulation of emotional balance.
3. An original psychodynamic approach was expanded by trauma-related treatment elements during the development of the treatment concept. The increasing focus on a trauma-specific approach evolved in the run-up to the investigation in the course of preliminary studies. Stabilisation and confrontation are to be placed in an advantageous relation to one another under a psychodynamic as well as trauma-related perspective. The final treatment concept seeks to optimise this tension. Finding this optimum also poses a challenge of psychotherapeutic treatment among HIV-infected persons today. The recent biographical experiences, particularly regarding HIV infection, remain psychotherapeutically untreated as a "trauma scheme", with the constant risk of getting into an uncontrollable experiential situation with overwhelming feelings. The "trauma-compensatory scheme" revises the different components of traumatic experience and is directed against those psychological structures which retain the experiential constellations in memory (Fischer & Riedesser, 1998). Between both schemata there is an unstable balance in the traumatic process. The therapeutic approach consists in the treatment of the distorted defence with simultaneous strengthening of healthy functions and structures of personality and targets activation, working through and integration of incompatible experiences.

HIV Infection/Illness as a Stressor

HIV infection constitutes a massive and repeating distortion of the biopsychosocial balance and is therefore invasive in every respect. This threat mobilises physical and psychological stress reactions, which on the one hand are supposed to serve the best possible adaptation to severe and permanent stress but on the other hand can even benefit or exacerbate the onset of psychological disorders and somatic illnesses due to their repeated and chronic occurrence and thus contribute to disease progression. What is supposed to help you can, therefore, also make you ill. Activations in the course of stress and emotional reactions are associated with the release of hormones (cortisol, etc.), which have a very general immunological effect and engender differential effects on the immune system (McEwen, 2007). Psychoimmunological studies deal with associations between psychosocial variables of coping with illness, immune status and in the event of HIV infection with disease progression (Scott-Sheldon, Kalichman, Carey, & Fielder, 2008).

In psychoimmunological terms, it can be shown that stress—depending on the duration of its effect—has immunosuppressive (weakening) as well as immunoexpressive (strengthening) effects on the immune system. There are indications that stress management can also be attributed to mediating effects on the immune system, i.e. ineffective stress management is depicted in weakened immune functions (e.g. increased susceptibility to infection, accelerated course of disease). So the psychological processing of a somatic illness has an influence with regard to how permanent stress can be experienced and stress reactions can be mitigated and reduced in their frequency of occurrence. An individual's coping with disease, such as "coming to terms with the situation and at the same time recognising and exploiting their opportunities to have an effect on the stress" has a decisive impact with regard to how self-esteem, well-being and quality of life are to be preserved and ensured despite persistent stress.

The psychological processing of an HIV infection can be characterised as a recurrent alternation between anxiety and anxiety defence. Aggressive, offensive behaviour towards the perceived threat as well as evasive behaviour for dosing perceptible anxieties can be conducive to a process of abnegation and working through and promote adaptation. In contrast—as coping research has proven (Moskowitz, Hult, Bussolari, & Acree, 2009; Weinel, 2017)—feelings of guilt and rumination in terms of a persistent, agonising tendency to brood about the HIV infection with resignation and self-recrimination prove to be clearly maladaptive. Perceived social support through important attachment figures seems to be helpful among homosexual and bisexual men, and a successful "coming out" for gaining a positive homosexual identity also contributes significantly to a positive self-concept (Chida & Vedhara, 2009; Moskowitz et al., 2009).

Our Own Investigation

In the **main study** (Study 1), it was examined to what extent a temporary group therapy intervention has a favourable effect on coping with disease (emotional state, illness behaviour, preventive behaviour) and the somatic course of disease (immune status, disease progression) with regard to HIV-positive homosexual and bisexual men in a relatively early disease stage, i.e. Walter Reed stage 1–3 (Schaefer, 1998; Schaefer et al., 1995).

In the **therapy group** (TG), a total of 15 HIV patients continuously took part in a 4-month group therapy programme. Coping with disease was examined with relevant psychological testing procedures at the beginning, after completion of therapy and after another 4 months (catamnesis date). The survey of clinically relevant functional parameters of the immune system occurred simultaneously. Among other things, the number of CD4 cells—which provides information about the functionality of cellular defence—was determined, and the p24 antigen was measured, which allows conclusions to be drawn about the spread of the HI virus in the body. The individual disease progression was operationalised at the respective **time of measurement** (TOM) via the exact classification in line with the Walter Reed staging classification.

The **comparison group** (CG1) consisted of 30 HIV patients who did not receive any psychotherapeutic intervention but were examined at the times of measurement analogous to TG. The research design enabled a consideration in the longitudinal view: "Have the findings within the study groups changed over the monitored eight months?" And in the cross section: "Are there any differences found between the two study groups at the three times of measurement?"

Under **extended questioning** (Study 2), it was examined whether the success of group therapy can also be substantiated by means of an altered handling of HIV patients with an acute psychosocial stressor, i.e. in a stress interview (Breukel, Elbers, Noack, Schaefer, & Stäcker, 1994, 1995). In addition, a mild stress interview was conducted with the TG before the beginning and after completion of 4-month group therapy. It was anticipated that temporary stress-related changes in the current immune status can be mitigated as a result of participation in the group. HIV-negative homosexual and bisexual men who did not have any severe pre-existing conditions in the case history served as **control group** (CG2, $N = 31$). No changes in the pre-post comparison were anticipated here.

A topic currently classified by respective study participants as "considerable" to "highly burdensome" was addressed in the 30-min stress interview. With the TG it concerned a topic "related to one's own HIV infection", and with the CG2 it concerned such a topic "dealing with one's own homosexuality". Blood samples were analysed after an initial relaxation period (t1) immediately after the interview (t2) and after a second relaxation period (t3) for examination of immunological effects. Circulating lymphocyte subpopulations—which are of relevance for AIDS (CD4 and CD8 cells, CD4/CD8 ratio and NK cells)—were measured.

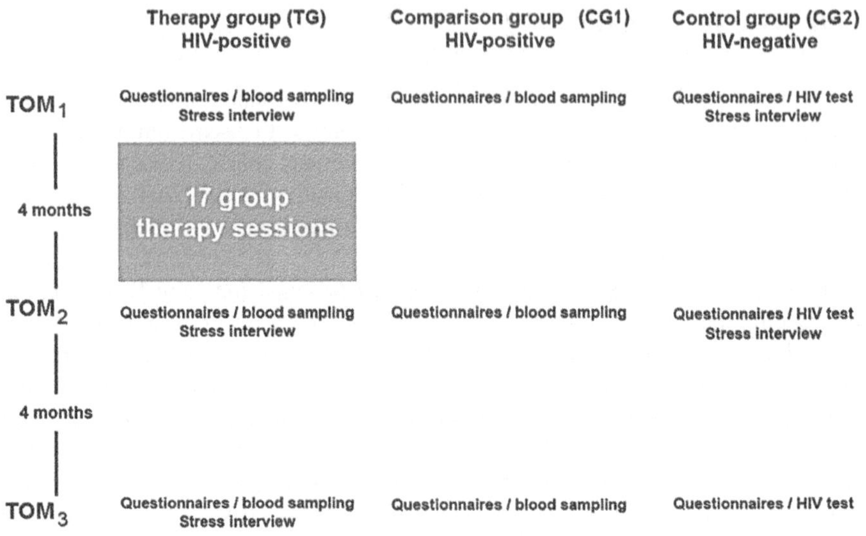

Fig. 9.1 Interconnection of Study 1 and 2

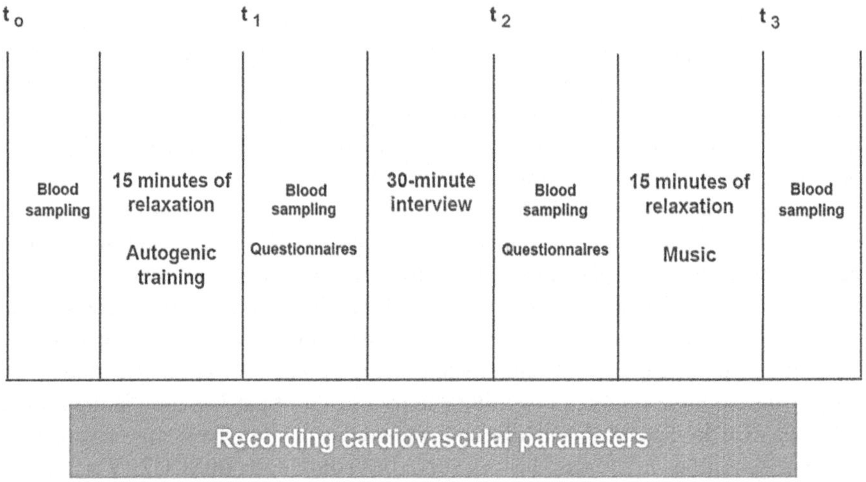

Fig. 9.2 Research design of stress interview (Study 2)

Emotional stress management strategies (positive self-instructions, resignation and self-pity) and the current state (general well-being, emotional irritability and anxiety) were surveyed at t1 and t2 to record the psychological stress effect of the interview among the study participants.

The interconnection of both studies (Fig. 9.1) and the research design of the stress interview (Study 2, Fig. 9.2) are graphically depicted for better understanding of the overall investigation.

The **group concept** for the TG was tailored to the needs of people infected with HIV and aimed at strengthening the psychological level of adaptation. The focus of the supportive-cognitive treatment concept was the handling of the adaptation of participants to their current situation in life. External experts were consulted in three sessions to convey specific information (medicine, nutrition, psychosocial services). In addition to group cohesiveness and "recognising oneself in others", the therapists actively promoted the current coping attempts and thereby strengthened the self-help potential of participants.

Individual therapeutic objectives were developed in individual discussions with each participant. A group (each max. 9 participants) encompassed 16 sessions (120 min each) and an introductory meeting (180 min each). The opposite-sex therapist couple had years of group experience: one therapist had psychoanalytical experience, while the other had behavioural therapy experience. So the therapist couple covered different therapeutic orientations. The sessions started with a relaxation exercise, and a "lightning round" was always conducted at the beginning and end of sessions.

Results

The HIV patients (TG and CG1) were on average in their mid-30s, relatively well-educated and socioeconomically secure. The HIV-negative study participants (CG2) were significantly younger (M = 28 years); their level of education and their socio-economic status did not differ. TG and CG1 knew about their HIV infection for 3.2 years on average. Participation in group therapy was free of charge.

Study 1 Significant differences between the two study groups became apparent. The psychological state significantly improved in the TG, and the immune status remained stable. In comparison to the CG1, the TG turned out to be stressed more severely in psychological and immunological terms at the outset (differences in the baseline values), but the psychological levels of stress in the TG diminished significantly at the end of therapy and decreased to the level of the CG1. These improvements immediately upon completion of therapy remained stable or even partially strengthened at the catamnesis date. A significant reduction of "depression" and "anxiety" appeared with the TG; the same is applied to the tendency towards "self-blame". The health-related preventive behaviour (medication compliance, nutrition, exercise and other factors) tended to improve. At the second and third time of measurement (TOM), the TG also reported significantly more often about self-initiated positive life events than the GG1. Immediately after the end of therapy, 80% of the TG indicated having social contacts with other group members outside the group setting; 87% reported about this on the catamnesis date. Satisfaction with the group offer increased from "considerable" to "strong" on the catamnesis date. Altogether the social inclusion, health behaviour and life satisfaction improved overall under psychotherapeutic treatment. In the CG1 there were no changes of psychological state and coping with illness in the investigation period. In contrast, changes appeared in the immune status (CD8 cells, beta-2 microglobulin, free p24 antigen, Walter Reed stage), which indicated a progression of the HIV infection.

Even in this early study, the efficacy of a brief outpatient psychotherapeutic intervention was shown among men infected with HIV. This was substantiated despite relatively small samples, a rather short observation period and limited immunological measurement methodology (e.g. the "viral load" could not be determined yet at that time). The progression differences between TG and CG1—even if weak overall—are indicative of a psychoimmunological cause-effect correlation between psychotherapeutic intervention and disease prevention.

Study 2 During the stress interview, a result contrary to expectation was found in the somatic reaction to the psychological stressor: TG and CG2 responded in conformity and equally sensitive to the addressed contents on the immunological level in the 4-month longitudinal view. Statistically significant differences appeared neither in the cross section nor in the longitudinal view among the two experimental groups. Both groups responded similarly with statistically significant redistributions in the subpopulations of lymphocytes over the measurement phases (each with a significant increase of CD8 and NK cells at t2 in comparison to t1 and t3). In comparison to the initial and concluding relaxation phase, a significant increase in the heart rate as well as systolic and diastolic blood pressure was observed in both groups during the 30-min interview. As a result, they showed a stress reaction which could not be reduced to a physiological correlate of speech activity (cf. Linden, 1987; McCann et al., 1993). The stress interview, therefore, proved to be a stressor that was responded to with a sympathetically controlled adaptation reaction, which presumably resulted in catecholamine-mediate, short-term redistribution responses in the lymphocyte subpopulations.

With regard to coping with disease (trait level), a protective effect of the group offer became apparent with the TG. Immediately at the end of therapy and shortly before the start of the interview (t1), the TG indicated a tendency to respond to stress situations less with resignation (second TOM < first TOM), yet at the same time, their general well-being had significantly increased (second TOM > first TOM). A protective effect of group therapy was also substantiated during the psychological reaction (state level) to the stress interview: before start of therapy (first TOM), the members of the TG reacted to the stress interview significantly more anxious and with a tendency to be more irritated (t2 > t1). In contrast, statistically significant effects were no longer displayed after therapy (second TOM). In the HIV-negative GC2, significant changes were shown neither over the investigation phases (t1, t2) nor in the pre-post comparison (first vs. second TOM) with regard to the current emotional state.

Overall there was a protective effect of group therapy with regard to coping with disease, which was also substantiated on the level of current emotional reactions to a short-term psychosocial stressor. However, the originally formulated hypothesis concerning psychoimmunological cause-effect correlation with regard to short-term psychosocial stress could not be retained and had to be reformulated. The short-term immunological reactions in the form of reversible lymphocyte redistributions can rather be understood as an adaptive and therefore functional reaction to a current psychological threat scenario. The immune system is apparently still capable in an early stage of HIV infection (WR 1–3). Moreover, the HIV-positive as well as the HIV-negative study participants reacted somatically more sensitive to psychosocial stress as they could consciously perceive emotionally. This is of crucial importance for the understanding of somatisation processes and possibly can be explained on a neurophysiological level with the nonconscious processing of emotional stimuli in the limbic system already interconnected via the thalamus, which takes place faster than conscious prefrontal processing (LeDoux, 1998).

After all, a group therapy intervention can help—i.e. with less effort—to process a current psychosocial stressor, even if this does not apply to immune responses. Measurable short-term immunological effects possibly also do not represent any suitable predictor for such a complex disease process as HIV infection. The problem lies in the recording of characteristics such as patient and therapist variables as well as somatic parameters of different systems in the form of time samples. It is crucial whether the "sampling frequency" with which the measurements occur are in a meaningful ratio to the self-dynamic of recorded systems (Schiepeck, 2015).

Steps in the Development to a Therapeutic Group Offer

The patients were not easy to win over for participation in the group but—despite the time-consuming corollary surveys—reliably participated in the sessions. Previous positive experiences with (semi) professional help, a rather biopsychosocial understanding of disease and a successful "acknowledgement" regarding infection with significant individuals proved to be beneficial for a commitment to the group.

The patient evaluation of therapeutic elements rendered if anything a rejection of relaxation sessions but a high approval regarding the information units. Patients appreciate it when the therapists were active and the session was well-structured. They also evaluated the preparatory and follow-up individual sessions as helpful.

The preference of psychoeducational treatment components—whereby less was geared towards the immediate experience of relaxation than rather was given to rational, intellectualising, emotional detachment enabling preference to information—already became apparent in the preliminary studies to the investigation and determined the development of the final treatment concept. This development shall be briefly exemplified in the following by the observable defensive behaviour of patients (Schaefer, 1989; Schaefer & Paar, 1992).

The homosexual men diagnosed as HIV-positive showed defensive behaviour of coping with anxiety that can be attributed to the poles of repressive/evasive avoidance of attention (repression) from the threat vs. highly sensitive directing of attention (sensitisation) towards the illness (Lazarus, Eriksen, & Fonda, 1951).

Based on the repressive anxiety defence, denial, avoidance and displacement are paramount. For example, a patient who for weeks insisted on not being infected with HIV, but with cancer instead, exhibited extreme **denial**. He could only allow his HIV infection to become an inner reality in the course of group discussions and then also admit the reality of his illness in a private environment, which he experienced as relieving and constructive afterwards. Sexualised behavioural patterns can be categorised as **avoidance/displacement**. Group members frequently flirted with each other and made eroticising innuendos with regard to the female group therapist. This could be interpreted as an escape from threatening topics and thereby limited the discussion. The tendency to remain among themselves and not to confront themselves with the menacing progressing of the illness was scenically depicted in a separation referred to as **psychosocial split-off**. The interest in an openly arranged self-help group for HIV patients was very high, so that the participants should split into two group rooms. The groups formed spontaneously, depending on the stage of illness. In the further course of events, constructive group processes became apparent in the group of patients in the early stage of disease, whereas the other group of more severely ill patients soon chose to meet noncommittally to have coffee and cake and to ignore possible discussions about illness, infirmity and death as they were burdensome.

Some patients stood out by seeking to ward off precisely this latent threat by means of *intensified directing of attention*. For example, after notification of diagnosis, one patient immediately bought a gravesite with the little money he had. He worried about having to die soon and was afraid that his family—who did not know about his homosexuality yet—would refuse to bury him. When he managed to "out himself" with regard to his sexual orientation and his HIV infection, he sold the gravesite again. Some patients exhibited a correspondingly **sensitive degree of coping with anxiety** already in the first group sessions when they drastically reported the death of their companion in life, which overburdened the group members, created a paralysing climate and led to the early dissolution of one group.

These examples illustrate which tensions can build up solely through witnessing various forms of coping with anxiety (retreat from danger vs. flight forward). Consequently, it was easily comprehensible that under the acute threat of AIDS, the feedback of patients showed that they wished less attention to their emotional experience rather than called for structuring, regulative intervention which made coping with everyday life easier. The helpful relationship with the group leadership was therefore less sought in an empathetic understanding of the suffering than rather in stabilising interventions which support mature defence mechanisms and enable an objectifying attitude in dealing with impairments due to illness. So the group leadership had to provide itself as a "helping ego" in order to avoid being overwhelmed with anxiety and to make dealing with anxiety more manageable. Accordingly, the promotion of group cohesiveness existed less in the mutual identification with the suffering rather than in the task to support mutual identification with active coping behaviour. Therefore the patients could remain easier in the "window of tolerance", so that they could improve to handle the traumatic experience of being HIV-positive (Porges & Carter 2010). Correspondingly, the goal of the psychotherapeutic intervention consisted of a mixture of focus and defence with simultaneous activation of bonding behaviour. In this respect there was no "trauma-focused" group concept but rather a "present-centred" group concept, because the group dealt with present problems (Spiegel, Classen, Thurston, & Butler, 2004).

How Has the Treatment of HIV Patients Developed Further?

With the introduction of HAART, HIV has become a treatable chronic disease for many people, although it is at times linked with high rates of medicinal adverse effects. Nevertheless, the prevalence of HIV infections has increased among the mentally ill. At the same time, higher comorbidity with psychological disorders is found among people infected with HIV. By now, age cohorts have grown up; these people have been infected with HIV for many years and have to deal with other chronic problems than in former times, such as age-related processes, cognitive impairments and dementia (Beck et al., 2010; Clifford et al., 2017).

According to a cohort study, the survival prognosis has gradually improved from 1996 to 2013. Estimates concerning life expectancy with a 20-year-old European man who starts antiretroviral therapy between 2008 and 2010 (and has a sufficient number of CD4 cells) predict a life expectancy of 78.0 years (The Antiretroviral Therapy Cohort Collaboration, 2017). After diagnosis, the confrontation with a life-threatening disease and the adaptation to a complex treatment regimen also persist today. The enforced regular intake of medication, dealing with adverse effects, the permanent concern about failure of therapy, anxieties about the future and social isolation can repeatedly shake self-esteem and lead to mood instability or depressions (van der Heijden & Abrahams, 2013). The challenge now is to maintain a high degree of adherence in order to achieve maximum efficacy.

HIV as a chronic disease requires various adaptation processes comparable to those of other chronic diseases. The task in terms of care/treatment is phase-appropriate support, whereby—depending on personality style—advantageous defensive patterns are supported and dysfunctional patterns are critically examined (Novalis, Rojcewicz, & Peele, 1993).

Despite the improved medical treatment of HIV infection, the search for effective psychotherapeutic/psychosocial interventions for patients consequently remains. On the one hand, the psychoimmunological associations found under earlier forms of medical treatment can also be confirmed in the HAART era (Belanoff et al., 2000). Psychosocial factors have decisive influence on the biomarkers of HIV infection, i.e. they predict changes in the CD4 cells and the viral load (e.g. Ironson et al., 2005). On the other hand, HIV patients still respond variable to new treatment. Secured interventions which slow down the disease progression and have a favourable effect on the immune status as well as the psychological adaptation, i.e. in terms of protecting health, reducing risk behaviour and ensuring compliance with therapy are still to be found (Gonzales, Batchelder, Psaros, & Safren, 2011).

Psychological interventions can be geared towards a reduction of negative factors such as depressive symptoms, stress experience and adverse stress management (e.g. evasive coping) as well as the strengthening of positive factors such as optimism, the experience of self-efficacy and favourably active coping. As various longitudinal studies substantiate (Carrico & Antoni, 2008), both classes of interventions have a decelerating effect on disease prevention but only if it is possible to successfully improve the psychological adaptation. The extent of change in the psychological adaptation therefore determines the effects on the somatic level, i.e. biomarkers of immune status and neuroendocrine regulation. In turn, an improved psychological adaptation has positive effects on compliance with therapy. At the same time, the range of examined interventions is quite large (van Luenen et al., 2017): **symptom-oriented interventions** (cognitive behavioural therapy, stress management, interpersonal therapy), **supportive interventions** (support, psychoeducation), **meditative interventions** (mindfulness, meditation, relaxation) and **physical exercise**. These effective interventions were even extensively taken into account in our own work.

The advantage of group-related interventions lies in the chance to share experienced and feared isolation with people who have to live with the same diagnosis, to reduce feelings of difference and to develop a feeling of commonly shared solidarity. Group membership conveys a benefit in terms of psychosocial and motivational support, presumably in comparable disease stages.

So with HIV infection, there are verifiable psychosomatic associations, which is indicative of earlier as well as subsequent studies. Based on the substantiated longer lifetime with the disease, more extensive topics to be therapeutically treated could be anticipated. A recent meta-analytic study shows that according to available investigations, therapeutic doses of 12–18 h render the largest effect size. Moreover, influences on the professional qualification of therapists on treatment results can be found (van Luenen et al., 2017). It is even more gratifying that already short, possibly recurrent psychological aids which provide support in finding meaning and hope may be sufficient to favourably influence adaptation and thereby the course of disease. However, booster session should follow in order to stabilise active effects on a long-term basis, as this has been shown in treatments of depression.

Acknowledgements We would like to thank our scientific colleagues from the Clinic for Dermatology, Venerology and Allergology (Professor Dr. med. M. Goos, PD Dr. med. N.H. Brockmeyer, Dr. med. L. Mertins), the Centre for Internal Medicine (Prof. Dr. med. G. Brittinger, Dr. med. H.-P. Böck), the Institute of Immunology (Prof. Dr. med. H. Grosse-Wilde) and the Clinic for Psychotherapy and Psychosomatic Medicine (Prof. Dr. med. W. Senf) for their active support in the implementation of the research project.

References

Beck, B. J., Freudenreich, O., & Worth, J. L. (2010). Patients with human immunodeficiency virus infection and acquired immunodeficiency syndrome. In T. A. Stern, G. L. Friccione, N. Cassem, M. S. Jellinek, & J. F. Rosenbaum (Eds.), *Massachusetts General Hospital: Handbook of general hospital psychiatry* (6th ed.). (pp. 353–370). Philadelphia: Saunders Elsevier.

Belanoff, J. K., Sund, B., Koopmann, C., Blasey, C., Flamm, J., Schatzberg, A. F., & Spiegel, D. (2000). A randomized trial of group therapy in changing viral load and CD4 counts in individuals living with HIV infection. *The International Journal of Psychiatry in Medicine, 35*, 349–362.

Breukel, M., Elbers, G., Noack, R., Schaefer, A., & Stäcker, K.-H. (1994). *Reproducible changes in emotional, cardiovascular and immunological parameters on an acute psychosocial stressor in HIV-positive and HIV-negative homosexual men*. Unpublished manuscript, pp. 1–34.

Breukel, M., Elbers, G., Noack, R., Schaefer, A., & Stäcker, K.-H. (1995). Therapiebedingte Veränderung der emotionalen und immunologischen Reaktion auf einen akuten emotionalen Stressor bei HIV-infizierten homosexuellen Männern. In G. Hüsler (Ed.), *HIV und Psychoimmunologie—Stand der Forschung in Deutschland und in der Schweiz* (pp. 82–105). Bern: Stämpfli*Cie AG.

Brodt, H. R., Helm, E. B., Werner, A., Joetten, A., Bergmann, L., Klüver, A., & Stille, W. (1986). Spontanverlauf der LAV/HTLV-III-Infektion: Verlaufsbeobachtungen bei Personen aus AIDS-Risikogruppen. *Deutsche Medizinische Wochenschrift, 31*(32), 1175–1180.

Carrico, A. W., & Antoni, M. H. (2008). The effects of psychological interventions on neuroendocrine hormone regulation and immune status in HIV-positive persons. *Psychosomatic Medicine, 70*(5), 575–584.

Chida, Y., & Vedhara, K. (2009). Adverse psychosocial factors predict poorer prognosis in HIV disease. A meta-analytic review for prospective investigations. *Brain, Behavior, and Immunity, 23*, 434–445.

Clifford, K., Samboju, V., Cobigo, Y., Milanini, B., Marx, G., Hellmuth, J., … Valcour, V. (2017). Progressive brain atrophy despite viral suppression in HIV patients older than 60 years. *Journal of Acquired Immune Deficiency Syndromes, 76*(3), 289–297.

Fätkenheuer, G. (2015, May 6). *HIV-Therapie: Je früher, desto besser*. Pressemitteilung des Deutschen Zentrums für Infektionsforschung.

Fischer, G., & Riedesser, P. (1998). *Lehrbuch der Psychotraumatologie*. (pp. 120–179). München: Ernst Reinhard.

Gonzales, J. S., Batchelder, A. W., Psaros, C., & Safren, S. A. (2011). Depression and HIV/AIDS treatment nonadherence: A review and metanalysis. *Journal of Acquired Immune Deficiency Syndromes, 58*(2), 181–187.

Ironson, G., O'Cleirigh, C., Fletscher, M. A., Laurenceau, J. P., Balbin, E., Klima, N., … Solomon, G. (2005). Psychosocial factors predict CD4 and viral load change in men and women with human immunodeficiency virus in the era of highly active antiretroviral treatment. *Psychosomatic Medicine, 67*(/6), 1013–1014.

Lazarus, R. S., Eriksen, C. W., & Fonda, C. P. (1951). Personality dynamics and auditory perceptual recognition. *Journal of Personality, 19*, 471–482.

LeDoux, J. (1998). *Das Netz der Gefühle—Wie Emotionen entstehen*. (pp. 163–191). München: Carl Hanser.

Linden, W. A. (1987). A microanalysis of autonomic activity during speech. *Psychosomatic Medicine, 49*, 562–578.

McCann, B. S., Carter, J., Vaughan, M., Raskind, M., Wilkinson, C. O. W., & Veith, R. (1993). Cardiovascular and neuroendocrine responses to extended laboratory challenge. *Psychosomatic Medicine, 55*, 497–504.

McEwen, B. S. (2007). Physiology and neurobiology of stress and adaption: Central role of the brain. *Physiology Reviews, 87*(3), 873–904.

Moskowitz, J. T., Hult, J. R., Bussolari, C., & Acree, M. (2009). What works in coping with HIV? A meta-analysis with implications for coping with serious illness. *Psychological Bulletin, 135*, 121–141.

Novalis, P. N., Rojcewicz, S. J., & Peele, R. (1993). *Clinical manual of supportive psychotherapy*. Washington: American Psychiatric Press.

Porges, S. W., & Carter, C. S. (2010): Neurobiological Basis of Social Behavior across the Life Span. In: M.E. Lamb & A.M. Freund (Eds.): *The Handbook of Life-Span Development. Volume 2: Social and Emotional Development*. (pp.9–50). Hoboken: John Wiley.

Schaefer, A. (1989). Begleitete Selbsthilfe—Psychotherapeutische Gruppenarbeit mit HIV-Infizierten, deren Angehörigen und Partnern. In S. R. Dunde (Ed.), *Psychotherapie bei HIV-Infektionen und AIDS* (pp. 30–35). Bonn: Deutscher Psychologen Verlag GmbH.

Schaefer, A. (1998). *Zum Einfluss ambulanter Gruppentherapie auf das psychische und körperliche Wohlbefinden von HIV-positiven homo- und bisexuellen Männern im Krankheitsstadium WR 1–3*. (pp. 103–222). Dissertation an der Universität-Gesamthochschule-Essen.

Schaefer, A., Noack, R., Elbers, G., Breukel, M., Paar, G., & Stäcker, K.-H. (1995). Psychosoziale und immunologische Veränderungen nach ambulanter Gruppentherapie bei homo- und bisexuellen HIV-Infizierten Männern. In G. Hüsler (Ed.), *HIV und Psychoimmunologie—Stand der Forschung in Deutschland und in der Schweiz* (pp. 134–170). Bern: Stämpfli*Cie AG.

Schaefer, A., & Paar, G. (1992). Ambulante Gruppentherapie mit HIV-Infizierten. In M. Ermann & B. Waldvogel (Eds.), *HIV-Betroffene und ihr Umfeld* (pp. 181–189). Berlin: Springer.

Schiepeck, G. (2015). Der psychotherapeutische Prozess—Einblicke in die Selbstorganisation bio-psycho-sozialer Systeme. In C. Schubert (Ed.), *Psychoneuroimmunologie und Psychotherapie* (pp. 395–417). Stuttgart: Schattauer.

Scott-Sheldon, L. A. J., Kalichman, S. C., Carey, M. P., & Fielder, R. L. (2008). Stress management interventions for HIV + adults. A meta-analysis of randomized controlled trials, 1989 to 2006. *Health Psychology, 27*, 129–139.

Spiegel, D., Classen, C., Thurston, E., & Butler, L. (2004). Trauma-focused versus present-focused models of group therapy for women sexually abused in childhood. In L. J. Koenig, L. S. Doll, A. O'Leary, & W. Pequenat (Eds.), *From child sexual abuse to adult sexual risk: Trauma, revictimization, and intervention* (pp. 251–268). Washington, DC: American Psychological Association Press.

The Antiretroviral Therapy Cohort Collaboration. (2017). Survival of HIV-positive patients starting antiretroviral therapy between 1996 and 2013: A collaborative analysis of cohort studies. *Lancet HIV, 4*, e349–e356.

van der Heijden, I., & Abrahams, N. (2013, 2013). Psychosocial group interventions for improving quality of life in adults living with HIV. *Cochrane Database of Systematic Reviews*, (11), CD010806, 1–7.

van Luenen, S., Garnefski, N., Spinhoven, P., Spaan, P., Dusseldorp, E., & Kraaij, V. (2017). The benefits of psychosocial interventions for mental health in people living with HIV: A systematic review and meta-analysis. *AIDS and Behaviour, 22*(1), 9–42.

Weber, C. S., Atanackovic, D., & Deter, H. C. (2015). Einfluss von Stressmanagement auf Elemente des Immunsystems. In C. Schubert (Ed.), *Psychoneuroimmunology und Psychotherapie* (pp. 303–325). Stuttgart: Schattauer.

Weinel, E. (2017). HIV-Infektion und Aids. In T. von Uexküll (Ed.), *Psychosomatische Medizin* (8. Auflage, (pp. 935–946). Urban & Fischer: München.

Chapter 10
Accept Pain for a Vital Life: Acceptance and Commitment Therapy for the Treatment of Chronic Pain

Maria Karekla, Marianna Zacharia, and Maria Koushiou

What Is Chronic Pain?

A frequently cited and widely adopted definition of chronic pain is provided by the International Association for the Study of Pain (IASP) and defines chronic pain as an "unpleasant physical and emotional experience, a combination of real and virtual tissue damage, that can last for longer than the expected time needed for the damage to heal" (Merskey & Bogduk, 1994, pp. 210–211). Chronic pain is characterized by a long duration (i.e., months or years), subsequent to a potential illness, or is related to tissue damage that despite the passage of time has not healed (IASP, 1994). The typical tissue healing time is considered to be 3 months (Chou et al., 2009; IASP, 1994).

Chronic pain arises in the context of various illnesses and syndromes (Gureje, Von Korff, Simon, & Gater, 1998; Verhaak, Kerssens, Dekker, Sorbi, & Bensing, 1998). A wide range of common conditions with diverse psychophysiologies involve chronic pain (e.g., fibromyalgia, migraine, osteoarthritis, cancer, diabetic neuropathy, degenerative spine disease, postherpetic neuralgia, and human immunodeficiency virus; Fine, 2011). The most common causes of chronic pain according to the Pain Proposal Patient Survey (2010) are back pain (55%), joint pain (46%), neck pain (34%), and headache (22%).

M. Karekla (✉) · M. Zacharia
Department of Psychology, University of Cyprus, Nicosia, Cyprus
e-mail: mkarekla@ucy.ac.cy

M. Koushiou
Department of Social Sciences, University of Nicosia, Nicosia, Cyprus
e-mail: koushiou.m@unic.ac.cy

C. Charis, G. Panayiotou (eds.), *Somatoform and Other Psychosomatic Disorders*,
https://doi.org/10.1007/978-3-319-89360-0_10

Chronic Pain: A Complex Experience

Chronic pain is a complex multifaceted phenomenon that incorporates both physical and psychological components (Gatchel, 1999). More specifically, patients' experience of chronic pain constitutes a subjective sensory and emotional experience (IASP, 1994), which may be affected by the patient's biological, social, environmental, and psychological factors (Gaikwad, Vanlint, Moseley, Mittinty, & Stocks, 2017). These factors along with expectations and belief systems influence individual experiences and treatment outcomes (Gaikwad et al., 2017; Oliver, 1993; Williams, 1994). Thus, it is vital to acknowledge that physical and psychological factors usually exist and overlap in chronic pain conditions, accentuating the significance of a quality-based physical examination prior to characterizing the problem as merely psychological (Feinberg & Brigham, 2013). Nevertheless, it is also vital to consider the social and psychological dimensions of the chronic pain experience.

Prevalence of Chronic Pain

A systematic review of 15 epidemiological studies of adults with chronic pain demonstrated prevalence estimates ranging from 2 to 40% (Verhaak et al., 1998). A qualitative systematic review of chronic pain that incorporated 17 epidemiological studies indicated prevalence estimates ranging from 7 to 55% (Nickel & Raspe, 2001). Additionally, a systematic review of 13 studies published between 1991 and 2002 indicated chronic pain prevalence rates from 12 to 55% of the population (Ospina & Harstall, 2002). A more recent study shows prevalence estimates of chronic pain between 8 and 48% in the general population and a weighted average prevalence of 22% (Andrew, Derry, Taylor, Straube, & Phillips, 2014).

Approximately 100 million Americans are living with chronic pain, suggesting that around half of American adults have a chronic pain condition (Institute of Medicine of the National Academies Report, 2011; Milton, 2013). A study of chronic pain in Europe demonstrated that 1 in 5 individuals older than 18 years old experiences chronic pain for more than 6 months (Breivik, Collett, Ventafridda, Cohen, & Gallacher, 2006). Similarly, a more recent systematic review of chronic noncancer pain in Europe indicates that the 1-month prevalence of moderate-to-severe pain is 19% (Reid et al., 2011). Almost 50% of individuals experiencing chronic pain report suffering with pain for more than 10 years, and of those, 66% report experiencing moderate pain, 34% severe pain, and 46% constant pain compared to 54% who report intermittent pain (Breivik et al., 2006). Thus one-third of chronic pain sufferers rate their pain intensity as severe, and almost half of them experience pain constantly.

The most frequent site of chronic pain is the lower back, and the most commonly reported cause is arthritis (Breivik et al., 2006). Chronic low back pain accounts for more disability compared to any other condition (Gatchel & Okifuji, 2006). With

1-year prevalence rates exceeding 60–70% and lifetime prevalence rates reaching more than 80%, back pain now constitutes one of the leading health problems in the adult population (Schmidt & Kohlmann, 2005; Schumacher & Brähler, 1999; Wenig, Schmidt, Kohlmann, & Schweikert, 2009).

Moreover, it is important to emphasize that the prevalence of chronic pain tends to be higher in women (16.5–21.5%) and the elderly (23.9–31.3%), with women older than 65 years old representing the majority of pain sufferers (26.0–34.2%; Reitsma, Tranmer, Buchanan, & Vandenkerkhof, 2011). Also, the prevalence of neuropathic pain is estimated at a range between 3 and 18% (Bouhassira, Lantéri-Minet, Attal, Laurent, & Touboul, 2008; Torrance, Smith, Bennett, & Lee, 2006), and the weighted average prevalence is 7% (Andrew et al., 2014).

Chronic Pain Consequences

Chronic pain is associated with significant disability and constitutes a considerable burden not only to the patient but also to the healthcare system and to society in general (Aronoff, 1991; Henry, 2008). In fact, chronic pain constitutes the most common cause of disability, as it impacts mood, mental health, sleep, quality of life, physical, work, social, sexual, and family functioning and has direct and indirect costs on healthcare systems (Dueñas, Ojeda, Salazar, Mico, & Failde, 2016; Fine, 2011; Green, Ndao-Brumblay, & Hart-Johnson, 2009). The aforementioned consequences of chronic pain are elucidated below.

Impact on Mood, Mental Health, and Sleep

Several studies demonstrate that chronic pain patients are more likely to develop mental health problems compared to individuals without chronic pain (Fine, 2011; Gureje et al., 1998). Chronic pain is related to increased rates of sleep disturbance, anxiety, depression (Green et al., 2009; Greenberg, Leong, Birnbaum, & Robinson, 2003; Ohayon & Schatzberg, 2003), suicidal ideation, and twice more suicide attempts than nonpain individuals (Ratcliffe, Enns, Belik, & Sareen, 2008; Tang & Crane, 2006). Around 21% of chronic pain patients are diagnosed with depression, and 35.1% have an anxiety disorder compared to respective 9.3% of depression and 18.1% of anxiety in the general population (Breivik et al., 2006; McWilliams, Cox, & Enns, 2003).

A noteworthy study by Demyttenaere et al. (2007) has examined the prevalence of mental disorders in chronic back and neck pain patients by employing the Composite International Diagnostic Interview across 17 countries globally. Results demonstrated elevated prevalence of anxiety disorders (i.e., generalized anxiety disorder, panic disorder), mood disorders, and alcohol abuse/dependence in chronic pain patients compared to nonpain individuals both in developing and developed countries. Similarly, a study by Kroenke et al. (2013) assessed the relationship between anxiety and health-related quality of life in patients with chronic musculoskeletal pain, and the results demonstrated that almost half of the chronic pain patients have one or more anxiety disorders. Also, chronic pain patients with comorbid anxiety and pain were adversely associated with diminished quality of life and significant functional impairment in relation to either of these populations alone, even when controlling for depression. Moreover, empirical evidence suggests that pain, anxiety, and depression often co-occur and lead to additional and more adverse effects on functional impairment, health-associated quality of life, as well as treatment response (Bair, Robinson, Katon, & Kroenke, 2003; Bair, Wu, Damush, Sutherland, & Kroenke, 2008; Löwe et al., 2008).

Furthermore, the emotional experience of chronic pain patients is mostly characterized by sadness, fear, and anger, contrary to otherwise healthy populations who encounter frequent positive emotions (i.e., happiness; Finucane, Dima, Ferreira, & Halvorsen, 2012). Anger and frustration are the strongest and most common feelings reported by chronic pain patients, particularly for those whose future objectives are reliant on pain alleviation (Bruehl, Chung, & Burns, 2003; Carson et al., 2005, 2005; Greenwood, Thurston, Rumble, Waters, & Keefe, 2003; Morley, Davies, & Barton, 2005; Okifuji, Turk, & Curran, 1999). According to Okifuji et al. (1999), extended deterioration in functioning, a sense of hopelessness, and perception of pain as a key aspect of one's life enhance frustration resulting in higher levels of negative attributions regarding oneself. In fact, empirical studies indicate that chronic pain is related to anger and hostility toward oneself and toward others (Greenwood et al., 2003; Okifuji et al., 1999), self-criticism (Rudich, Lerman, Gurevich, Weksler, & Shahar, 2008), self-blame (Cedraschi et al., 2013), diminished acceptance of one's physical restraints (Risdon, Eccleston, Crombez, & McCracken, 2003), as well as frustration and disappointment with pain (Dow, Roche, & Ziebland, 2012). Additionally, anger in chronic pain patients is associated with poor response to pain treatment (Burns, Higdon, Mullen, Lansky, & Wei, 1999; Burns, Johnson, Devine, Mahoney, & Pawl, 1998).

Often co-occurring with chronic pain are sleep disturbances, since they are reported by 50–89% of patients (Fine, 2011; Marty et al., 2008; McCracken & Iverson, 2002; Morin, Gibson, & Wade, 1998). Sleep disorders can augment stress levels and impair patients' cognitive ability and performance of simple everyday tasks both at the workplace and at home (Tüzün, 2007). The extent of sleep disturbance is found to directly associate with pain severity (Alsaadi, McAuley, Hush, & Maher, 2011; Marin, Cyhan, & Miklos, 2006). A bidirectional relationship is demonstrated between sleep and pain, with a night of sleep disturbance being followed by an amplification in pain intensity the next day, and vice versa, forming a vicious cycle (O'Brien et al., 2011). Sleep problems in pain patients can further contribute to more psychopathologies and problems in a patients' life, including decreases in quality of life, which we turn to next.

Impact on Quality of Life

Chronic pain menaces the quality of life of individuals (Green, Hart-Johnson, & Loeffler, 2011). Patients experiencing frequent and severe pain have a lower quality of life than those who experience less frequent pain and with moderate intensity (Langley, Pérez Hernández, Margarit Ferri, Ruiz Hidalgo, & Lubián López, 2011). Diminished quality of life is found in both the physical and mental dimensions compared to patients experiencing acute pain or those with no pain (Lopez-Silva, Sanchez de Enciso, Rodriguez-Fernandez, & Vazquez-Seijas, 2007; McCarberg, Nicholson, Todd, Palmer, & Penles, 2008). Significant declines in all quality of life aspects are demonstrated in conditions such as low back pain, rheumatoid arthritis, and fibromyalgia (Campos & Vázquez, 2012; Carmona, Ballina, Gabriel, & Laffon, 2001).

Impact on Physical, Work, Social, Family, and Sexual Functioning

A strong association exists between chronic pain and diminished physical activity (Azevedo, Costa-Pereira, Mendonça, Dias, & Castro-Lopes, 2012; Lerman, Rudich, Brill, Shalev, & Shahar, 2015). The majority of patients with chronic pain suffer various difficulties, especially regarding their capacity to preserve an independent lifestyle, exercise, execute domestic tasks, and engage in social events and activities (Breivik et al., 2006).

Chronic pain deleteriously impacts the workplace of the patient. As a result of pain symptoms, patients exhibit problems of absenteeism, modify their occupational posts and duties, and may also lose their occupation (Blyth, March, Nicholas, & Cousins, 2003; Breivik et al., 2006; Patel et al., 2012). When examining the impact of diverse types of pain on work, it is demonstrated that the majority of sick leave days were found in back pain and pain due to rheumatic diseases (Burton, Morrison, Maclean, & Ruderman, 2006; Connolly, Fitzpatrick, O'Toole, Doran, & O'Shea, 2015; Tornero, Atance, Grupeli, & Vidal, 1998). In fact, low back pain constitutes one of the most commonly reported causes of job loss (Watson, Main, Waddell, Gales, & Purcell-Jones, 1998). A Spanish study indicated that nearly half of fibromyalgia patients lost their ability to work, 23% had a permanent disability pension due to recognized inability to work, and 30% had adaptations at work (Collado et al., 2014). As a result of pain, 61% of chronic pain patients state that their job performance was affected, 29% worry about the possibility of losing their job, 21% feel they are incapable of working, and 19% have lost their jobs due to their condition (Breivik et al., 2006; Pain Proposal, 2010). Also, "presenteeism" at work is a problem as even if patients attend work while being in pain, this leads to decreases in productivity and efficiency (Langley, Ruiz-Iban, Molina, De Andres, & Castellón, 2011), which is intensified as pain intensity augments (Patel et al., 2012).

Chronic pain also influences patients' social interactions (Porter, Keefe, Wellington, & de Williams, 2008), constraining their social contacts and attendance in family events and leisure activities (Moulin, Clark, Speechley, & Morley-Forster, 2002). The Pain Proposal Survey (2010) exhibits that 27% of patients report feeling isolated, 50% worry about the impact of their condition on their relationships, and 36% state that pain had a negative effect on their friends and families. Nearly half of chronic pain patients have less interaction with their families, 23% report low satisfaction levels with their family life, and 59% state numerous difficulties in their romantic relationships (Collado et al., 2014). Additionally, negative feelings of anger and irritability frequently affecting chronic pain patients also tend to have a deleterious effect on stress levels in families and on interpersonal relationships (Henwood & Ellis, 2004). Both the patients and their family members report that factors having the most adverse effects on family are mood swings, decrease in leisure activities, and the perception of sadness in the family (Ojeda et al., 2014).

Furthermore, an elevated prevalence of sexual dysfunction is found in chronic pain patients, with 54–63% reporting such impairments (Ambler, de C Williams, Hill, Gunary, & Cratchley, 2001; Ryan, Hill, Thwaites, & Dawes, 2008). Problems with performance, arousal, sexual positions, confidence, relationships, and fear of pain aggravation, all are commonly reported by patients (Ambler et al., 2001). Ryan et al. (2008) demonstrated that fibromyalgia adversely influences sexual relationships by alleviating sexual intercourse's enjoyment and frequency. The reported contributing factors of sexual difficulties were physical symptoms related with the condition, such as pain, fatigue, perceived joint stiffness, diminished movement, and low mood. Findings suggest that sexual dysfunction in chronic pain patients is not just associated with mood (Ambler et al., 2001).

Overall, it is evident that chronic pain can adversely affect mood, mental health, sleep, quality of life, as well as physical, work, social, sexual, and interpersonal functioning.

Direct and Indirect Costs of Chronic Pain

In addition to the above consequences of pain, there is ample evidence showing that chronic pain causes a significant economic burden and has substantial direct and indirect costs. Direct costs of chronic pain entail costs related to medication or treatments, unsuccessful interventions (i.e., additional doctor visits), costs resulting from a lack of suitable facilities locally (endured by patients, their families, and health services), and costs stemming from preventing adverse events that arise due to prescribing decisions (i.e., certain medications; Pain Proposal, 2010 ; Phillips, 2001). Patients with severe pain visit their doctor on average 13 times in 6 months, which is twice the average in the general population doctor visits (National Health and Wellness Survey, 2014). Direct costs of chronic pain are estimated annually to €187 million in Belgium (Van Zundert & Van Kleef, 2005), €289 million ($368 million) in the Netherlands (Van Tulder, Koes, & Bouter, 1995), and €1.9 billion (£1.6 billion) in the UK (Maniadakis & Gray, 2000). The total annual costs of chronic pain in the USA are over half a trillion dollars (Institute of Medicine of the National Academies Report, 2011). Medical costs associated with chronic pain surpass the costs of cancer, heart disease, and AIDS combined (Manchikanti, 2006).

The indirect costs of chronic pain entail costs of disability benefits, lost productivity and work absenteeism, family burden (i.e., home care and loss of earnings), social security benefits, and decreased quality of life for the patients and their families (Pain Proposal, 2010; Phillips, 2001). Chronic pain reductions in work productivity and labor market participation as well as increases in absenteeism from work result in 1.2–7.8 times higher costs than in nonpain individuals (Andrew et al., 2014; Davis, Robinson, Le, & Xie, 2011; Langley et al., 2010).

The total yearly cost of the most prominent sources of chronic pain (both direct and indirect costs), like musculoskeletal disorders and back pain, may vary between €1.1 billion in Finland and almost €50 billion in Germany (Mäntyselkä, Kumpusalo, Ahonen, & Takala, 2002). The average annual costs of back pain per person are €1322 (95% CI [1173–1487]; Wenig et al., 2009). The total cost of chronic pain across Europe is estimated at around €300 billion annually (Wenig et al., 2009).

Pain vs. Suffering

A conclusion that can be drawn from the information discussed in the previous section is that chronic pain accounts for substantial healthcare expenditure. Also, concerns are raised regarding the effectiveness of medical interventions. It appears that the available medical interventions do not reliably alleviate the severity of pain or ameliorate functioning, as 38% of European chronic pain patients state that their pain is not sufficiently managed by typical medical interventions (Pain Proposal, 2010). Thus, despite the availability of treatment options, chronic pain still severely affects the quality of life of patients as almost half of them do not attain sufficient pain management (Breivik et al., 2006). Additionally, the path via the healthcare system may be long, complicated, and ineffective for chronic pain patients as it includes contradictory advice and numerous interventions (Breivik et al., 2006; Dewar, Gregg, White, & Lander, 2009). Many treatments and medications are prescribed and tested in order to alleviate the pain to a tolerable degree, which is often not achieved (Hylands-White, Duarte, & Raphael, 2017). In fact, when analgesic medication (first-line intervention for pain) is given, patients rarely attain lasting pain relief (Hylands-White et al., 2017), with on average only 30% decrease in pain from opioids (Kalso, Edwards, Moore, & McQuay, 2004). Also, several studies indicate that both patients and physicians struggle with pain management, and a feeling of inadequacy is emphasized regarding the provision of optimal treatment among doctors (Green, Wheeler, Marchant, LaPorte, & Guerrero, 2001; Potter et al., 2001; Upshur, Luckmann, & Savageau, 2006). This contributes to patient dissatisfaction regarding the treatments provided (Turk, Wilson, & Cahana, 2011) and raises the questions of "what exactly are health professionals treating? Pain or suffering?" and "which one should they focus on in order to achieve better pain management and improve the quality of life of chronic pain patients?"

Traditional psychotherapeutic approaches (i.e., cognitive-behavioral therapy) to chronic pain emphasized pain control prior to mobilizing the patient to start moving and living (Hylands-White et al., 2017; McCracken & Vowles, 2006), treating mainly symptoms and attempting to reduce the severity of pain (similar to the goal of pharmacotherapy). Two Cochrane reviews of psychological therapies for the management of chronic pain in adults demonstrated that CBT has some small to moderate positive effects for pain, disability, and mood at posttreatment when compared to wait list or treatment as usual (Eccleston, Williams, & Morley, 2009; Williams, Eccleston, & Morley, 2012). Nevertheless, these treatment gains were not sustained at the 6-month follow-up, apart from a small effect of CBT on mood (Williams et al., 2012). The RCTs entailed in the reviews report findings with reference to statistical instead of clinical significance, raising the question as to the amount of chronic pain patients successfully treated by CBT (Eccleston et al., 2009). Overall, it appears that not all patients respond to CBT which has demonstrated only weak effectiveness in chronic pain.

Research stemming from the area of acceptance and commitment therapy (ACT) proposes that the emphasis on symptom reduction as a means to achieve well-being is unhelpful as it is impossible to directly control one's inner world (thoughts, emotions, sensations, memories, etc.) associated with the experience of pain (Hayes & Duckworth, 2006). McCracken and colleagues demonstrated that avoidance and the struggle to control pain (experiential avoidance) constitute the most significant, reliable, and independent predictor of greater disability, distress, suffering, depression, avoidance, hindered functioning, poorer activity, and worse pain in chronic pain patients (McCracken, Eccleston, & Bell, 2005; McCracken, Gauntlett-Gilbert, & Vowles, 2007). Individuals engaging in experiential avoidance have lower pain tolerance and endurance, and their recovery time is extended as they recover more slowly (Feldner et al., 2006).

Additionally, numerous studies indicate that acceptance of chronic pain, more specifically willingness to encounter pain without struggling or avoidance and persistence with pursuing activities, is associated with lower depression and anxiety levels and ameliorated daily functioning (McCracken, 1998; McCracken et al., 2005, 2007; McCracken & Eccleston, 2003). Empirical evidence also suggests that ACT is efficacious for treatment-resistant patients (Gloster et al., 2015) and is associated with lower dropout rates (Karekla, Constantinou, Ioannou, Gloster, & Kareklas, under review).

Numerous health professionals still focus on alleviating pain severity, attempting to change the form, content, and frequency of maladaptive cognitions and modify physical sensations in chronic pain patients. Nevertheless, empirical evidence elucidated above suggests that focusing on the aforementioned has not been considerably effective in ameliorating pain management and overall functioning in this particular population. Therefore, it is accentuated that there is a need to shift the treatment goal from one of reducing pain (i.e., intensity and severity) through control-oriented strategies to one of improving disability, suffering, life functioning, and quality of life through acceptance and valued living. Chronic pain patients may not have a choice as to whether they will experience pain or not, but they do have a choice as to whether they will suffer. It is the struggle with the pain, emotions, thoughts, and sensations, which seems to become the problem rather than pain itself. Thus, in chronic pain, suffering and impairments in functioning stem from attempts at controlling pain and its symptoms (Karekla, Karademas, & Gloster, 2018). This will be further expanded in the following section through the description of the theoretical framework of ACT.

Theoretical Framework of ACT and the Psychological Flexibility Model

ACT is a relatively new therapeutic approach rooted in radical behaviorism, based on relational frame theory (RFT, a behavioral theory of language and cognition; for more details see Blackledge, 2003) and the philosophy of functional contextualism (Hayes, Barnes-Holmes, & Wilson, 2012). ACT focuses on skills that foster acceptance and self and present-moment awareness while concurrently promoting valued actions (Hayes, Strosahl, & Wilson, 2011).

According to ACT, human suffering including problems with health conditions and psychopathology directly stems from context incongruent and inflexible behavioral patterns (Karekla et al., 2018). More specifically, problematic behaving is grounded on abstract rules formulated by the individual, instead of what is functional in this situation. The individual utilizes certain learned and rule-governed ways of addressing hardships, irrespective of the current context and whether these actions will bring about the desired outcomes. For example, a person may avoid attending a family gathering for fear that his/her pain will get worse, whereas the suffering (pain exacerbated by thoughts of missed opportunities and feelings such as guilt, sadness, frustration, etc.) may be immensely greater than (or exacerbate) the physical pain that would have been experienced. Thus, the individual responds in old habitual ways that may be ineffective and keep him/her "stuck" in his/her current situation. When the desired outcome (e.g., pain alleviation) is not achieved, individuals appraise the situation as hopeless and problematic, view themselves as ineffective, and experience augmented negative emotional reactions (i.e., sadness, distress, frustration). This can result in reproducing further ineffective actions (i.e., incorrect use of medicines, avoiding doctor's advice), creating a vicious cycle that for patients is difficult to break on their own (Karekla et al., 2018).

ACT aims to influence the individual's relationship with cognitions and emotions so as to reduce their impact on behavior (Hayes, Strosahl, & Wilson, 1999). This is achieved by regarding the experience of the individual within a context of personal values; encouraging acceptance of one's thoughts, emotions, and sensations; and committing to behavior change consistent with one's values (Hayes & Lillis, 2012). In doing so, ACT promotes psychological flexibility, which is its primary goal. Psychological flexibility is defined as the capacity to adapt to internal or external situational demands, "shift mindsets or behavioral repertoires when these strategies compromise personal or social functioning, maintain balance among important life domains, and be aware, open and committed to behaviors that are congruent with deeply held values" (Kashdan & Rottenberg, 2010, p. 865).

Psychological inflexibility is the opposite of psychological flexibility and is considered as the primary cause of psychopathology (Hayes, Luoma, Bond, Masuda, & Lillis, 2006). Psychological flexibility is comprised of six interrelated core skills developed to each address the contributors to psychological inflexibility (see Hayes et al., 2006, 2011): acceptance (vs. experiential avoidance), cognitive defusion (vs. cognitive fusion), contact with the present moment (vs. dominance of the conceptualized past and future), self as context (vs. attachment to a conceptualized self), values (vs. confusion about what is important for the person, behavior incongruous to one's values), and committed action (vs. inaction, impulsivity, or persistent avoidant behaving). Each of these skills is targeted in ACT and is elucidated below:

Acceptance vs. Experiential Avoidance

Experiential avoidance is the attempt to modify or control situational sensitivity, frequency, and form of internal experiences, such as emotions, memories, sensations, and thoughts, even in cases where such avoidance can lead to behavioral problems and contribute to suffering (Hayes, Wilson, Gifford, Follette, & Strosahl, 1996). Efforts to avoid painful private events are also verbal in nature and are associated with conceptualized adverse consequences, which contribute to narrowing of potential behavioral choices, since numerous behaviors can induce the dreaded private events (Hayes et al., 2006).

Experiential avoidance is associated with pathological physical, mental, and behavioral outcomes (Gloster, Meyer, & Lieb, 2017; Hayes et al., 2006). For instance, a chronic pain patient may try hard to avoid encountering any symptoms related to their condition (i.e., discomfort or pain) or may attempt to escape unwanted internal events, such as thoughts related to a disease (i.e., "Why me?"), and can engage in several ineffective actions (i.e., avoiding social events or exercise, taking excessive analgesic medicines) so as to accomplish this (Karekla et al., 2018). These attempts instead increase the unwanted private events, which further elicit more unhelpful actions (i.e., rumination, using substances, giving up, not going on vacations) as a way of avoiding contact with negative stimuli.

As a means of dealing with experiential avoidance, ACT proposes active acceptance of private events (Hayes et al., 2006). Acceptance entails actively embracing all private events (i.e., thoughts, emotions, sensations, memories) without attempting to alter their form, frequency, or content (Hayes et al., 2006). For instance, chronic pain patients are taught methods that promote letting go of their struggle with pain. Acceptance in ACT is promoted as a way of augmenting values-based action and does not constitute an end in itself. Methods utilized incorporate exercises that promote flexible interaction with experiences that were avoided in the past. Exposure exercises utilized aim to increase willingness to respond flexibly even in the face of strong emotions, worrisome thoughts, or pain (Luoma, Hayes, & Walser, 2007). ACT suggests observing these thoughts and feelings via a detective mindset. For instance, "What can I do when I treat this thought as just a thought and I do what is important to me even if it present without struggling with it?" instead of "What can I do when I treat this thought as a literal truth?" (Karekla et al., 2018). This enables the patient to explore thoughts and feelings, understand their function, and recognize them just as thoughts and feelings and not for what they say they are (i.e., menacing cognitive representations or beliefs about the illness). This aids to remove the "suffering" aspect of the pain experience.

Cognitive Defusion vs. Cognitive Fusion

Cognitive fusion pertains to extreme or inappropriate regulation of behavior through verbal processes (e.g., rules) and derived relational networks (Hayes et al., 1999). When behavior is controlled by certain verbal rules, it tends to become inflexible and rigid (Hayes, 1989). From an ACT perspective, the problem is not the utilization of an incorrect rule but instead that a verbally interpreted event that appears to be one thing is actually two things, namely, the event as well as the interpretation of the event (Luoma et al., 2007). What is problematic is *not what patients think* but *how patients relate to what they think*. Patients tend to forget that they are interacting with thoughts instead of the actual event. Thus, in cognitive fusion, cognitive/verbal formations replace direct contact with events (Luoma et al., 2007).

Cognitive defusion is the ability to observe inner private events (cognitions and emotions) from a distance in order to gradually realize that they do not constitute rules or facts that govern behavior but rather ways a person represents the world (and may be ineffective ways; Gillanders, Sinclair, MacLean, & Jardine, 2015). Numerous cognitive defusion techniques have been developed and include repeating a bothersome thought out loud until the only thing remaining is its sound; or physicalizing the thought by attributing to it a color, form, size, shape, or speed (Hayes et al., 2006); or thanking one's mind for having an "interesting" thought; or describing the process of thinking (e.g., "I am having the thought that nothing I do can help me with my symptoms"). In this way, the patient can watch what the mind says, without being a slave to it, and he/she can understand that it is only a thought/belief and not a fact (Harris, 2009). All these defusion exercises seek to decrease the literal quality of the thought, thus becoming more psychologically flexible in the process (Luoma et al., 2007). Therefore, cognitive defusion offers a new way of addressing dysfunctional illness representations by teaching patients to hold evaluations and thoughts lightly rather than fighting with them (Karekla et al., 2018).

Contact with the Present Moment vs. Dominance of the Conceptualized Past and Future

Contact with the present moment declines as a result of avoidance and cognitive fusion. Consequently, the continuing, flexible awareness of feelings, thoughts, sensations, and memories in the moment is diminished, since such an awareness will enable contact with experiences of pain, sadness, anger, and so on (Hayes et al., 2006). The conceptualized past and future takes over the present and gains regulatory control over behavior, further promoting psychological inflexibility. Specifically, behavior tends to be directed by previously programmed thoughts and responses, bringing about the same behavior that happened in the past, thus foreclosing novel possibilities (Luoma et al., 2007).

ACT promotes present-moment awareness. The purpose is to experience the world, including environmental and psychological events nonjudgmentally and directly as they unfold. In this way, patients' behavior becomes more flexible, and consequently their actions are more in line with their values (Hayes et al., 2006). Contact with the present moment is promoted through mindfulness exercises. Numerous mindfulness exercises exist and can be adapted for specific clients and their set of difficulties. In our recent pain protocols, we expand mindfulness exercises to include exposure to bothersome sensations (e.g., pain) where the therapist guides an individual through a mindfulness exercises and at the same time asks the person to focus their attention on the pain, to "dive into" the pain site, and in general to introduce new more appetitive relations with previously avoided sensations (see ALGEA study protocol; Karekla, Vasiliou, & Karademas, 2013).

Self as Context vs. Attachment to a Conceptualized Self

Conceptualized self is the term used to describe how a person describes and analyzes his/her attributes (Hayes et al., 1999). As the stories about the self become more stable over time, interpretations, expectations, and evaluations regarding the self are formed. For example, a person may conceptualize him/herself in association with a specific characteristic (e.g., "I am good person", "I am smart," etc.). When a person becomes "fused" with such attributes, especially ones related to a chronic health condition (e.g., "I am a migrainer," "I am a problem for others," "I am no good," etc.), there is a narrowing in the way the person regards themselves leading to inflexible behavioral patterns on the bases of these conceptualizations (termed also as "self as content"; Luoma et al., 2007). The specific experiences encountered when a person regards the world limit other experiences and aspects of the self to be expressed at the same time (e.g., "I am chronic pain patient" may interfere with "I am a good wife"). All this results in an attachment to a damaged conceptualized self.

In ACT, the skill of self as context is promoted so as to counter problematic. That is, rather than viewing the self as an experience, the self is viewed more like "a context or arena for experience" (Luoma et al., 2007, p. 19). The self as context is vital because an individual can be aware of his/her own flow of experiences without being attached to them or investing solely in specific experiences that occur. Therefore, acceptance and defusion are encouraged (Hayes et al., 2006). Experiential exercises and metaphors are employed to enable contact the sense of self as context. The purpose is to assist patients in developing a more solid sense of self as observers, independent of the specific experience they have at a particular moment ("I am more than my illness/my pain"; Luoma et al., 2007).

Lack of Values Clarity/Contact vs. Valued Directions

According to Wilson and Murrell (2004), values are the response to the question "In a world where you could choose to have your life be about something, what would you choose?" (p. 135). Values constitute long-term desired qualities of life; they cannot be attained as an object and "can be instantiated moment by moment" (Hayes et al., 2006, p. 9). When values are replaced by more immediate goals of looking and feeling good, protecting a conceptualized self, being right, etc., there is lack of values clarity (Hayes et al., 2006). That is, patients lose contact with what they want in life.

ACT employs various exercises to aid patients in choosing valued life directions in several domains, such as health, spirituality, career, and family. Additionally, ACT weakens verbal processes that lead to choices grounded on social compliance (e.g., "My father wants me to value X'), fusion (e.g., "A nice person would value Y"), or avoidance (e.g., "I would feel embarrassed if I did not value Z"; Hayes et al., 2006). A case study of a cancer patient receiving ACT has demonstrated that identifying and employing the patient's family and spiritual values facilitated acceptance of the illness facts (i.e., hair loss as part of a chosen treatment that could save her life and not as a punishment for not being a good Christian as her mind was telling her) and enabled better coping with the illness and living a meaningful life (Karekla & Constantinou, 2010).

Inaction, Impulsivity, or Avoidant Persistence vs. Committed Action

Patterns of action that are detached from patient's long-term values occur and progressively dominate in the patient's repertoire. As a result, behavioral repertoires become constricted and less sensitive to the options for valued-based action in the current context. Rigid persistence or impulsivity is exhibited rather than flexible behavior consistent with long-term values (Hayes et al., 2006). For example, when goals are not consistent with values, the patient is less likely to follow instructions of healthcare providers just because they told them to act in a certain way or simply because they have to (Karekla et al., 2018).

In ACT, the development of greater patterns of effective action associated with chosen values is strongly encouraged. More specifically, according to ACT in order to achieve successful behavior change and improved quality of life, it is important to initially clarify the patient's values, which are frequently unclear due to living with the disease and symptoms and because of cognitive fusion (Hayes et al., 2006). Subsequently, it is important to set health-related and other goals consistent with personal values (i.e., "I will walk for fifteen minutes per day in the service of my health, because I value being healthy" as opposed to "I have to walk for 15 minutes"; Karekla et al., 2018). Then, patients can commit to specific actions in order to reach these valued goals (Hayes et al., 2006; Karekla & Constantinou, 2010). Empirical evidence demonstrates that increasing valued behaviors precedes alleviations in suffering (Gloster et al., 2017), which accentuates the need for identifying personal value-driven goals for each patient. ACT protocols include several behavioral change methods, such as goal setting, exposure, shaping methods, and skills acquisition. When patients attempt behavior change that incorporates psychological barriers, these barriers are tackled via other ACT processes (acceptance, defusion, etc.; Hayes et al., 2006).

The six skills of ACT are interconnected and overlapping. Each skill supports the other, and all of them aim for psychological flexibility. They are allocated into two groups, mindfulness and acceptance as well as commitment and behavior change. Mindfulness and acceptance include acceptance, defusion, contact with the present moment, and self as context. Commitment and behavior change include contact with the present moment, self as context, values, and committed action (Hayes et al., 2006).

Overall, ACT encourages patients to view their entire experience with chronic pain as a whole (Karekla et al., 2018), that is, to accept and make room for things they cannot change (i.e., thoughts, feelings, memories, bodily sensations, a limitation that will be prevalent for a long time) and simultaneously commit to taking action so as to alter what can be changed (i.e., change a health behavior in the service of achieving a value-driven goal). Consequently, this is expected to lead to changes in the way the patient experiences and reacts to his/her condition, symptoms, and other difficulties (i.e., challenging private events; Karekla et al., 2018). This thorough discussion of the ACT framework raises the question of why might ACT be useful for this specific population.

Why Might ACT Be Useful in Chronic Pain?

Distress and negative beliefs about illness can be realistic in long-term conditions, like chronic pain at certain times (Graham, Gouick, Krahé, & Gillanders, 2016). The ACT intervention model can potentially be more effective as it focuses on value-directed actions and on accepting feelings and thoughts instead of making efforts to directly modify them, as proposed in traditional CBT (Graham, Simmons,

Stuart, & Rose, 2015; Low et al., 2012). Therefore, ACT acknowledges the normality of negative emotions and thoughts. Additionally, in contrast to traditional CBT interventions, ACT focuses on altering the relationship between illness representations and resulting behaviors instead of changing the content of these representations. According to Gloster et al. (2015), the aforementioned may constitute a salient reason explaining why ACT is particularly beneficial for treatment-resistant patients who do not respond to prior treatments. Also, with its additional constituents and alternative philosophy, ACT constitutes a broader approach to treatment that seems promising in offering further ameliorated treatment effects (Hulbert-Williams, Storey, & Wilson, 2015). In fact, empirical evidence suggests that ACT techniques are extensively employed by health professionals working within the field of long-term conditions (Thewes et al., 2014).

Empirical Research: The Broad Applicability of ACT

Based on the current literature, the effects of ACT on various psychological symptoms seem promising (Abad, Bakhtiari, Kashani, & Habibi, 2016). The effectiveness of ACT has been demonstrated across a wide variety of populations, including individuals experiencing several psychological symptoms and patients with chronic health conditions.

More specifically, research has indicated that ACT is an effective treatment for depression (Forman, Herbert, Moitra, Yeomans, & Geller, 2007), psychosis (Bach & Hayes, 2002; Bach, Hayes, & Gallop, 2012), and several anxiety disorders (Dalrymple & Herbert, 2007), including obsessive-compulsive disorder (Twohig et al., 2010) and posttraumatic stress disorder (Orsillo & Batten, 2005). Benefits of ACT are related to improved self-management in diabetes (Gregg, Callaghan, Hayes, & Glenn-Lawson, 2007); ameliorated quality of life in epilepsy (Lundgren, Dahl, Melin, & Kies, 2006; Lundgren, Dahl, Yardi, & Melin, 2008); improved quality of life, fewer cravings and less emotional eating, and experiential avoidance in obesity (Forman et al., 2007; Forman, Butryn, Hoffman, & Herbert, 2009; Lillis, Hayes, Bunting, & Masuda, 2009); ameliorated depression, anxiety, distress, psychological flexibility, and quality of life in cancer patients (Feros, Lane, Ciarrochi, & Blackledge, 2013; Mohabbat-Bahar, Maleki-Rizi, Akbari, & Moradi-Joo, 2015; Najvani, Neshatdoost, Abedi, & Mokarian, 2015; Rost, Wilson, Buchanan, Hildebrandt, & Mutch, 2012); and reduced pain interference and better pain management in chronic pain (Wetherell et al., 2011).

The Efficacy of ACT in Chronic Pain

ACT is considered by the American Psychological Association's Division 12 as an empirically supported intervention with strong empirical support for chronic pain (Society of Clinical Psychology, 2011).

Randomized Clinical Trials of ACT in Chronic Pain

Several randomized clinical trials (RCTs) provide support for employing ACT in chronic pain patients (Buhrman et al., 2013; Dahl, Wilson, & Nilsson, 2004; Thorsell et al., 2011; Wetherell et al., 2011; Wicksell, Ahlqvist, Bring, Melin, & Olsson, 2008; Wicksell et al., 2013). Chronic pain patients receiving acceptance and commitment-based Internet-delivered intervention exhibited improvements in pain-related distress and depressive and anxiety symptoms at posttreatment and at a 6-month follow-up (Buhrman et al., 2013). Also, those receiving ACT showed fewer average days of sick leave use compared to those receiving medical treatment as usual (Dahl et al., 2004). Chronic pain patients in an ACT condition demonstrated greater ameliorations in satisfaction with life, higher level of function, and reduced pain intensity compared to those in an applied relaxation condition (Thorsell et al., 2011). Chronic pain patients receiving ACT showed improved pain-related anxiety, depression, and pain interferences (Wetherell et al., 2011). Even though there were no significant differences on these outcome measures between patients in the ACT and CBT conditions, those receiving ACT reported greater satisfaction than those in the CBT condition.

Additionally, chronic pain patients in an ACT-based condition exhibited significant ameliorations in life satisfaction, depression, pain disability, fear of movements, and psychological flexibility compared to a waiting list condition, at both posttreatment and a 7-month follow-up (Wicksell et al., 2008). Another more recent RCT comparing an ACT group intervention with a waiting list condition demonstrated significant improvements in depression, anxiety, quality of life, pain-related functioning, impact of the disease, self-efficacy, and psychological inflexibility, in favor of ACT (Wicksell et al., 2013). Also, results demonstrated that psychological inflexibility mediated pre- to 3-month follow-up improvements in these outcome variables. Similarly, Wicksell, Olsson, and Hayes (2010) found that psychological flexibility significantly mediates treatment effects of ACT on life satisfaction and disability in chronic pain patients. Recently, another RCT has been conducted in order to examine the effectiveness of ACT in chronic pain, and the project's name is "ALGEA."

The ALGEA Project

Algea in the ancient Greek mythology symbolized pain of the psychic and the somatic. Pain as the son of Eris and grandson of Night was considered as a dark and mystic phenomenon that was eventually inevitable. Despite the efforts to treat, minimize, or even vanish any pain experience, pain is still an inevitable truth in peoples' lives from the ancient years until today.

The "ALGEA" project (www.algea.com.cy) aimed to develop and examine the effects of the new third-wave CBT therapy, namely, ACT (Hayes et al., 1999) for patients with chronic pain (CP) and their families. The specific objectives of the "ALGEA" project include (a) understanding the contributing factors involved in the experience of pain in individuals with CP conditions, their dyadic interactions with their partners, and differences with individuals suffering from other chronic illnesses not involving pain; (b) designing a culturally sensitive intervention based on new empirical findings stemming from third-wave CBTs for use in clinical settings (i.e., CP organizations, CP rehabilitation and outpatients units, etc.); (c) evaluating via randomized clinical trials the acceptability and effectiveness of this intervention especially in reducing suffering, interference of pain, and medical utilization in various CP conditions; (d) training interested health professionals in this new approach and widely disseminating it into clinical settings; and (e) translating the intervention into a digitally based intervention so as to be more accessible and reach a wider audience of CP sufferers. This was a collaborative project between the University of Cyprus, the University of Crete, and the Cyprus Institute of Neurology and Genetics and was funded by "The European Territorial Cooperation programs – INTERREG IV C interregional programme, Greece-Cyprus."

This integrative biopsychosocial intervention utilized ACT, which focuses on alleviating suffering and the sociopsychological consequences of the experience of pain, thus aiming to help patients to embrace pain and identify and follow a meaningful and valued life even when pain is present. Patients and especially those with CP often report the need to avoid any experience of pain (such as physical and mental distress) and thus might find themselves in a continuous and often futile effort to control pain (McCracken & Morley, 2014; Wicksell, Dahl, Magnusson, & Olsson, 2005). Such pain reduction efforts might provide short-term relief however; on the long run, they become their main behavioral repertoire at the expense of other meaningful activities and valuable relationships. Patients report leaving aside aspects of themselves since their lives are consumed in attempts to reduce, alter, or control pain (Vowles & McCracken, 2008). Therefore, the aim of this project was not the direct reduction of pain symptoms but rather the facilitation of patients' adjustment to their pain experience, which was expected to result in higher psychological flexibility, less suffering, and life interference, associated with CP.

Description of the "ALGEA" Protocol

ACT skills and exercises were encompassed in the protocol that was developed for the psychosocial intervention administered to chronic pain patients in a group format. Firstly, group cohesion was achieved through ACT-consistent metaphors such as *the two mountains metaphor* that could help group members identify the similarities among them (e.g., climbing up their own mountain that has many dangerous places on it) and recognize how one's perspective can help the other. In addition, icebreaker exercises, values identification through discussions in dyads, and experiential exercises such as breathing exercises and self as observer were used to build group cohesion and trust in an ACT-based context.

One of the main aims of the protocol was to help CP patients understand the illusion of their control agenda, and for this purpose, experiential as well as more explicit exercises were used. The matrix exercise engaged patients through asking them to identify what was important for them, what stands on their way to moving toward their values, and lastly how they manage their pain (how many hours and efforts they spend in controlling and managing their pain). Through this exercise symptom control was challenged and assessed against one's values. In addition, during experiential exercises patients were invited to try to induce specific sensations to part of their bodies, e.g., try to make their left leg completely numb, and thus realize that they cannot control how they feel or at least have less control than they would like to have. Culturally relevant metaphors were also used such as Hercules choice of one of two paths either the hardest path leading to virtue or the easiest path full of pleasures enticing him to the vice.

Another integral part of the protocol was mindfulness, perspective taking, and exposure to pain. Through breathing and mindfulness exercises, participants were invited to gradually expose themselves to pain, increase their willingness to experience their pain, be aware of it, accept, and embrace it. Different exercises with a similar exposure focus were administered each week as homework. These exercises provided an opportunity for participants to practice mindfulness in their everyday life and a way to develop an open and more accepting stand toward pain experience.

Activities aiming to develop participants' skill to contact the present moment were also incorporated in the protocol. CP patients focus on the problematic aspects of living or negative consequences of their health state. This often sends them to the past and entangles them into a narrow understanding of themselves and of the world. The antidote used is getting out of living in their mind. To this end, exercises promoting living in the present were employed as part of the specific protocol.

Value clarification was promoted through exercises such as making one's lifeline and acting out at one's own funeral. Exercises as the ones mentioned help patients to identify what is important for them and what they want their life to stand for. In addition, barriers to achieving one's meaningful goals were explored, while well-being and self-care were enhanced with a focus on the importance of physical activity and improvements in dietary and sleeping habits.

Self-compassion and self as context were instigated through exercises such as writing a love letter to one's self and defusion from the conceptualized self. Experiential exercises for facilitating acceptance and acceptance-based metaphors such as the Passengers on the Bus Metaphor were used to further cultivate acceptance, willingness, and openness to experience.

Lastly, a session with significant others was also implemented as part of the protocol. This session aimed to validate significant other's reaction to the partner's pain and examine the long-term negative consequences of reinforcing pain behaviors. Significant others were taught which behaviors to reinforce in order to facilitate patient's effort to identify and lead a meaningful and valuable life.

"ALGEA" Trial: Patient Perspectives

Based on patients' self-reports, the protocol and the group format, which facilitated the sharing of experiences among patients, provided new perspectives for them. Patients also expressed their pleasure from mindfulness homework and the experiential exercises performed during the group sessions. Among their favorite exercises were the funeral exercise and the Passengers on the Bus Metaphor. However, they disliked completing the large set of questionnaires and the fact that they had novice therapists that they mainly relied on manuals. They also reported that they wanted more discussion time and that they found mindfulness exercises too long while they felt "pushed" to open up to pain.

Preliminary Results from the ALGEA Project

Study 1: The role of psychological flexibility in predicting pain behaviors In the first study, we run multiple regression analyses to investigate the role of psychological flexibility in predicting pain behaviors in a heterogeneous sample of 40 pain patients in Cyprus (91% females; age range, 25–74 years; $M_{age} = 50.08$, SD = 12.31) with a mean of 13.17 years (SD = 8.86) since they were first diagnosed. The 50% of the sample had a college education or higher, and most of them (75%) were married. Pain behaviors were inserted as the outcome measure and were assessed via self-reported facial expressions of pain, body movements associated with pain and vocalization of pain. Psychological flexibility including experiential avoidance and mindfulness was entered as predictors.

Vocalization of pain was significantly associated with more experiential avoidance (lower psychological flexibility) and lower mindfulness (present-moment awareness). The results of the regression indicated that psychological flexibility and more specifically low experiential avoidance significantly predicted pain vocalization ($R^2 = .42$, $\beta = .42$; $F = 4.64$, $p = .04$) but no other pain behaviors. Mindfulness significantly predicted body movements associated with pain ($R^2 = .21$, $\beta = -.46$; $F = 5.75$, $p = .03$) and vocalizations of pain ($R^2 = .39$, $\beta = -.62$; $F = 13.95$, $p = .001$). In a subsequent two-step regression analyses, mindfulness and psychological flexibility were inserted as predictors of assessment of pain vocalization. The model was significant ($F = 6.80$, $p = .01$), but psychological flexibility did not significantly contribute with additional variance (R^2 change = .01). In conclusion, psychological flexibility and mindfulness are significantly associated with certain pain behaviors, such as pain vocalization, in CP patients.

Study 2: Pain interference and pain outcomes: the mediating effects of acceptance and cognitive fusion The aim of the second study was to examine the mediating effects of acceptance and cognitive fusion between pain interference and pain-related outcomes in a heterogeneous sample of 153 CP patients in Cyprus. All patients met the inclusion criteria of the study, that is, being 18 years of age or older and having a primary chronic nonmalignant pain diagnosis for a minimum of 6 months (assessed via medical records). The majority of the samples were female patients (81.4%) with a mean age of 56.8 years (SD = 13). Most of the patients had either high school or university level education, they were married (72.4%), and they were prescribed pain medication (67%).

In the various models tested, both direct and mediating effects were examined. More specifically the effects examined were (a) the direct effects of pain interference on pain outcomes, (b) the mediating effects of acceptance parameters between pain interference and pain outcomes, and (c) the mediating effects of acceptance and cognitive fusion (open response style) between pain interference and pain outcomes.

Study 3: A randomized controlled trial of acceptance and commitment therapy vs. medical treatment as usual for chronic head pain The third study aimed to compare the medical treatment as usual (MTAU) to the randomized controlled trial of acceptance and commitment therapy (ACT+MTAU) for chronic head pain. It is important to note that MTAU was used as a wait list control group that would receive the ACT treatment after the termination of the experimental group's treatment. A total of 94 patients were randomized to one of the two conditions (47 in each; M_{age} = 43.9 years old, SD = 10.35; 84% female; 37% had completed high school). The mean years since their head pain onset was 18 years (SD = 10; range 1–46 years), and the mean duration of their head pain was 9 days per month. Seventy-one percent of them were prescribed headache medication. The two groups were equal on all measures of the study prior to the intervention.

Repeated measures of ANOVA were conducted to examine the differences between the two groups prior to the randomized controlled trial, immediately after the termination of the trial and at 3-month follow-up on headache general disability (HGD) and quality of life (QoL) levels.

Based on the study's results, ACT+MTAU reported significantly lower disability immediately following treatment (${F_{(1.59)}}^2 = 7.43$, $\eta^2 = .11$, $p \leq 0.05$) and at 3-month follow-up (${F_{(1.59)}}^2 = 9.92$, $\eta^2 = .14$, $p \leq 0.05$) as well as a significant increase in functioning and quality of life (immediately following treatment, ${F_{(1.59)}}^2 = 12.53$, $\eta^2 = .17$, $p \leq 0.001$; at 3-month follow-up, ${F_{(1.59)}}^2 = 17.88$, $\eta^2 = .23$, $p \leq 0.001$) in comparison to the WL-MTAU group (ITT analyses). All effect sizes were medium and in some cases (e.g., QoL, avoidance of pain and pain acceptance) were large at the 3-month follow-up. Treatment did not reduce pain severity, consistent with the ACT theoretical framework based on which effective daily functioning is possible in the context of continuing pain, but instead increased functionality. Finally, these preliminary findings support ACT for a mixed headache population and further add to the limited empirical findings of ACT for headache management (Dindo, Recober, Marchman, O'Hara, & Turvey, 2015; Dindo, Recober, Marchman, Turvey, & O'Hara, 2012; Mo'tamedi, Rezaiemaram, & Tavallaie, 2012).

Next Steps

Following technological advances in the service of mental health, a digital adaptation of ALGEA program is currently under preparation ("ALGEApp"; www.alegeapp.com, in Greek). The digital ALGEA program will be disseminated to CP patients in remote areas that might not otherwise have the chance to benefit from such psychosocial interventions. The digital adaptation of ALGEA that will be tested and compared for its effectiveness and usefulness with the standard (face-to-face) program is expected to offer a wider coverage of patients by addressing accessibility issues due to geography, mental ill health, physical disability, and financial barriers. The development of this web-based psychological intervention that is grounded in theory and empirical evidence uses the persuasive system design methodology to provide an attractive content for the users, capture their interest, and facilitate their engagement in treatment conducted at their own time, location, and pace. The development and implementation of such web-based interventions are promising significant advancements, not otherwise achieved with traditional face-to-face psychotherapies and other conventional methods.

In conclusion, the ALGEA project provides an innovative patient-centered context where CP patients are invited to effectively manage their pain symptoms, alter their relation to pain behaviors, and minimize interference of pain experience with their own stated values (such as maintaining close relationships with loved ones even when pain is present) and daily activities. Based on the preliminary results presented here, the ALGEA project appears effective in reducing disability and enhancing quality of life among patients with chronic head pain as compared to the medical treatment as usual. The results from the entire ALGEA project (analysis currently under way) will provide significant insights as to the mechanisms underlying ACT for CP that will further aid our understanding of patients' pain experience and adjustment and help us optimize the existing intervention protocols.

References

Abad, A. N. S., Bakhtiari, M., Kashani, F. L., & Habibi, M. (2016). The comparison of effectiveness of treatment based on acceptance and commitment with cognitive-behavioral therapy in reduction of stress and anxiety in cancer patients. *International Journal of Cancer Research and Prevention, 9*(3), 229–246.

Alsaadi, S. M., McAuley, J. H., Hush, J. M., & Maher, C. G. (2011). Prevalence of sleep disturbance in patients with low back pain. *European Spine Journal, 20*, 737–743.

Ambler, N., de C Williams, A. C., Hill, P., Gunary, R., & Cratchley, G. (2001). Sexual difficulties of chronic pain patients. *The Clinical Journal of Pain, 17*(2), 138–145.

Andrew, R., Derry, S., Taylor, R. S., Straube, S., & Phillips, C. J. (2014). The costs and consequences of adequately managed chronic non-cancer pain and chronic neuropathic pain. *Pain Practice, 14*(1), 79–94.

Aronoff, G. M. (1991). Chronic pain and the disability epidemic. *The Clinical Journal of Pain, 7*(4), 330–338.

Azevedo, L. F., Costa-Pereira, A., Mendonça, L., Dias, C. C., & Castro-Lopes, J. M. (2012). Epidemiology of chronic pain: A population-based nationwide study on its prevalence, characteristics and associated disability in Portugal. *The Journal of Pain, 13*(8), 773–783.

Bach, P., & Hayes, S. C. (2002). The use of acceptance and commitment therapy to prevent the rehospitalization of psychotic patients: A randomized controlled trial. *Journal of Consulting and Clinical Psychology, 70*(5), 1129–1138.

Bach, P., Hayes, S. C., & Gallop, R. (2012). Long-term effects of brief acceptance and commitment therapy for psychosis. *Behavior Modification, 36*(2), 165–181.

Bair, M. J., Robinson, R. L., Katon, W., & Kroenke, K. (2003). Depression and pain comorbidity: A literature review. *Archives of Internal Medicine, 163*(20), 2433–2445.

Bair, M. J., Wu, J., Damush, T. M., Sutherland, J. M., & Kroenke, K. (2008). Association of depression and anxiety alone and in combination with chronic musculoskeletal pain in primary care patients. *Psychosomatic Medicine, 70*(8), 890–897.

Blackledge, J. T. (2003). An introduction to relational frame theory: Basics and applications. *The Behavior Analyst Today, 3*(4), 421–434.

Blyth, F. M., March, L. M., Nicholas, M. K., & Cousins, M. J. (2003). Chronic pain, work performance and litigation. *Pain, 103*(1), 41–47.

Bouhassira, D., Lantéri-Minet, M., Attal, N., Laurent, B., & Touboul, C. (2008). Prevalence of chronic pain with neuropathic characteristics in the general population. *Pain, 136*(3), 380–387.

Breivik, H., Collett, B., Ventafridda, V., Cohen, R., & Gallacher, D. (2006). Survey of chronic pain in Europe: Prevalence, impact on daily life, and treatment. *European Journal of Pain, 10*(4), 287–333.

Bruehl, S., Chung, O. Y., & Burns, J. W. (2003). Differential effects of expressive anger regulation on chronic pain intensity in CRPS and non-CRPS limb pain patients. *Pain, 104*(3), 647–654.

Buhrman, M., Skoglund, A., Husell, J., Bergström, K., Gordh, T., Hursti, T., … Andersson, G. (2013). Guided internet-delivered acceptance and commitment therapy for chronic pain patients: A randomized controlled trial. *Behaviour Research and Therapy, 51*(6), 307–315.

Burns, J. W., Higdon, L. J., Mullen, J. T., Lansky, D., & Wei, J. M. (1999). Relationships among patient hostility, anger expression, depression, and the working alliance in a work hardening program. *Annals of Behavioral Medicine, 21*(1), 77–82.

Burns, J. W., Johnson, B. J., Devine, J., Mahoney, N., & Pawl, R. (1998). Anger management style and the prediction of treatment outcome among male and female chronic pain patients. *Behaviour Research and Therapy, 36*(11), 1051–1062.

Burton, W., Morrison, A., Maclean, R., & Ruderman, E. (2006). Systematic review of studies of productivity loss due to rheumatoid arthritis. *Occupational Medicine, 56*(1), 18–27.

Campos, R. P., & Vázquez, M. I. R. (2012). Health-related quality of life in women with fibromyalgia: Clinical and psychological factors associated. *Clinical Rheumatology, 31*(2), 347–355.

Carmona, L., Ballina, J., Gabriel, R., & Laffon, A. (2001). The burden of musculoskeletal diseases in the general population of Spain: Results from a national survey. *Annals of the Rheumatic Diseases, 60*(11), 1040–1045.

Carson, J. W., Keefe, F. J., Goli, V., Fras, A. M., Lynch, T. R., Thorp, S. R., & Buechler, J. L. (2005). Forgiveness and chronic low back pain: A preliminary study examining the relationship of forgiveness to pain, anger, and psychological distress. *The Journal of Pain, 6*(2), 84–91.

Carson, J. W., Keefe, F. J., Lynch, T. R., Carson, K. M., Goli, V., Fras, A. M., & Thorp, S. R. (2005). Loving-kindness meditation for chronic low back pain: Results from a pilot trial. *Journal of Holistic Nursing, 23*(3), 287–304.

Cedraschi, C., Girard, E., Luthy, C., Kossovsky, M., Desmeules, J., & Allaz, A. F. (2013). Primary attributions in women suffering fibromyalgia emphasize the perception of a disruptive onset for a long-lasting pain problem. *Journal of Psychosomatic Research, 74*(3), 265–269.

Chou, R., Fanciullo, G. J., Fine, P. G., Adler, J. A., Ballantyne, J. C., Davies, P., … Gilson, A. M. (2009). Clinical guidelines for the use of chronic opioid therapy in chronic noncancer pain. *The Journal of Pain, 10*(2), 113–130.

Collado, A., Gomez, E., Coscolla, R., Sunyol, R., Solé, E., Rivera, J., ... Castells, X. (2014). Work, family and social environment in patients with Fibromyalgia in Spain: An epidemiological study: EPIFFAC study. *BMC Health Services Research, 14*(1), 513.

Connolly, D., Fitzpatrick, C., O'Toole, L., Doran, M., & O'Shea, F. (2015). Impact of fatigue in rheumatic diseases in the work environment: A qualitative study. *International Journal of Environmental Research and Public Health, 12*(11), 13807–13822.

Dahl, J., Wilson, K. G., & Nilsson, A. (2004). Acceptance and commitment therapy and the treatment of persons at risk for long-term disability resulting from stress and pain symptoms: A preliminary randomized trial. *Behavior Therapy, 35*(4), 785–801.

Dalrymple, K. L., & Herbert, J. D. (2007). Acceptance and commitment therapy for generalized social anxiety disorder a pilot study. *Behavior Modification, 31*(5), 543–568.

Davis, J. A., Robinson, R. L., Le, T. K., & Xie, J. (2011). Incidence and impact of pain conditions and comorbid illnesses. *Journal of Pain Research, 4*, 331–345.

Demyttenaere, K., Bruffaerts, R., Lee, S., Posada-Villa, J., Kovess, V., Angermeyer, M. C., ... Lara, C. (2007). Mental disorders among persons with chronic back or neck pain: Results from the World Mental Health Surveys. *Pain, 129*(3), 332–342.

Dewar, A. L., Gregg, K., White, M. I., & Lander, J. (2009). Navigating the health care system: Perceptions of patients with chronic pain. *Chronic Diseases in Canada, 29*(4), 162–168.

Dindo, L., Recober, A., Marchman, J., O'Hara, M., & Turvey, C. (2015). Depression and disability in migraine: The role of pain acceptance and values-based action. *International Journal of Behavioral Medicine, 22*(1), 109–117.

Dindo, L., Recober, A., Marchman, J. N., Turvey, C., & O'Hara, M. W. (2012). One-day behavioral treatment for patients with comorbid depression and migraine: A pilot study. *Behaviour Research and Therapy, 50*(9), 537–543.

Dow, C. M., Roche, P. A., & Ziebland, S. (2012). Talk of frustration in the narratives of people with chronic pain. *Chronic Illness, 8*(3), 176–191.

Dueñas, M., Ojeda, B., Salazar, A., Mico, J. A., & Failde, I. (2016). A review of chronic pain impact on patients, their social environment and the health care system. *Journal of Pain Research, 9*, 457–467.

Eccleston, C., Williams, A. D. C., & Morley, S. (2009). Psychological therapies for the management of chronic pain (excluding headache) in adults. *Cochrane Database of Systematic Reviews, 2*. Retrieved from https://www.ncor.org.uk/wp-content/uploads/2012/11/eccleston-2009-Psych-interventions-for-chronic-pain.pdf

Feinberg, S. D., & Brigham, C. R. (2013). Assessing disability in the pain patient. In T. R. Deer, M. S. Leong, A. Buvanendran, V. Gordin, P. S. Kim, S. J. Panchal, & A. L. Ray (Eds.), *Comprehensive treatment of chronic pain by medical, interventional, and integrative approaches: The American Academy of Pain Medicine textbook on patient management* (pp. 1031–1043). New York, NY: Springer.

Feldner, M. T., Hekmat, H., Zvolensky, M. J., Vowles, K. E., Secrist, Z., & Leen-Feldner, E. W. (2006). The role of experiential avoidance in acute pain tolerance: A laboratory test. *Journal of Behavior Therapy and Experimental Psychiatry, 37*(2), 146–158.

Feros, D. L., Lane, L., Ciarrochi, J., & Blackledge, J. T. (2013). Acceptance and Commitment Therapy (ACT) for improving the lives of cancer patients: A preliminary study. *Psycho-Oncology, 22*(2), 459–464.

Fine, P. G. (2011). Long-term consequences of chronic pain: Mounting evidence for pain as a neurological disease and parallels with other chronic disease states. *Pain Medicine, 12*(7), 996–1004.

Finucane, A. M., Dima, A., Ferreira, N., & Halvorsen, M. (2012). Basic emotion profiles in healthy, chronic pain, depressed and PTSD individuals. *Clinical Psychology and Psychotherapy, 19*(1), 14–24.

Forman, E. M., Butryn, M. L., Hoffman, K. L., & Herbert, J. D. (2009). An open trial of an acceptance-based behavioral intervention for weight loss. *Cognitive and Behavioral Practice, 16*(2), 223–235.

Forman, E. M., Herbert, J. D., Moitra, E., Yeomans, P. D., & Geller, P. A. (2007). A randomized controlled effectiveness trial of acceptance and commitment therapy and cognitive therapy for anxiety and depression. *Behavior Modification, 31*(6), 772–799.

Forman, E. M., Hoffnan, K. L., MeGrath, K. B., Herbert, J. D., Brandsma, L. L., & Lowe, M. R. (2007). A comparison of acceptance- and control-based strategies for coping with food cravings: An analog study. *Behaviour Research and Therapy, 45*, 2372–2386.

Gaikwad, M., Vanlint, S., Moseley, G. L., Mittinty, M. N., & Stocks, N. (2017). Understanding patient perspectives on management of their chronic pain–online survey protocol. *Journal of Pain Research, 10*, 31–35.

Gatchel, R. J. (1999). Perspectives on pain: A historical overview. In R. J. Gatchel & D. C. Turk (Eds.), *Psychosocial factors in pain. Critical perspectives* (pp. 3–17). New York: The Guilford Press.

Gatchel, R. J., & Okifuji, A. (2006). Evidence-based scientific data documenting the treatment and cost-effectiveness of comprehensive pain programs for chronic nonmalignant pain. *The Journal of Pain, 7*(11), 779–793.

Gillanders, D. T., Sinclair, A. K., MacLean, M., & Jardine, K. (2015). Illness cognitions, cognitive fusion, avoidance and self-compassion as predictors of distress and quality of life in a heterogeneous sample of adults, after cancer. *Journal of Contextual Behavioral Science, 4*(4), 300–311.

Gloster, A. T., Meyer, A. H., & Lieb, R. (2017). Psychological flexibility as a malleable public health target: Evidence from a representative sample. *Journal of Contextual Behavioral Science, 6*(2), 166–171.

Gloster, A. T., Sonntag, R., Hoyer, J., Meyer, A. H., Heinze, S., Ströhle, A., … Wittchen, H. U. (2015). Treating treatment-resistant patients with panic disorder and agoraphobia using psychotherapy: A randomized controlled switching trial. *Psychotherapy and Psychosomatics, 84*(2), 100–109.

Graham, C. D., Gouick, J., Krahé, C., & Gillanders, D. (2016). A systematic review of the use of Acceptance and Commitment Therapy (ACT) in chronic disease and long-term conditions. *Clinical Psychology Review, 46*, 46–58.

Graham, C. D., Simmons, Z., Stuart, S. R., & Rose, M. R. (2015). The potential of psychological interventions to improve quality of life and mood in muscle disorders. *Muscle & Nerve, 52*(1), 131–136.

Green, C. R., Hart-Johnson, T., & Loeffler, D. R. (2011). Cancer-related chronic pain. *Cancer, 117*(9), 1994–2003.

Green, C. R., Ndao-Brumblay, S. K., & Hart-Johnson, T. (2009). Sleep problems in a racially diverse chronic pain population. *The Clinical Journal of Pain, 25*(5), 423–430.

Green, C. R., Wheeler, J. R., Marchant, B., LaPorte, F., & Guerrero, E. (2001). Analysis of the physician variable in pain management. *Pain Medicine, 2*(4), 317–327.

Greenberg, P. E., Leong, S. A., Birnbaum, H. G., & Robinson, R. L. (2003). The economic burden of depression with painful symptoms. *The Journal of Clinical Psychiatry, 64*, 17–23.

Greenwood, K. A., Thurston, R., Rumble, M., Waters, S. J., & Keefe, F. J. (2003). Anger and persistent pain: Current status and future directions. *Pain, 103*(1–2), 1–5.

Gregg, J. A., Callaghan, G. M., Hayes, S. C., & Glenn-Lawson, J. L. (2007). Improving diabetes self-management through acceptance, mindfulness, and values: A randomized controlled trial. *Journal of Consulting and Clinical Psychology, 75*(2), 336–343.

Gureje, O., Von Korff, M., Simon, G. E., & Gater, R. (1998). Persistent pain and well-being: A World Health Organization study in primary care. *JAMA, 280*(2), 147–151.

Harris, R. (2009). *ACT made simple: An easy-to-read primer on acceptance and commitment therapy*. Oakland, CA: New Harbinger Publications.

Hayes, S. C. (1989). *Rule-governed behavior: Cognition, contingencies, and instructional control*. New York, NY: Plenum Press.

Hayes, S. C., Barnes-Holmes, D., & Wilson, K. G. (2012). Contextual behavioral science: Creating a science more adequate to the challenge of the human condition. *Journal of Contextual Behavioral Science, 1*, 1), 1–1),16.

Hayes, S. C., & Duckworth, M. P. (2006). Acceptance and commitment therapy and traditional cognitive behavior therapy approaches to pain. *Cognitive and Behavioral Practice, 13*(3), 185–187.

Hayes, S. C., & Lillis, J. (2012). *Acceptance and commitment therapy*. Washington, DC: American Psychological Association.

Hayes, S. C., Luoma, J. B., Bond, F. W., Masuda, A., & Lillis, J. (2006). Acceptance and commitment therapy: Model, processes and outcomes. *Behaviour Research and Therapy, 44*(1), 1–25.

Hayes, S. C., Strosahl, K. D., & Wilson, K. G. (1999). *Acceptance and commitment therapy: An experiential approach to behavior change*. New York, NY: Guilford Press.

Hayes, S. C., Strosahl, K. D., & Wilson, K. G. (2011). *Acceptance and commitment therapy: The process and practice of mindful change*. New York, NY: Guildford Press.

Hayes, S. C., Wilson, K. G., Gifford, E. V., Follette, V. M., & Strosahl, K. (1996). Experiential avoidance and behavioral disorders: A functional dimensional approach to diagnosis and treatment. *Journal of Consulting and Clinical Psychology, 64*(6), 1152–1168.

Henry, J. L. (2008). The need for knowledge translation in chronic pain. *Pain Research and Management, 13*(6), 465–476.

Henwood, P., & Ellis, J. A. (2004). Chronic neuropathic pain in spinal cord injury: The patient's perspective. *Pain Research and Management, 9*(1), 39–45.

Hulbert-Williams, N. J., Storey, L., & Wilson, K. G. (2015). Psychological interventions for patients with cancer: Psychological flexibility and the potential utility of Acceptance and Commitment Therapy. *European Journal of Cancer Care, 24*(1), 15–27.

Hylands-White, N., Duarte, R. V., & Raphael, J. H. (2017). An overview of treatment approaches for chronic pain management. *Rheumatology International, 37*(1), 29–42.

Institute of Medicine of the National Academies Report (IOM). (2011). *Relieving pain in America: A blueprint for transforming prevention, care, education, and research.* Washington, DC: The National Academies Press. Retrieved from https://www.ncbi.nlm.nih.gov/books/NBK91497/

International Association for the Study of Pain (IASP). (1994). Task force on taxonomy, part III. Pain terms. A current list with definitions and notes on usage. In H. Merskey & N. Bogduk (Eds.), *Classification of chronic pain* (pp. 209–214). Seattle, WA: International Association for the Study of Pain Press.

Kalso, E., Edwards, J. E., Moore, R. A., & McQuay, H. J. (2004). Opioids in chronic non-cancer pain: Systematic review of efficacy and safety. *Pain, 112*(3), 372–380.

Karekla, M., & Constantinou, M. (2010). Religious coping and cancer: Proposing an acceptance and commitment therapy approach. *Cognitive and Behavioral Practice, 17*(4), 371–381.

Karekla, M., Constantinou, P., Ioannou, M., Gloster, A., & Kareklas, I. (under review). Meta-analysis of third wave cognitive behavioral treatment dropouts.

Karekla, M., Karademas, E. C., & Gloster, A. T. (2018). The Common Sense Model of Self-Regulation and Acceptance and Commitment Therapy: integrating strategies to guide interventions for chronic illness. Health psychology review, 1–14.

Karekla, M., Vasiliou, V., & Karademas, E. (2013). ALGEA study treatment protocol for therapists to deal with chronic pain. Unpublished protocol.

Kashdan, T. B., & Rottenberg, J. (2010). Psychological flexibility as a fundamental aspect of health. *Clinical Psychology Review, 30*(7), 865–878.

Kroenke, K., Outcalt, S., Krebs, E., Bair, M. J., Wu, J., Chumbler, N., & Yu, Z. (2013). Association between anxiety, health-related quality of life and functional impairment in primary care patients with chronic pain. *General Hospital Psychiatry, 35*(4), 359–365.

Langley, P., Müller-Schwefe, G., Nicolaou, A., Liedgens, H., Pergolizzi, J., & Varrassi, G. (2010). The impact of pain on labor force participation, absenteeism and presenteeism in the European Union. *Journal of Medical Economics, 13*(4), 662–672.

Langley, P., Pérez Hernández, C., Margarit Ferri, C., Ruiz Hidalgo, D., & Lubián López, M. (2011). Pain, health related quality of life and healthcare resource utilization in Spain. *Journal of Medical Economics, 14*(5), 628–638.

Langley, P. C., Ruiz-Iban, M. A., Molina, J. T., De Andres, J., & Castellón, J. R. G. E. (2011). The prevalence, correlates and treatment of pain in Spain. *Journal of Medical Economics, 14*(3), 367–380.
Lerman, S. F., Rudich, Z., Brill, S., Shalev, H., & Shahar, G. (2015). Longitudinal associations between depression, anxiety, pain, and pain-related disability in chronic pain patients. *Psychosomatic Medicine, 77*(3), 333–341.
Lillis, J., Hayes, S. C., Bunting, K., & Masuda, A. (2009). Teaching acceptance and mindfulness to improve the lives of the obese: A preliminary test of a theoretical model. *Annals of Behavioral Medicine, 37*(1), 58–69.
Lopez-Silva, M. C., Sanchez de Enciso, M., Rodriguez-Fernandez, M. C., & Vazquez-Seijas, E. (2007). Cavidol: Quality of life and pain in primary care. *Revista-Sociedad Espanola Del Dolor, 14*(1), 9–19.
Low, J., Davis, S., Drake, R., King, M., Tookman, A., Turner, K., … Jones, L. (2012). The role of acceptance in rehabilitation in life-threatening illness. *Journal of Pain and Symptom Management, 43*(1), 20–28.
Löwe, B., Spitzer, R. L., Williams, J. B., Mussell, M., Schellberg, D., & Kroenke, K. (2008). Depression, anxiety and somatization in primary care: Syndrome overlap and functional impairment. *General Hospital Psychiatry, 30*(3), 191–199.
Lundgren, T., Dahl, J., Melin, L., & Kies, B. (2006). Evaluation of acceptance and commitment therapy for drug refractory epilepsy: A randomized controlled trial in South Africa: A pilot study. *Epilepsia, 47*(12), 2173–2179.
Lundgren, T., Dahl, J., Yardi, N., & Melin, L. (2008). Acceptance and commitment therapy and yoga for drug-refractory epilepsy: A randomized controlled trial. *Epilepsy & Behavior, 13*(1), 102–108.
Luoma, J. B., Hayes, S. C., & Walser, R. D. (2007). *Learning ACT: An acceptance & commitment therapy skills-training manual for therapists*. Oakland, CA: New Harbinger Publications.
Manchikanti, L. (2006). Prescription drug abuse: What is being done to address this new drug epidemic? Testimony before the Subcommittee on Criminal Justice, Drug Policy and Human Resources. *Pain Physician, 9*(4), 287–321.
Maniadakis, N., & Gray, A. (2000). The economic burden of back pain in the UK. *Pain, 84*(1), 95–103.
Mäntyselkä, P. T., Kumpusalo, E. A., Ahonen, R. S., & Takala, J. K. (2002). Direct and indirect costs of managing patients with musculoskeletal pain—Challenge for health care. *European Journal of Pain, 6*(2), 141–148.
Marin, R., Cyhan, T., & Miklos, W. (2006). Sleep disturbance in patients with chronic low back pain. *American Journal of Physical Medicine & Rehabilitation, 85*(5), 430–435.
Marty, M., Rozenberg, S., Duplan, B., Thomas, P., Duquesnoy, B., Allaert, F., & Section Rachis de la Société Française de Rhumatologie. (2008). Quality of sleep in patients with chronic low back pain: A case-control study. *European Spine Journal, 17*(6), 839–844.
McCarberg, B. H., Nicholson, B. D., Todd, K. H., Palmer, T., & Penles, L. (2008). The impact of pain on quality of life and the unmet needs of pain management: Results from pain sufferers and physicians participating in an Internet survey. *American Journal of Therapeutics, 15*(4), 312–320.
McCracken, L. M. (1998). Learning to live with the pain: Acceptance of pain predicts adjustment in persons with chronic pain. *Pain, 74*(1), 21–27.
McCracken, L. M., & Eccleston, C. (2003). Coping or acceptance: What to do about chronic pain? *Pain, 105*(1), 197–204.
McCracken, L. M., Eccleston, C., & Bell, L. (2005). Clinical assessment of behavioral coping responses: Preliminary results from a brief inventory. *European Journal of Pain, 9*(1), 69–78.
McCracken, L. M., Gauntlett-Gilbert, J., & Vowles, K. E. (2007). The role of mindfulness in a contextual cognitive-behavioral analysis of chronic pain-related suffering and disability. *Pain, 131*(1), 63–69.
McCracken, L. M., & Iverson, G. L. (2002). Disrupted sleep patterns and daily functioning in patients with chronic pain. *Pain Research and Management, 7*(2), 75–79.

McCracken, L. M., & Morley, S. (2014). The psychological flexibility model: A basis for integration and progress in psychological approaches to chronic pain management. *The Journal of Pain, 15*(3), 221–234.

McCracken, L. M., & Vowles, K. E. (2006). Acceptance of chronic pain. *Current Pain and Headache Reports, 10*(2), 90–94.

McWilliams, L. A., Cox, B. J., & Enns, M. W. (2003). Mood and anxiety disorders associated with chronic pain: An examination in a nationally representative sample. *Pain, 106*(1), 127–133.

Merskey, H., & Bogduk, N. (1994). *Classification of chronic pain, IASP Task Force on Taxonomy*. Seattle, WA: International Association for the Study of Pain Press.

Milton, J. (2013). Caring for patients with chronic pain: Pearls and pitfalls. *The Journal, 113*(8), 620–627.

Mohabbat-Bahar, S., Maleki-Rizi, F., Akbari, M. E., & Moradi-Joo, M. (2015). Effectiveness of group training based on acceptance and commitment therapy on anxiety and depression of women with breast cancer. *Iranian Journal of Cancer Prevention, 8*(2), 71–76.

Morin, C. M., Gibson, D., & Wade, J. (1998). Self-reported sleep and mood disturbance in chronic pain patients. *The Clinical Journal of Pain, 14*(4), 311–314.

Morley, S., Davies, C., & Barton, S. (2005). Possible selves in chronic pain: Self-pain enmeshment, adjustment and acceptance. *Pain, 115*(1), 84–94.

Mo'tamedi, H., Rezaiemaram, P., & Tavallaie, A. (2012). The effectiveness of a group-based acceptance and commitment additive therapy on rehabilitation of female outpatients with chronic headache: Preliminary findings reducing 3 dimensions of headache impact. *Headache: The Journal of Head and Face Pain, 52*(7), 1106–1119.

Moulin, D. E., Clark, A. J., Speechley, M., & Morley-Forster, P. K. (2002). Chronic pain in Canada-prevalence, treatment, impact and the role of opioid analgesia. *Pain Research and Management, 7*(4), 179–184.

Najvani, B. D., Neshatdoost, H. T., Abedi, M. R., & Mokarian, F. (2015). The effect of acceptance and commitment therapy on depression and psychological flexibility in women with breast cancer. *Zahedan Journal of Research in Medical Sciences, 17*(4), 29–33.

National Health and Wellness Survey. (2014). The global health and wellness report. *Kantar Health.* Retrieved from http://www.kantarhealth.com/docs/ebooks/global-health-and-wellness-report.pdf

Nickel, R., & Raspe, H. H. (2001). Chronischer schmerz: Epidemiologie und inanspruchnahme. *Der Nervenarzt, 72*(12), 897–906.

O'Brien, E. M., Waxenberg, L. B., Atchison, J. W., Gremillion, H. A., Staud, R. M., McCrae, C. S., & Robinson, M. E. (2011). Intraindividual variability in daily sleep and pain ratings among chronic pain patients: Bidirectional association and the role of negative mood. *The Clinical Journal of Pain, 27*(5), 425–433.

Ohayon, M. M., & Schatzberg, A. F. (2003). Using chronic pain to predict depressive morbidity in the general population. *Archives of General Psychiatry, 60*(1), 39–47.

Ojeda, B., Salazar, A., Dueñas, M., Torres, L. M., Micó, J. A., & Failde, I. (2014). The impact of chronic pain: The perspective of patients, relatives, and caregivers. *Families, Systems, & Health, 32*(4), 399.

Okifuji, A., Turk, D. C., & Curran, S. L. (1999). Anger in chronic pain: Investigations of anger targets and intensity. *Journal of Psychosomatic Research, 47*(1), 1–12.

Oliver, R. L. (1993). Cognitive, affective, and attribute bases of the satisfaction response. *Journal of Consumer Research, 20*(3), 418–430.

Orsillo, S. M., & Batten, S. V. (2005). Acceptance and commitment therapy in the treatment of posttraumatic stress disorder. *Behavior Modification, 29*(1), 95–129.

Ospina, M., & Harstall, C. (2002). *Prevalence of chronic pain: An overview.* Edmonton: Alberta Heritage Foundation for Medical Research, Health Technology Assessment. Retrieved from http://citeseerx.ist.psu.edu/viewdoc/download?doi=10.1.1.510.5502&rep=rep1&type=pdf

Pain Proposal. (2010). Improving the current and future management of chronic pain. *A European Consensus Report*. Retrieved from http://www.dgss.org/fileadmin/pdf/Pain_Proposal_European_Consensus_Report.pdf

Patel, A. S., Farquharson, R., Carroll, D., Moore, A., Phillips, C. J., Taylor, R. S., & Barden, J. (2012). The impact and burden of chronic pain in the workplace: A qualitative systematic review. *Pain Practice, 12*(7), 578–589.

Phillips, C. J. (2001). The real cost of pain management. *Anaesthesia, 56*(11), 1031–1033.

Porter, L. S., Keefe, F. J., Wellington, C., & de Williams, A. (2008). Pain communication in the context of osteoarthritis: Patient and partner self-efficacy for pain communication and holding back from discussion of pain and arthritis-related concerns. *The Clinical Journal of Pain, 24*(8), 662–668.

Potter, M., Schafer, S., Gonzalez-mendez, E., Gjeltema, K., Lopez, A., Wu, J., … Croughan-minihane, M. (2001). Opioids for chronic nonmalignant pain. *Journal of Family Practice, 50*(2), 145–145.

Ratcliffe, G. E., Enns, M. W., Belik, S. L., & Sareen, J. (2008). Chronic pain conditions and suicidal ideation and suicide attempts: An epidemiologic perspective. *The Clinical Journal of Pain, 24*(3), 204–210.

Reid, K. J., Harker, J., Bala, M. M., Truyers, C., Kellen, E., Bekkering, G. E., & Kleijnen, J. (2011). Epidemiology of chronic non-cancer pain in Europe: Narrative review of prevalence, pain treatments and pain impact. *Current Medical Research and Opinion, 27*(2), 449–462.

Reitsma, M. L., Tranmer, J. E., Buchanan, D. M., & Vandenkerkhof, E. G. (2011). The prevalence of chronic pain and pain-related interference in the Canadian population from 1994 to 2008. *Chronic Diseases and Injuries in Canada, 31*(4), 157–164.

Risdon, A., Eccleston, C., Crombez, G., & McCracken, L. (2003). How can we learn to live with pain? A Q-methodological analysis of the diverse understandings of acceptance of chronic pain. *Social Science & Medicine, 56*(2), 375–386.

Rost, A. D., Wilson, K., Buchanan, E., Hildebrandt, M. J., & Mutch, D. (2012). Improving psychological adjustment among late-stage ovarian cancer patients: Examining the role of avoidance in treatment. *Cognitive and Behavioral Practice, 19*(4), 508–517.

Rudich, Z., Lerman, S. F., Gurevich, B., Weksler, N., & Shahar, G. (2008). Patients' self-criticism is a stronger predictor of physician's evaluation of prognosis than pain diagnosis or severity in chronic pain patients. *The Journal of Pain, 9*(3), 210–216.

Ryan, S., Hill, J., Thwaites, C., & Dawes, P. (2008). Assessing the effect of fibromyalgia on patients' sexual activity. *Nursing Standard, 23*(2), 35–41.

Schmidt, C. O., & Kohlmann, T. (2005). Was wissen wir über das Symptom Rückenschmerz? *Zeitschrift für Orthopädie und Ihre Grenzgebiete, 143*(03), 292–298.

Schumacher, J., & Brähler, E. (1999). Prävalenz von Schmerzen in der deutschen Bevölkerung. *Der Schmerz, 13*(6), 375–384.

Society of Clinical Psychology, American Psychological Association, Division 12. (2011). *Acceptance and commitment therapy for chronic pain.* Retrieved from http://www.div12.org/PsychologicalTreatments/treatments/chronicpain_act.html

Tang, N. K., & Crane, C. (2006). Suicidality in chronic pain: A review of the prevalence, risk factors and psychological links. *Psychological Medicine, 36*(05), 575–586.

Thewes, B., Brebach, R., Dzidowska, M., Rhodes, P., Sharpe, L., & Butow, P. (2014). Current approaches to managing fear of cancer recurrence; a descriptive survey of psychosocial and clinical health professionals. *Psycho-Oncology, 23*(4), 390–396.

Thorsell, J., Finnes, A., Dahl, J., Lundgren, T., Gybrant, M., Gordh, T., & Buhrman, M. (2011). A comparative study of 2 manual-based self-help interventions, acceptance and commitment therapy and applied relaxation, for persons with chronic pain. *The Clinical Journal of Pain, 27*(8), 716–723.

Tornero, M., Atance, M., Grupeli, B. E., & Vidal, F. (1998). Economic and social impact of rheumatic short-term work disability in Guadalajara. *Revista Espanola de Reumatismo, 25*(9), 340–345.

Torrance, N., Smith, B. H., Bennett, M. I., & Lee, A. J. (2006). The epidemiology of chronic pain of predominantly neuropathic origin. Results from a general population survey. *The Journal of Pain, 7*(4), 281–289.

Turk, D. C., Wilson, H. D., & Cahana, A. (2011). Treatment of chronic non-cancer pain. *The Lancet, 377*(9784), 2226–2235.
Tüzün, E. H. (2007). Quality of life in chronic musculoskeletal pain. *Best Practice & Research Clinical Rheumatology, 21*(3), 567–579.
Twohig, M. P., Hayes, S. C., Plumb, J. C., Pruitt, L. D., Collins, A. B., Hazlett-Stevens, H., & Woidneck, M. R. (2010). A randomized clinical trial of acceptance and commitment therapy versus progressive relaxation training for obsessive-compulsive disorder. *Journal of Consulting and Clinical Psychology, 78*(5), 705–716.
Upshur, C. C., Luckmann, R. S., & Savageau, J. A. (2006). Primary care provider concerns about management of chronic pain in community clinic populations. *Journal of General Internal Medicine, 21*(6), 652–655.
van Tulder, M. W., Koes, B. W., & Bouter, L. M. (1995). A cost-of-illness study of back pain in The Netherlands. *Pain, 62*(2), 233–240.
Van Zundert, J., & Van Kleef, M. (2005). Low back pain: From algorithm to cost-effectiveness? *Pain Practice, 5*(3), 179–189.
Verhaak, P. F., Kerssens, J. J., Dekker, J., Sorbi, M. J., & Bensing, J. M. (1998). Prevalence of chronic benign pain disorder among adults: A review of the literature. *Pain, 77*(3), 231–239.
Vowles, K. E., & McCracken, L. M. (2008). Acceptance and values-based action in chronic pain: A study of treatment effectiveness and process. *Journal of Consulting and Clinical Psychology, 76*(3), 397.
Watson, P. J., Main, C. J., Waddell, G., Gales, T. F., & Purcell-Jones, G. (1998). Medically certified work loss, recurrence and costs of wage compensation for back pain: A follow-up study of the working population of Jersey. *Rheumatology, 37*(1), 82–86.
Wenig, C. M., Schmidt, C. O., Kohlmann, T., & Schweikert, B. (2009). Costs of back pain in Germany. *European Journal of Pain, 13*(3), 280–286.
Wetherell, J. L., Afari, N., Rutledge, T., Sorrell, J. T., Stoddard, J. A., Petkus, A. J., ... Atkinson, J. H. (2011). A randomized, controlled trial of acceptance and commitment therapy and cognitive-behavioral therapy for chronic pain. *Pain, 152*(9), 2098–2107.
Wicksell, R. K., Ahlqvist, J., Bring, A., Melin, L., & Olsson, G. L. (2008). Can exposure and acceptance strategies improve functioning and life satisfaction in people with chronic pain and Whiplash-Associated Disorders (WAD)? A randomized controlled trial. *Cognitive Behaviour Therapy, 37*(3), 169–182.
Wicksell, R. K., Dahl, J., Magnusson, B., & Olsson, G. L. (2005). Using acceptance and commitment therapy in the rehabilitation of an adolescent female with chronic pain: A case example. *Cognitive and Behavioral Practice, 12*(4), 415–423.
Wicksell, R. K., Kemani, M., Jensen, K., Kosek, E., Kadetoff, D., Sorjonen, K., ... Olsson, G. L. (2013). Acceptance and commitment therapy for fibromyalgia: A randomized controlled trial. *European Journal of Pain, 17*(4), 599–611.
Wicksell, R. K., Olsson, G. L., & Hayes, S. C. (2010). Psychological flexibility as a mediator of improvement in Acceptance and Commitment Therapy for patients with chronic pain following whiplash. *European Journal of Pain, 14*(10), 1059–10e1.
Williams, B. (1994). Patient satisfaction: A valid concept? *Social Science & Medicine, 38*(4), 509–516.
Williams, A. C., Eccleston, C., & Morley, S. (2012). Psychological therapies for the management of chronic pain (excluding headache) in adults. *Cochrane Database of Systematic Reviews, 11*, 1–108.
Wilson, K. G., & Murrell, A. R. (2004). Values work in acceptance and commitment therapy: Setting a course for behavioral treatment. In S. C. Hayes, V. M. Follette, & M. M. Linehan (Eds.), *Mindfulness and acceptance: Expanding the cognitive-behavioral tradition* (pp. 120–151). New York, NY: Guilford.

Chapter 11
Health Anxiety: A Cognitive-Behavioral Framework

Lauren Rutter, Jacob A. Nota, Miryam Yusufov, and Thröstur Björgvinsson

Defining Health Anxiety

Health anxiety (HA) is characterized by a preoccupation with the inaccurate belief that one has, or is in danger of developing, a serious medical illness. HA is not a disorder within our current diagnostic classification system but, nonetheless, is costly for health services and is associated with considerably increased sick-related benefits, posing a social burden (Eilenberg, Kronstrand, Fink, & Frostholm, 2013). With the most recent *Diagnostic and Statistical Manual of Mental Disorders* (*DSM-5*; American Psychiatric Association [APA], 2013), clinically interfering HA symptoms have been classified into two distinct diagnoses: illness anxiety disorder and somatic symptom disorder. Illness anxiety disorder is characterized by at least 6 months of obsessive fears regarding having or acquiring an illness while minimal somatic symptoms are present. Alternatively, somatic symptom disorder is defined by persistent physical complaints that accompany excessive, maladaptive thoughts and behaviors about the seriousness of the symptoms for at least 6 months. In this chapter, we used the term "HA" to refer to clinically interfering and/or distressing symptoms of illness anxiety disorder and somatic symptom disorder. Additionally, we used HA to capture what was historically diagnosed as hypochondriasis. However, if a particular study examined "hypochondriasis," we will use that term when discussing the study for purposes of consistency.

L. Rutter · J. A. Nota · M. Yusufov · T. Björgvinsson (✉)
McLean Hospital, Belmont, MA, USA

Harvard Medical School, Boston, MA, USA
e-mail: lrutter@mclean.harvard.edu; jnota@mclean.harvard.edu; Miryam_Yusufov@dfci.harvard.edu; tbjorgvinsson@mclean.harvard.edu

C. Charis, G. Panayiotou (eds.), *Somatoform and Other Psychosomatic Disorders*,
https://doi.org/10.1007/978-3-319-89360-0_11

Illness anxiety disorder was derived from the previous diagnosis of hypochondriasis, which does not exist in *DSM-5*. Both illness anxiety disorder and somatic symptom disorder are now classified within the "somatic symptom and related disorders" category. These reconceptualized diagnoses, based on the reorganized *DSM-IV* somatoform disorder diagnoses, were meant to be more useful to healthcare providers in primary care and other medical settings (APA, 2013). However, the validity of this recategorization has been met with debate among those who argue that hypochondriasis is best conceptualized as an anxiety disorder (Olatunji, Deacon, & Abramowitz, 2009). Advances in the conceptualization of HA and in evidence-based practice approaches provide insight into the most current treatments and their efficacy.

Diagnosis

A diagnosis of illness anxiety disorder is based on the following *DSM-5* criteria: (A) preoccupation with having or acquiring a serious illness, (B) somatic symptoms are not present or, if present, are only mild in intensity, (C) there is a high level of anxiety about health, and the individual is easily alarmed about personal health status, (D) the individual performs excessive health-related behaviors (e.g., repeatedly checks his or her body for signs of illness) or exhibits maladaptive avoidance (e.g., avoids doctor appointments and hospitals), (E) illness preoccupation is present for at least 6 months, but the specific illness that is feared may change over that period of time, and (F) the illness-related preoccupation is not better explained by another mental disorder (APA, 2013). Illness anxiety disorder is now specified by two subtypes: (1) care-seeking type and (2) care-avoidant type. With care-seeking type, medical care, including testing and physician visits, is frequently used. With care-avoidant type, medical care is rarely used.

Somatic symptom disorder is similar to an illness anxiety disorder, but with elevated levels of bodily complaints. To meet *DSM-5* criteria for a somatic symptom disorder, the individual must experience: (A) one or more distressing somatic symptoms that result in a significant disruption in daily life, (B) excessive thoughts, feelings, or behaviors related to the somatic symptoms or health concerns as manifested by at least one of the following: (1) persistent and disproportionate thoughts about the seriousness of symptoms, (2) persistent high anxiety about health, (3) excessive time and energy devoted to health or symptoms, and (C) although any one somatic symptom may not be continuous, the state of being symptomatic is persistent (typically for 6 months or more). Additional diagnostic specifiers listed for a somatic symptom disorder include "with predominant pain (previously pain disorder): for individuals whose somatic symptoms involve predominantly pain," and "persistent: characterized by severe symptoms, marked impairment, and long duration (more than 6 months)." In addition, a severity specifier exists whereby patients can be diagnosed with mild (only one of criterion B is fulfilled), moderate (two or more of criterion B fulfilled), or severe (two or more of criterion B fulfilled, plus multiple somatic complaints (or one very severe somatic symptom) (APA, 2013). Somatic symptom disorder is highly comorbid with medical disorders, anxiety disorders, and depressive disorders. When a medical illness is concurrently present, the degree of impairment must be more marked than expected from the physical illness alone (APA, 2013).

Treatment

Findings of early, psychodynamic interventions regarded hypochondriasis as a treatment-resistant condition (Taylor, Asmundson, & Coons, 2005). Drastic treatment approaches were employed, including prefrontal lobotomies (Bernstein, Callahan, & Jaranson, 1975). The emergence of a cognitive-behavioral model set the stage for a more humane, appropriate approach to treatment (Olatunji et al., 2014). According to Abramowitz, Deacon, and Valentiner's (2007) cognitive-behavioral model of hypochondriasis, dysfunctional beliefs about bodily symptoms play a significant role in the development of the disorder. The development of clinical hypochondriasis and other forms of HA is largely driven by mistaken beliefs about illnesses and is maintained by maladaptive coping strategies (safety behaviors). These safety behaviors prevent individuals from acquiring accurate information that could disconfirm their beliefs about illnesses.

Cognitive-behavioral therapy (CBT) for HA (formerly referred to as hypochondriasis) involves psychoeducation, exposure and response prevention, and stress management. Initial investigations using CBT for hypochondriasis have produced encouraging results. In an early RCT, patients with hypochondriasis were randomized to a scripted six-session individual CBT intervention and a consultation letter to their primary care physician or to a control condition (Barsky & Ahern, 2004). This brief intervention demonstrated a significant long-term effect on the symptoms of hypochondriasis. In a study comparing CBT to short-term psychodynamic psychotherapy to waitlist control (Sørensen, Birket-Smith, Wattar, Buemann, & Salkovskis, 2011), CBT performed significantly better on all measures relative to the waitlist and on a specific measure of health anxiety symptoms when compared to the psychodynamic psychotherapy group. Additionally, the psychodynamic psychotherapy group did not significantly differ from the waitlist group on any outcomes.

Meta-analyses have shown that CBT is effective in reducing HA/hypochondriasis symptoms (Cooper, Gregory, Walker, Lambe, & Salkovskis, 2017; Taylor et al., 2005; Thomson & Page, 2007). A recent meta-analysis of RCTs demonstrated that CBT is effective in reducing both disorder-specific and nonspecific (e.g., depression) symptoms of HA (Olatunji et al., 2014). Specifically, higher pretreatment HA was associated with larger effect sizes of symptom reduction at follow-up visits. Higher pretreatment depression severity was associated with a decrease in the advantage of CBT over control conditions at posttreatment (Olatunji et al., 2014), consistent with other findings showing that depressive symptoms at baseline were negatively related to improvement after Internet-based CBT for HA (Hedman et al., 2013). A greater number of CBT sessions were associated with larger effect sizes at posttreatment, suggesting that more sessions or longer, more intensive sessions, could be beneficial.

Therapist competence and therapeutic alliance are important in treating HA or hypochondriasis. In a study assessing therapist adherence, therapist competence, and therapeutic alliance via independent raters, patients, therapists, and supervisors across 68 treatments (cognitive therapy and exposure therapy), therapist competence and therapeutic alliance were associated with treatment outcome, and the relationship between therapist competence and treatment outcome was mediated by therapeutic alliance (Weck, Richtberg, Jakob, Neng, & Höfling, 2015). Thus, it is important to consider therapeutic alliance in HA treatment.

Despite the magnitude of recent studies offering empirical support for CBT in treating HA and hypochondriasis, studies investigating the potential treatment mechanisms are scarce. Investigating mechanisms and mediators of HA can lead to the development of more effective treatments. In a nonclinical sample, changes in health-related thoughts mediated the relationship between safety behaviors and increased HA (Olatunji, Etzel, Tomarken, Ciesielski, & Deacon, 2011). In a RCT of hypochondriasis/HA patients, the reduction of dysfunctional attributions of somatic symptoms mediated the treatment effect for both cognitive therapy and exposure therapy (Weck, Neng, Schwind, & Höfling, 2015). Mindfulness processes have also been shown to mediate the treatment effects of severe HA. Mindful non-reactivity is defined as the process of observing thoughts, feelings, and bodily sensations without responding to them (Baer, Smith, Hopkins, Krietemeyer, & Toney, 2006). In a recent RCT of mindful non-reactivity as a putative mediator in exposure-based CBT for severe HA, participants were randomized to receive exposure-based CBT or an active control condition that received behavioral stress management (BSM). Treatments were delivered via Internet, and the main study outcome revealed that CBT produced superior reductions in HA symptoms compared to BSM (Hedman et al., 2014). Additionally, mindful non-reactivity was shown to mediate the treatment effect of exposure therapy (Hedman et al., 2017). These results suggest that mindful non-reactivity may enhance HA exposure treatments, but do not indicate that mindfulness training should be the sole focus of treatment. Instead, mindfulness training may be used as a means to potentiate exposure.

Additional research has supported the use of third-wave CBT methods in treating HA. In an uncontrolled pilot study, 34 patients with severe HA were referred from their general practitioner or hospital department to receive ten sessions of acceptance and commitment (ACT) group therapy, followed by questionnaires for 6 months. ACT group therapy was associated with significant reductions in HA, somatic symptoms, and emotional distress compared to baseline (Eilenberg et al., 2013). Further RCTs are needed to determine if the positive outcomes are maintained over longer periods.

While CBT has been shown to be an effective treatment, it is not widely available because of lack of properly trained therapists (Shafran et al., 2009). Group CBT for HA is a potentially highly cost-effective treatment (Hedman et al., 2010). A prolonged baseline design was used to test the effects of a 10-week group-based CBT treatment for hypochondriasis. Results showed that medical and nonmedical costs were substantially lowered, and HA symptoms based on questionnaire scores showed significant improvement at posttreatment and 6-month follow-up (Hedman et al., 2010). Supporting evidence for the effectiveness of group CBT for HA has also been demonstrated in a larger study (Weck, Neng, et al., 2015; Weck, Richtberg, et al., 2015) in which patients who received group CBT showed large improvements at posttreatment and at a 12-month follow-up.

An additional way to increase access to CBT is via Internet-based CBT. Regarding the efficacy of Internet-based CBT for somatic disorders, a meta-analysis comparing the effects of therapist-guided Internet-based CBT to face-to-face CBT for psychiatric and somatic symptom disorders showed that the two treatments yielded similar effects (Andersson, Cuijpers, Carlbring, Riper, & Hedman, 2014). Participants with severe HA may be more likely to be compliant with an Internet-based treatment in the comfort of their own homes, due to their level of pain and discomfort. While Internet-based CBT has the promise to be an effective and cost-effective alternative and complement to face-to-face therapy, it is still relatively new and rapidly developing. Therefore, more studies are needed before firm conclusions can be drawn (Andersson et al., 2014).

Pharmacological Treatment

Until recently, just two RCTs have demonstrated the benefit of selective serotonin reuptake inhibitors (SSRI) for treating HA. The first compared CBT and paroxetine and found that that the two modalities were similar in treatment effect (Greeven et al., 2007). The other study was a double-blind placebo-controlled study of fluoxetine for hypochondriasis, and the results showed that fluoxetine was moderately effective and well-tolerated for treating hypochondriasis (Fallon et al., 2008). A recent RCT of medication and CBT for hypochondriasis (Fallon et al., 2017) tested whether joint treatment offers additional benefit. In this 24-week study, 195 adults with a *DSM-IV* hypochondriasis diagnosis were randomly assigned to 1 of 4 treatment conditions: fluoxetine plus medication management, placebo plus medication management, CBT, and joint treatment with fluoxetine and CBT. Treatment responder rates were as follows: joint treatment, 47.2%; single active treatment group, 41.8%; and placebo group, 29.6%. Responder rates for each active treatment were not significantly different from placebo, and secondary analyses showed that in comparing placebo and fluoxetine (but not CBT), fluoxetine was more effective in reducing hypochondriasis at week 24. Fluoxetine also was associated with significantly less anxiety and better quality of life than placebo. Higher dosing has been associated with greater improvement of OCD and depression symptoms and was associated with substantial improvement in this study. Overall, the joint treatment provided a small incremental benefit (Fallon et al., 2017).

HA in Patients with Comorbid Physical Illnesses

Treating HA is often complicated by a history of physical health diagnoses and treatments. Previous experiences with illness have often been thought of as substantial risk factors for developing HA. However, one study revealed that HA and comparison samples did not differ in total medical morbidity. Notably, within the hypochondriasis sample, no correlation was found between degree of hypochondriasis and extent of medical morbidity (Barsky, Wyshak, Latham, & Klerman, 1991). Nonetheless, identifying and treating HA in individuals with or without previous or current health diagnoses is critical to guiding appropriate intervention selection. Further, ruling out current health diagnoses is essential to establishing therapeutic rapport and alliance for HA treatment.

Cancer

Fear of cancer progression is a unique psychopathological phenomenon, but it does not differ from other forms of anxiety in its psychological and somatic burdens (Dinkel, Kremsreiter, Marten-Mittag, & Lahmann, 2014). An estimated *more than half* of cancer survivors have fear of cancer recurrence (FCR). However, only *21%* of clinical staff in oncology settings reported consistently referring FCR patients to psychosocial professionals. Psychosocial professionals reported that acceptance and commitment therapy and CBT were helpful in addressing FCR (Thewes et al., 2014). Sarkar et al. (2015) found that FCR was associated with unmet supportive care needs, underscoring the importance of psychological support for cancer survivors. A study of 231 cancer survivors found that higher FCR levels predicted a greater number of outpatient and ER visits (Lebel, Tomei, Feldstain, Beattie, & McCallum, 2013). In contrast to this, another study found that previous experiences with illness were not risk factors for hypochondriasis (Weck, Neng, Göller, & Müller-Marbach, 2014).

Individuals with a history of cancer are at heightened risk of HA. For example, cancer survivors often deal with unexplained symptoms, which often impact their functioning and well-being (Feuerstein, Bruns, Pollman, & Todd, 2010). Interestingly, perceived social support contributed significantly to differences in HA among women with early-stage breast cancer (Jones, Hadjistavropoulos, & Sherry, 2012). Further, cancer-related concerns encompass a specific form of HA, marked by fears of tumor development or progression. Notably, one study revealed a unique form of HA, specifically related to cancer (Trumbo, McComas, & Kannaovakun, 2007). Thus, rates of HA among patients with a history of cancer warrant treatment guidelines and recommendations.

Before discussing additional comorbid medical conditions and HA, we provide a case example to convey a CBT-based treatment for a patient with a history of oral cancer and current HA which manifests as FCR.

The Case of Mrs. C

Mrs. C, a 52-year-old female with oral cancer in remission, was referred by her oncologist for depressed mood, excessive worry, dizziness, chest pain, heart palpitations, anger, and interpersonal struggles. Mrs. C was certain that her symptoms were related to cancer recurrence. She continuously sought physical examinations, diagnostic tests, and requested biopsies. Her oncologist assured her and her behavioral health team that her cancer had been in remission for 2 years and that her symptoms appeared to be psychosomatic. However, Mrs. C had a history of invalidation, when she initially complained of pain on her tongue but was told that it was psychosomatic. The pain was only diagnosed as cancer when she sought a second opinion. Thus, Mrs. C had a history of having her physical symptoms dismissed, which ultimately led to a delay in her cancer diagnosis and treatment. Not surprisingly, Mrs. C's experience led to her eventual mistrust of medical professionals and their appraisal of her presenting symptoms.

This history of physical illness, physician invalidation, and misdiagnosis invariably complicated HA treatment. Mrs. C's initial treatment plan was to address adjustment to cancer, as well as her fear of cancer recurrence. The first three sessions focused on rapport building and validation of experiences with cancer. During the fourth session, Mrs. C discussed her first oncologist's dismissal of her oral pain, thus delaying her cancer diagnosis and treatment. Mrs. C ultimately revealed that this experience led to her mistrust of medical providers. This was addressed by having the patient complete a homework assignment of writing a letter to the oncologist, describing how the invalidation led to a delay of cancer treatment. Upon discussion, Mrs. C attributed her health anxiety to this experience.

In light of this revelation, session 5 focused on case reconceptualization and treatment planning. Mrs. C expressed interest in HA treatment and agreed to completing questionnaires to track her symptoms. Session 6 focused on HA psychoeducation, which Mrs. C described as being incredibly validating and helpful. Throughout treatment, rapport was crucial, as it was especially important to have Mrs. C's physical and emotional experiences be heard. Sessions 7 and 8 focused on self-monitoring, with an emphasis on recording physical symptoms in the context of emotional distress or stress. This data was used to further the case conceptualization, as the patient had increased physical sensations and negative emotions during or after stressful experiences (e.g., with family, work, friends). Over the next four sessions (9–12), Mrs. C reported a substantial decrease in anxiety and depression symptoms, along with somatic symptoms. Thus, she began to "buy in" to the association between anxiety/depression symptoms and HA. Interestingly, Mrs. C did not make any appointments with her oncologist throughout psychological treatment, despite not being instructed to resist. As her treatment evolved and symptoms improved, Mrs. C expressed interest in working on her marital and family issues, and the following 11 sessions were not at all focused on HA and fear of cancer recurrence. Rather, the sessions focused on her employment concerns, martial distress, and trauma history.

This case illustrates numerous factors important to HA treatment that overlap with much of the evidence-based recommendations for HA treatment. First, establishing and maintaining therapeutic alliance is essential and may be tracked with measures such as the WAI. Second, rapport may be maintained with frequent validation and acknowledgment of physical sensations, emotions, and thoughts associated with fear of cancer recurrence. Third, HA psychoeducation is helpful in normalizing the patient's experience. Fourth, establishing and maintaining communication with the patient's health provider (e.g., oncologist) to discuss the patients' physical and anxiety-based symptoms may demonstrate genuine concern for the patient's physical and emotional well-being. Together with the research on HA treatment, this case illustrates that HA may be successfully treated, even in patients with a history of life-threatening illness (e.g., cancer).

Diabetes

Given quality of life implications and prognosis for diabetes, the intersection of diabetes and HA complicates CBT. One study found that among adults with Type 1 or Type 2 diabetes, HA was associated with fear of diabetes complications, lower physical quality of life, and poor adherence to dietary and exercise self-care activities (Janzen Claude, Hadjistavropoulos, & Friesen, 2014). Additionally, Fazil, Akram, and Kapoor (2013) revealed that Type 2 diabetes patients demonstrated a higher prevalence of hypochondriasis, with temperament as the underlying mechanism driving increased hypochondriasis. Notably, diabetes often complicates treatment because patients' physical health makes it challenging to adhere to behavioral interventions. Given that poor diabetes management is associated with comorbid hypochondriasis or HA, psychological treatment is crucial to both mental and physical health outcomes.

Other Intersections of Health Conditions and HA

In addition to cancer and diabetes, several other intersections of physical health and HA exist. A study of 392 medical inpatients revealed a high prevalence of somatoform disorders (including hypochondriasis), particularly among younger women, and found that physicians detected only one-third of these cases (Fink, Hansen, & Oxhoj, 2004). Notably, severe HA may precede early-stage Lewy body dementia (Fujishiro et al., 2016). Further, one study of patients who survived a venous thrombotic embolism found that post-traumatic symptom scores were associated with development of HA. This study underscored the value of intervening on short- and long-term distress in this population (Bennett, Patterson, & Noble, 2016).

Pain

A review of 57 studies revealed that somatization and hypochondriasis were consistently related to chronic pain (Fishbain, Lewis, Gao, Cole, & Steele Rosomoff, 2009). For example, fibromyalgia patients reported a higher frequency of anxiety and depressive disorders, compared to controls without fibromyalgia (Fietta & Manganelli, 2007). An earlier study found that compared to 35 patients with organic gastrointestinal disease, 40 patients with irritable bowel syndrome (IBS) had higher depression, bodily preoccupation, hypochondriacal belief, and disease phobia scores. Thus, IBS was associated with abnormal illness attitudes (Gomborone, Dewsnap, Libby, & Farthing, 1995). Further, a qualitative study of 60 chronic pain patients with HA revealed concerns about pain appraisal, pain preoccupation, coping strategies, self-identity, and suicidal ideation. This study revealed the importance of matching CBT techniques for chronic pain patients to their psychological characteristics (Tang et al., 2009). In another study, migraine and non-migraine headaches were consistently associated with increased anxiety (Zwart et al., 2003). Additionally, a study of somatosensory amplification revealed that compared to 35 healthy individuals, 35 patients with HA continued to amplify somatic sensations despite normal coronary arteries (Korkmaz, Korkmaz, Yildiz, Gündoğan, & Atmaca, 2017). Collectively, these studies point to the strong association between somatic symptoms and HA.

Chronic Obstructive Pulmonary Disease (COPD)

Research has revealed a high prevalence of anxiety in COPD patients, underscoring the need for screening and management of anxiety disorders (Willgoss & Yohannes, 2013). A cross-sectional study of 172 veterans revealed that cognitive and perceptual factors were more concurrent with anxiety than disease severity (Thakur et al., 2018). Further, a qualitative study revealed that fear of suffocation and death-related fears were most salient in COPD patients (Strang, Ekberg-Jansson, & Henoch, 2014). Targeting disease-specific fear and anxiety in COPD patients can improve physiological and psychological outcomes. Cognitive-behavioral approaches, including cognitive restructuring and behavioral exposure, are commonly recommended treatment components (von Leupoldt & Janssens, 2016). Altogether, COPD patients benefit from anxiety management to address their disease concerns and adherence to COPD treatment recommendations. Collectively, these studies highlight the challenges and complications of treating HA in individuals with physical health diagnoses.

Utilization of Medical Services

Individuals with HA commonly overutilize medical services, including emergency departments, walk-in clinics, and primary care offices. For instance, Miles and Wardle (2006) found that health anxious individuals experienced *greater* reductions in anxiety and worry about cancer following colorectal cancer screening, but had *lower* levels of reassurance. Notably, incidence of hypochondriasis was elevated by 68% in patients after coronary angiography, compared to the normal population (Christoph et al., 2014). Thus, HA interventions are essential, as one study revealed that a CBT intervention for recurrent non-cardiac chest pain patients resulted in two to three times fewer hospital bed days (Tyrer et al., 2017).

Conceptualizing HA Treatment in a CBT Framework

As outlined above, CBT is the first-line treatment for HA. For many individuals with HA, maladaptive beliefs about health interact with health-related stimuli resulting in misinterpretations of these stimuli, aversive health-related images, and worry about health. The individual then attempts to cope with perceived health-related threats by seeking safety signals from the environment or employing safety behaviors. These efforts are aimed at reducing the anxiety experienced through these triggers, and may even be successful in the short-term, but ultimately prevent the individual from disconfirming their maladaptive health-related beliefs, increasing tolerance of uncertainty, and finding alternative methods of managing distress.

CBT for HA begins with the identification of maladaptive health-related beliefs and safety signals/behaviors. Subsequently, the patient is supported in removing safety signals/behaviors so that they might have the opportunity to test their health-related interpretations and beliefs. Specific interventions to achieve this goal typically include cognitive restructuring (where an individual examines assumptions in their thinking and evidence that supports different perspectives) and behavioral experiments (where an individual purposefully exposes themselves to situations that trigger health-related anxiety without safety signals/behaviors). To the extent that these beliefs and interpretations are not based in fact, the individual will have the opportunity to modify them based upon these experiences.

CBT for HA is conceptually similar to CBT for anxiety disorders, and exposure and response prevention treatment for obsessive-compulsive disorder, however, presents some unique characteristics and challenges. Treatment outcome literature documents that this treatment can be efficacious in a course of brief treatment (e.g., 16 sessions; Taylor & Asmundson, 2004). In practice, thoughtful development of an individual case conceptualization and flexibility in its application is necessary to inform the pacing, difficulty, and timing of interventions (Taylor, 2004). Herein an example case, a conglomerate of real individuals and descriptions from the literature, will be used to demonstrate case conceptualization and treatment of HA.

The Case of "Mrs. O"

Mrs. O is a 33-year-old married woman referred for assessment by her medical treaters. Mrs. O has been pursuing appointments and testing related to her vision and allergies. She reports that she experiences visual perceptual aberrations similar to "floaters" and regular headaches. She is concerned that she may have a brain tumor or may have experienced a stroke. Mrs. O also reports difficulty breathing when she is aware of nuts being in her vicinity and believes that she is allergic to nuts. Mrs. O has undergone testing related to these conditions (allergy testing, MRI, ophthalmological examination) and sought multiple opinions from medical professionals, and her medical treaters have found no evidence to support a major threat to her health. The presentation from medical treatment is typical for many individuals with HA (see *DSM-5*, APA, 2013). Indeed, individuals may have undergone extensive testing and/or sought medical professionals that were willing to conduct extensive testing before either considering psychological treatment or being "coerced" by family members to seek psychological treatment.

Introducing CBT for HA

The first stage of CBT for HA is focused on establishing a therapeutic relationship with the patient and building a case conceptualization. A warm, empathetic stance is important to join with the patient. Mrs. O had strained relationships with her medical treatment providers; she experienced their suggestion of a psychosomatic cause for her symptoms and the lack of confirmatory evidence for her fears as invalidating. It was important to validate her experiences of distressing and uncomfortable symptoms, as these experiences are real for Mrs. O, even if they are not related to a serious medical illness. The purpose of the treatment was framed as helping Mrs. O pursue her goal of "understanding the reasons she continues to have these symptoms."

The first step in this shared venture was asking Mrs. O to conduct self-monitoring and bring records of her observations to sessions. Specifically, she was asked to record changes and sensations in her body (e.g., headaches, "floaters") and her interpretations of these sensations (e.g., "I have a tumor pressing against my optic nerve"). Furthermore she was asked to record any accompanying health-related images (e.g., seeing herself bald and tired, going through radiation therapy) and behaviors she engaged in following these experiences (e.g., checking her vision by rubbing her eyes and looking at white paper; checking Internet articles about symptoms of brain tumors). Self-monitoring is useful for a number of reasons. First, this exercise demonstrates that the patient's experiences will be valued and considered. This is very important for building rapport with individuals who suffer with HA. Second, it sets the expectation that treatment will be a collaborative venture, where both patient and provider will work together to understand the patient's symptoms and what maintains them. Third, self-monitoring provides the data for building a case conceptualization. Self-monitoring can make patients aware of functional relationships between thoughts, feelings, and behaviors that were not previously salient. The various interpretations and feared outcomes that the patient holds are recorded. The obvious and subtle safety-oriented behaviors and signals are made clear to the therapist. Finally, this stage of treatment provides time for the therapeutic alliance to build and accurate empathy to be expressed toward the patient's physical symptoms and interpretations. For Mrs. O, self-monitoring also presented opportunities to begin questioning the effectiveness of safety behaviors. Mrs. O was able to acknowledge that the intensity of her headaches did not remit when she engaged in Internet searches of medical resources. Thus, the therapist was also able to introduce curiosity about the effect Mrs. O's rubbing of her eyes had on her perceptions of pain and aberrations in her vision without undermining her report of her symptoms.

These initial sessions, as well as examination of the self-monitoring data, enhanced the therapist understanding of the context surrounding Mrs. O's HA symptoms. Mrs. O reported that as a child, her parents had been highly responsive to any signs of symptoms of illness in Mrs. O and her siblings. While she perceived their reactions as hyperbolic at the time, she also recalls instances of having been frightened that she may be very ill. Further, she reported that her parents expressed doubts about the competence of her doctors. Mrs. O denied having persistent physical symptoms or difficulties interacting with medical providers until adulthood. Early learning experiences like these are often reported as potentially predisposing factors in individuals with HA (Taylor, 2004). Mrs. O reported that her physical symptoms and difficulty reaching satisfaction with her health began after her marriage, when she was 32 years old. Mrs. O and her husband had been discussing having children. Mrs. O acknowledged that this was an exciting and stressful prospect. She had concerns about the impact pregnancy would have on her body and the health of her potential children. Around this time, Mrs. O learned that her uncle, who had been apparently healthy, required an emergency surgery to treat a cardiovascular issue that was previously undetected. She described this as the time when she began noticing headaches and issues with her vision and began more regularly checking medical resources on the Internet. For many individuals with HA, onset is precipitated by changes in lifestyle or responsibility or unexpected health-related experiences with family or peers (Taylor, 2004).

Since this time, Mrs. O had struggled to maintain her performance in her work. She frequently took time to attend medical appointments. She describes difficulty completing her work due to headaches. She also avoided interacting with coworkers during break periods because of fears that she may encounter nuts and have an allergic reaction. Further, Mrs. O acknowledged that her physical symptoms and medical treatment-seeking had taken a toll on her relationship with her husband. She did not want to pursue having children, given her belief that she was seriously ill. These experiences contributed to Mrs. O's desperation and frustration with her physical symptoms, which contributed to her focus on these. Many individuals with HA become stuck in a similar situation where their efforts to "solve" their symptoms paradoxically seem to maintain the negative impact these symptoms have on their lives. Fortunately, the relatively acute onset, brief duration, and absence of secondary gain from physical symptoms were protective factors that improved Mrs. O's prognosis (APA, 2013).

At this point in CBT for HA, self-monitoring and contextual data are used to facilitate an examination of health-related beliefs. The goal is to clarify what beliefs the patient holds and how these are shaping their interpretations of physical experiences and informing their responses to them (Asmundson, Taylor, & Cox, 2001; Wells, 1997). For Mrs. O, her experiences with her parents were related to beliefs that she may be more vulnerable to illness than other people and that it is better to be safe rather than sorry. Her inability to move forward with her work and plans with her husband were related to beliefs that illnesses must be identified and treated or nothing else will matter. Mrs. O's self-monitoring data indicated a belief that unexpected physical stimuli are symptoms of disease that must be evaluated and that checking her body is an effective way to do so. Further, Mrs. O's excessive treatment-seeking and vicarious learning from her uncle related to beliefs that normal test results cannot be trusted and that doctors often make serious mistakes. It was critical to identify these beliefs but not to initially take a stance that these beliefs are maladaptive. Instead, a more Socratic approach to these beliefs was employed (e.g., "Checking your body *always* helps you identify a solution to your pain?"). At this point, building a therapeutic relationship is still the primary goal; therefore, these topics are raised as probes for a patient's insight, conviction about their health-related beliefs.

In addition to assessing health-related beliefs, evaluation of patients' motivation is indicated during the development of a case conceptualization and treatment planning. Many individuals with HA may have ambivalence about psychological treatment for their symptoms. Low insight is common in individuals with HA (APA, 2013) and they may feel coerced to attend treatment; however, most individuals will not have complete conviction about their health-related beliefs. Mrs. O's motivation for attending treatment was explored (e.g., "If you are 100% certain you have a tumor, why are you here?"). She was able to acknowledge that extensive testing suggested she was well. Mrs. O expressed dissatisfaction because she continued to have physical symptoms and she was motivated to understand what maintains them. Again, alternative explanations were explored for these physical symptoms that did not include serious illness using Socratic dialogue (e.g., "Have you ever been given an explanation for what causes these symptoms, if not serious disease?"). Mrs. O could not identify alternative explanations, and she had not previously considered that anxiety and selective attention to her body could actually maintain her symptoms.

Understanding what is valuable to a patient is critical for building motivation to engage in future interventions. Personally meaningful and fulfilling activities can also be important resources for distress tolerance and distraction from anxiety-provoking internal stimuli. For Mrs. O, her relationships with family were valuable. It was clear that her HA had an impact on her relationship with her husband and it interfered with their plans to grow their family. This was a crucial part of her engagement with treatment. In the course of these early sessions, Mrs. O also shared that she had previously spent much of her free time interacting with friends via text message, watching movies, and cooking. Her desire to return to these activities would prove an asset in planning alternative activities when she reduced her safety behaviors later in the treatment.

Another piece of the case conceptualization and treatment planning is a consultation with a patient's medical providers and social support network (i.e., family, friends, etc.). It is important that contact with collateral sources be negotiated with the patient. The importance of this contact should be emphasized, as individuals with HA may be reluctant to involve others, as they may not want to share details of the fact that they are now seeking psychological services for a problem they perceive as physical. Consultation with medical providers is also necessary to understand the motivations and conditions of any ongoing treatments and evaluations. For example, Mrs. O had scheduled evaluations with medical professionals concurrent with beginning CBT. When contact was made with these professionals, it became clear that the tests were only being conducted at Mrs. O's request and were not considered medically indicated. Consultation with friends and family is intended to understand the state of a patient's interpersonal relationships (Taylor, 2004). Individuals with HA often seek reassurance and are accommodated by their family members or friends, and thus, the reassuring individuals become "safety signals." When these safety signals are identified, it is important to address them directly. For Mrs. O, her husband often provided reassurance related to her health and had taken on many responsibilities that were previously managed by Mrs. O in order to reduce her anxiety. Further, Mrs. O noted that her employer had been accommodating of her many medical appointments but that she had received informal feedback that this might not continue and she was at risk of losing her job if she continued on this track.

Sharing the Case Conceptualization and Developing a Treatment Plan

With sufficient data to produce an initial case conceptualization and an established working alliance with the patient, the therapist in CBT for HA now begins to directly address the struggles that the patient is having with HA. The theme of collaboration continues as both parties contribute to the treatment plan. This requires sharing the case conceptualization with the patient and attaining the patient's "buy in" to taking part in treatment. This process includes psychoeducation about HA (which is a crucial part of any CBT intervention for reducing HA symptoms) and a collaborative application of Mrs. O's own data, collected during the initial sessions, and ongoing self-monitoring. It was crucially important to continuously validate that these distressing physical symptoms that Mrs. O was experiencing were absolutely "real" to her and could possibly be explained by a cause other than serious illness. Mrs. O was presented with the following:

> *"Mrs. O, you have done a great job collecting data about your physical symptoms and the thoughts and behaviors that are associated with them. We have also gotten to talk about how these distressing symptoms have had a huge impact on your relationship with your husband and pulled you away from so many things you usually like to do. It is clear to me that you are suffering immensely because of these headaches, the changes in your vision, and your difficulty breathing at times. You have been trying desperately to figure these problems out, so you can get back to your life! That determination is a strength and is really admirable. Unfortunately, it seems that, so far, your efforts have not reduced any of these physical symptoms. You said yourself that the pursuit of all these medical tests has only worn you down and left you frustrated.*
>
> *Based on all of the information we have gathered together, I believe that your physical symptoms (while very real) are being caused by something other than a serious physical illness. There is a pattern of feelings, thoughts, and behaviors that happens in 5–10% of people called somatic symptom disorder. This pattern involves physical sensations that are interpreted as very threatening. The interpretation of these sensations is based on individuals' beliefs about health. For example, one may feel they are more vulnerable to illness than others or that illnesses that are not identified and treated will lead to catastrophe. Events from your past, important experiences, may also be related to some of these health-related beliefs: like having a healthy relative have an unexpected serious illness. You told me about some similar experiences you had earlier in your life, and more recently, that seem to be related to the beliefs you hold about your health now. The way you were scared by your parents' reactions to your physical symptoms as a child. Your uncle's scare with the stent.*
>
> *In somatic symptom disorder, individuals seek out safety signals and act in ways to seek safety related to their physical health. For example, checking medical resources, going to doctors for tests, and limiting themselves from activities. You told me about many instances of doing the same. This makes total sense, because if you experience a physical symptom, interpret it as a serious threat, then of course you would take action to try to eliminate the threat! This is a normal reaction to these symptoms. However, in this pattern, there are some glitches that transform what makes sense most of the time into something that is actually not helpful. If there isn't a physical cause for these symptoms, the stress one experiences trying to eliminate the threat may work against them. In fact, the actions a person takes in order to try to eliminate their symptoms seem to maintain the very symptoms they want to eliminate. This happens because their anxiety keeps their attention on these symptoms, keeping their stress level high, and not allowing a person to find out that their initial interpretation of the symptoms as a sign of serious illness may not be true.*
>
> *What happens with this pattern is that a person gets stuck. When uncomfortable physical experiences happen, they feel terrifying, and thus we pay attention more to them, continue to try to solve them through one avenue (medical treatment). However, there isn't a physical illness causing the experiences and ultimately we have more of the symptoms because of stress and fatigue. This is ironic because many people are afraid of having a serious illness that will ruin their quality of life and their efforts to figure out the cause of their physical symptoms already does this! Luckily, this explanation gives us ideas about how to change the pattern. Taking time to examine the evidence for beliefs and assumptions that are made about physical symptoms can help a person to see alternatives to serious illness being the cause. This results in a less stressed reaction to the symptom, which may reduce their intensity. One can also learn that the feeling of distress and uncertainty that is associated with their physical symptoms does not last forever or that one can still live their life with that feeling along for the ride. Further, stopping the safety-seeking actions that have followed these symptoms will allow one the opportunity to build new beliefs that are based on experiences and focus energy on the things that are important to them in their life.*

This will be scary at first, as you won't fully know what is going to happen. But, the research that has been done suggests that in 16 weeks, you could experience meaningful changes in this pattern and back into your life. Having more meaningful interactions with your family. Spending time doing what you want, instead of constantly searching for a medical answer over and over again for the same symptoms. The research also suggests, that if you engage in the treatment fully, that you will likely be experiencing fewer of these physical symptoms. From my perspective, this seems to be in line with what you said you wanted: answers about these symptoms, relief, and to get back to your life. What do you think?"

The questions and concerns raised by the patient should be addressed, and the conceptualization should be updated in collaboration. It is not uncommon for questions about the etiology of physical symptoms to arise. Researchers have investigated whether individuals with HA have more "noisy" bodies (i.e., actually experience more physical sensations) or are more sensitive to internal stimuli; findings have been inconsistent. It may be satisfactory to relate that all bodies are unique and have unique abilities and difficulties. For example, many athletes experience regular pain in their bodies *and* are able to achieve exceptional feats. Unrealistic treatment goals (e.g., never having pain) should be identified and reframed with the patient. Further, a pragmatic evaluation of seeking further medical explanations for physical symptoms is indicated.

Cognitive Restructuring for HA

Once the patient and therapist agree on an initial conceptualization, the focus of treatment will shift to application of CBT interventions. Cognitive restructuring of health-related interpretations and beliefs can begin with self-monitoring data. The therapist should not take a stance that the CBT model is correct, but instead continue to use Socratic dialogue to encourage the patient to consider what evidence they have for their beliefs and how they are defining persuasive evidence. The therapist may ask questions that highlight patterns in the patient's thinking. For Mrs. O: "You have experienced headaches and difficulty breathing. What is the likelihood that these are related to two serious and undiagnosed illnesses?" The therapist may also reframe unsatisfactory experiences with medical evaluations as related to potential distortions in the logic being applied to the patient's physical symptoms (e.g., "What kind of evidence would persuade you that your symptoms are not related to a serious medical illness?" "Would you question the validity of medical test results that confirm you have a serious illness?"). The therapist could also ask the patient to consider how their own values and their beliefs relate (e.g., "If illness and death are realities of everyone's lives, how would you choose to spend your time; are your beliefs facilitating a life that you want?"). Mrs. O had relatively good insight and was responsive to cognitive restructuring. She acknowledged that she had not been living consistent with her own values. In particular, the impact her safety behaviors had on her family were clear to her. Mrs. O described that she rejected medical test results because she continued to experience uncomfortable physical symptoms and did not have a satisfactory explanation for them. She was willing to entertain the possibility that stress and anxiety were maintaining her symptoms, but expressed that she was not yet convinced. Mrs. O's increased willingness to consider the CBT for HA model following cognitive restructuring enabled the addition of exposure and safety behavior prevention interventions.

Exposures for HA

The goal of exposure in CBT for HA is the activation of physical symptoms that are typically interpreted as threatening without simultaneous safety signals and the prevention of safety behaviors, allowing the patient to learn from experience the consequences of these symptoms. This is conceptually very similar to exposure and response prevention for obsessive-compulsive disorder (Foa & Kozak, 1986). Mrs. O engaged in exposures where she worked on tasks that required concentration (e.g., her work) and resisted checking her eyesight and rubbing her eyes. Using a graduated hierarchy of exposures, she approached situations related to her difficulty breathing in the presence of nuts. For example, early exposures included spending time in the breakroom at her job while her coworkers ate meals that may contain nuts. Mrs. O then prepared items that contained nuts. Eventually, she ate meals that she could not confirm nor deny contained nuts (increasing uncertainty) and that she knew contained nuts. Throughout this process, Mrs. O and the therapist created a plan to resist seeking reassurance from checking medical resources on the Internet or from her husband. This included communication with her husband about treatment-consistent ways of responding to her at times when she sought reassurance. Input from her medical providers was also sought to clarify that these activities would involve minimal legitimate risk to her health based on their understanding.

Exposure plans are highly individualized to a patient's particular symptoms and must be treated as living documents that are constantly updated based on the patient's experiences in each exposure, opportunities that arise due to unforeseen circumstances, and the patient's willingness from day to day. For Mrs. O, a refrain that was emphasized in treatment was to "find a way forward everyday." This translated to reframing situations that trigger HA as opportunities to continue testing beliefs and never abandoning exposure when she felt it was too overwhelming to carry out her plan, but instead to identify a way that she did feel willing to test her beliefs. Indeed, over the course of treatment, the therapist transitioned from a coaching role (taking more control over what exposures are carried out) to a cheerleading role (providing support and reinforcement for exposures that the patient identified herself). Therapists using a CBT for HA approach plan from the beginning of treatment for their patients to become their own therapists and provide scaffolding for this.

The cognitive restructuring and exposure portion of CBT for HA typically lasts 12 weeks. This is considered sufficient time for an individual to make significant changes in their safety behaviors and increase the flexibility in their health-related beliefs. A linear decrease in both of these should not be expected. Individuals may see step-wise and recursive patterns in their distress and interference due to HA. Mrs. O completed 14 sessions of CBT for HA. Twice in the course of these sessions, she and the therapist spent portions of their meetings discussing exposure experiences that Mrs. O initially considered failures and evidence that she could not continue in treatment. The therapist took time to validate Mrs. O's distress and simultaneously use curiosity and Socratic dialogue to allow her to reframe these "failures" as learning opportunities. Mrs. O increasingly viewed her increases in distress as consistent with the CBT for HA model and was able to continue her treatment plan without support.

Relapse Prevention

The final stage of CBT for HA involves efforts to maintain gains and to anticipate future risk factors for a return to maladaptive health-related beliefs and safety behaviors. Mrs. O and the therapist created behavioral schedules that included valued activities (e.g., work, spending time with her husband, interacting with friends on social media). Explicit plans for appropriate medical care were also arranged in consultation with Mrs. O's medical providers. Specifically, Mrs. O informed her providers about the unhelpful effects of reassurance and unnecessary medical testing. She worked together with them to clarify symptoms that do not require emergency medical appointments and to arrange a regimen for treatment that was appropriate for her age. At the conclusion of treatment, Mrs. O was not yet ready to consider having a child; however, she and her husband did resume having conversations about these plans, including the rewards and challenges this would pose for Mrs. O and for their family.

Summary

HA, as we have defined it here, is a set of symptoms characterized by preoccupation with beliefs that one has or will develop a physical illness. HA is often accompanied by physical symptoms that contribute to these anxious preoccupations. HA can be effectively treated with a CBT framework, as we have outlined. The treatment becomes significantly more complicated when the patient currently has a comorbid medical illness. Ultimately, a primary goal of HA treatment is to guide a patient to challenge their own dysfunctional beliefs about illness and physical symptoms through exposing themselves to the very thoughts that trigger and maintain their anxiety. This enables the patient to act in a manner consistent with their values and goals, rather than one that is dictated by their anxieties and compulsive pursuit of safety signals.

References

Abramowitz, J. S., Deacon, B. J., & Valentiner, D. P. (2007). The short health anxiety inventory: Psychometric properties and construct validity in a non-clinical sample. *Cognitive Therapy and Research, 31*(6), 871–883.

American Psychiatric Association. (2013). *Diagnostic and statistical manual of mental disorders* (5th ed.). Washington, DC: Author.

Andersson, G., Cuijpers, P., Carlbring, P., Riper, H., & Hedman, E. (2014). Internet-based vs. face-to-face cognitive behaviour therapy for psychiatric and somatic disorders: A systematic review and meta-analysis. *World Psychiatry, 13*, 288–295.

Asmundson, G. J. G., Taylor, S., & Cox, B. J. (Eds.). (2001). *Health anxiety: Clinical and research perspectives on hypochondriasis and related disorders*. New York: Wiley.

Baer, R. A., Smith, G. T., Hopkins, J., Krietemeyer, J., & Toney, L. (2006). Using self-report assessment methods to explore facets of mindfulness. *Assessment, 13*, 27–45.

Barsky, A. J., & Ahern, D. K. (2004). Cognitive behavior therapy for hypochondriasis: A randomized controlled trial. *JAMA: Journal of the American Medical Association, 291*(12), 1464–1470.

Barsky, A. J., Wyshak, G., Latham, K. S., & Klerman, G. L. (1991). The relationship between hypochondriasis and medical illness. *Archives of Internal Medicine, 151*(1), 84–88.

Bennett, P., Patterson, K., & Noble, S. (2016). Predicting post-traumatic stress and health anxiety following a venous thrombotic embolism. *Journal of Health Psychology, 21*(5), 863–871.

Bernstein, I. C., Callahan, W. A., & Jaranson, J. M. (1975). Lobotomy in private practice: Long-term follow-up. *Archives of General Psychiatry, 32*(8), 1041–1047.

Christoph, M., Christoph, A., Dannemann, S., Poitz, D., Pfluecke, C., Strasser, R. H., … Ibrahim, K. (2014). Mental symptoms in patients with cardiac symptoms and normal coronary arteries. *Open Heart, 1*(1), e000093.

Cooper, K., Gregory, J. D., Walker, I., Lambe, S., & Salkovskis, P. M. (2017). Cognitive behaviour therapy for health anxiety: A systematic review and meta-analysis. *Behavioural and Cognitive Psychotherapy, 45*(2), 110–123.

Dinkel, A., Kremsreiter, K., Marten-Mittag, B., & Lahmann, C. (2014). Comorbidity of fear of progression and anxiety disorders in cancer patients. *General Hospital Psychiatry, 36*(6), 613–619.

Eilenberg, T., Kronstrand, L., Fink, P., & Frostholm, L. (2013). Acceptance and commitment group therapy for health anxiety—Results from a pilot study. *Journal of Anxiety Disorders, 27*(5), 461–468.

Fallon, B. A., Ahern, D. K., Pavlicova, M., Slavov, I., Skritskya, N., & Barksy, A. J. (2017). A randomized controlled trial of medication and cognitive-behavioral therapy for psychochondriasis. *American Journal of Psychiatry, 174*, 756–764.

Fallon, B. A., Petkova, E., Skritskaya, N., Sanchez-Lacay, A., Schneier, F., Vermes, D., … Liebowitz, M. R. (2008). A double-masked, placebo-controlled study, of fluoxetine for hypochondriasis. *Journal of Clinical Psychopharmacology, 28*(6), 638–645.

Fazil, M., Akram, M., & Kapoor, P. (2013). General hypochondriasis in diabetes mellitus type-II (DM-II): Implications for clinicians. *Global Journal of Medicine and Public Health, 2*(3), 1–11.

Feuerstein, M., Bruns, G. L., Pollman, C., & Todd, B. L. (2010). Management of unexplained symptoms in survivors of cancer. *Journal of Oncology Practice, 6*(6), 308–311.

Fietta, P., & Manganelli, P. (2007). Fibromyalgia and psychiatric disorders. *Acta Bio Medica Atenei Parmensis, 78*(2), 88–95.

Fink, P., Hansen, M. S., & Oxhoj, M. L. (2004). The prevalence of somatoform disorders among internal medical inpatients. *Journal of Psychosomatic Research, 56*(4), 413–418.

Fishbain, D. A., Lewis, J. E., Gao, J., Cole, B., & Steele Rosomoff, R. (2009). Is chronic pain associated with somatization/hypochondriasis? An evidence-based structured review. *Pain Practice, 9*(6), 449–467.

Foa, E. B., & Kozak, M. J. (1986). Emotional processing of fear: Exposure to corrective information. *Psychological Bulletin, 99*(1), 20–35.

Fujishiro, H., Iritani, S., Sekiguchi, H., Habuchi, C., Torii, Y., Matsunaga, S., … Fujita, K. (2016). Hypochondriasis as an early manifestation of dementia with Lewy bodies: An autopsied case report. *Psychogeriatrics, 16*(2), 139–144.

Gomborone, J., Dewsnap, P., Libby, G., & Farthing, M. (1995). Abnormal illness attitudes in patients with irritable bowel syndrome. *Journal of Psychosomatic Research, 39*(2), 227–230.

Greeven, A., van Balkom, A. M., Visser, S., Merkelbach, J. W., van Rood, Y. R., van Dyck, R., … Spinhoven, P. (2007). Cognitive behavior therapy and paroxetine in the treatment of hypochondriasis: A randomized controlled trial. *The American Journal of Psychiatry, 164*(1), 91–99.

Hedman, E., Axelsson, E., Görling, A., Ritzman, C., Ronnheden, M., El Alaoui, S., … Ljótsson, B. (2014). Internet-delivered exposure-based cognitive–behavioural therapy and behavioural stress management for severe health anxiety: Randomised controlled trial. *The British Journal of Psychiatry, 205*(4), 307–314.

Hedman, E., Lindefors, N., Andersson, G., Andersson, E., Lekander, M., Rück, C., & Ljótsson, B. (2013). Predictors of outcome in Internet-based cognitive behavior therapy for severe health anxiety. *Behaviour Research and Therapy, 51*(10), 711–717.

Hedman, E., Ljótsson, B., Andersson, E., Rück, C., Andersson, G., & Lindefors, N. (2010). Effectiveness and cost offset analysis of group CBT for hypochondriasis delivered in a psychiatric setting: An open trial. *Cognitive Behaviour Therapy, 39*(4), 239–250.

Hedman, E., Ljótsson, B., Axelsson, E., Andersson, G., Rück, C., & Andersson, E. (2017). Health anxiety in obsessive compulsive disorder and obsessive compulsive symptoms in severe health anxiety: An investigation of symptom profiles. *Journal of Anxiety Disorders, 4*, 580–586.

Janzen Claude, J. A., Hadjistavropoulos, H. D., & Friesen, L. (2014). Exploration of health anxiety among individuals with diabetes: Prevalence and implications. *Journal of Health Psychology, 19*(2), 312–322.

Jones, S. L., Hadjistavropoulos, H. D., & Sherry, S. B. (2012). Health anxiety in women with early-stage breast cancer: What is the relationship to social support? *Canadian Journal of Behavioural Science/Revue canadienne des sciences du comportement, 44*(2), 108.

Korkmaz, H., Korkmaz, S., Yildiz, S., Gündoğan, B., & Atmaca, M. (2017). Determination of health anxiety, anxiety, and somatosensory amplification levels in individuals with normal coronary angiography. *Psychiatry Research, 252*, 114–117.

Lebel, S., Tomei, C., Feldstain, A., Beattie, S., & McCallum, M. (2013). Does fear of cancer recurrence predict cancer survivors' health care use? *Supportive Care in Cancer, 21*(3), 901–906.

Miles, A., & Wardle, J. (2006). Adverse psychological outcomes in colorectal cancer screening: Does health anxiety play a role? *Behaviour Research and Therapy, 44*(8), 1117–1127.

Olatunji, B. O., Deacon, B. J., & Abramowitz, J. S. (2009). Is hypochondriasis an anxiety disorder? *The British Journal of Psychiatry, 194*(6), 481–482.

Olatunji, B. O., Etzel, E. N., Tomarken, A. J., Ciesielski, B. G., & Deacon, B. (2011). The effects of safety behaviors on health anxiety: An experimental investigation. *Behaviour Research and Therapy, 49*(11), 719–728.

Olatunji, B. O., Kauffman, B. Y., Meltzer, S., Davis, M. L., Smits, J. J., & Powers, M. B. (2014). Cognitive-behavioral therapy for hypochondriasis/health anxiety: A meta-analysis of treatment outcome and moderators. *Behaviour Research and Therapy, 58*, 65–74.

Sarkar, S., Sautier, L., Schilling, G., Bokemeyer, C., Koch, U., & Mehnert, A. (2015). Anxiety and fear of cancer recurrence and its association with supportive care needs and health-care service utilization in cancer patients. *Journal of Cancer Survivorship, 9*(4), 567–575.

Shafran, R., Clark, D. M., Fairburn, C. G., Arntz, A., Barlow, D. H., Ehlers, A., … Salkovskis, P. M. (2009). Mind the gap: Improving the dissemination of CBT. *Behaviour Research and Therapy, 47*(11), 902–909.

Sørensen, P., Birket-Smith, M., Wattar, U., Buemann, I., & Salkovskis, P. (2011). A randomized clinical trial of cognitive behavioural therapy versus short-term psychodynamic psychotherapy versus no intervention for patients with hypochondriasis. *Psychological Medicine, 41*(2), 431–441.

Strang, S., Ekberg-Jansson, A., & Henoch, I. (2014). Experience of anxiety among patients with severe COPD: A qualitative, in-depth interview study. *Palliative and Supportive Care, 12*(6), 465–472.

Tang, N. K., Salkovskis, P. M., Hodges, A., Soong, E., Hanna, M. H., & Hester, J. (2009). Chronic pain syndrome associated with health anxiety: A qualitative thematic comparison between pain patients with high and low health anxiety. *British Journal of Clinical Psychology, 48*(1), 1–20.

Taylor, S. (2004). Understanding and treating health anxiety: A cognitive-behavioral approach. *Cognitive and Behavioral Practice, 11*(1), 112–123.

Taylor, S., & Asmundson, G. J. G. (2004). *Treating health anxiety: A cognitive-behavioral approach*. New York: The Guilford Press.

Taylor, S., Asmundson, G. J. G., & Coons, M. J. (2005). Current directions in the treatment of hypochondriasis. *Journal of Cognitive Psychotherapy, 19*(3), 285–304.

Thakur, E. R., Sansgiry, S., Petersen, N. J., Stanley, M., Kunik, M. E., Naik, A. D., & Cully, J. A. (2018). Cognitive and perceptual factors, not disease severity, are linked with anxiety in COPD: Results from a cross-sectional study. *International Journal of Behavioral Medicine, 25*(1), 74–84.

Thewes, B., Brebach, R., Dzidowska, M., Rhodes, P., Sharpe, L., & Butow, P. (2014). Current approaches to managing fear of cancer recurrence; A descriptive survey of psychosocial and clinical health professionals. *Psychooncology, 23*(4), 390–396.

Thomson, A. B., & Page, L. A. (2007). Psychotherapies for hypochondriasis. *Cochrane Database of Systematic Reviews, 4*, CD006520.

Trumbo, C. W., McComas, K. A., & Kannaovakun, P. (2007). Cancer anxiety and the perception of risk in alarmed communities. *Risk Analysis, 27*(2), 337–350.

Tyrer, P., Tyrer, H., Morriss, R., Crawford, M., Cooper, S., Yang, M., … Barrett, B. (2017). Clinical and cost-effectiveness of adapted cognitive behaviour therapy for non-cardiac chest pain: A multicentre, randomised controlled trial. *Open Heart, 4*(1), e000582.

von Leupoldt, A., & Janssens, T. (2016). Could targeting disease specific fear and anxiety improve COPD outcomes? *Expert Review of Respiratory Medicine, 10*(8), 835–837.

Weck, F., Neng, J. M., Göller, K., & Müller-Marbach, A. M. (2014). Previous experiences with illness and traumatic experiences: A specific risk factor for hypochondriasis? *Psychosomatics, 55*(4), 362–371.

Weck, F., Neng, J. B., Schwind, J., & Höfling, V. (2015). Exposure therapy changes dysfunctional evaluations of somatic symptoms in patients with hypochondriasis (health anxiety). A randomized controlled trial. *Journal of Anxiety Disorders, 34*, 1–7.

Weck, F., Richtberg, S., Jakob, M., Neng, J. B., & Höfling, V. (2015). Therapist competence and therapeutic alliance are important in the treatment of health anxiety (hypochondriasis). *Psychiatry Research, 228*(1), 53–58.

Wells, A. (1997). *Cognitive therapy of anxiety disorders: A practice manual and conceptual guide*. Chichester, UK: Wiley.

Willgoss, T. G., & Yohannes, A. M. (2013). Anxiety disorders in patients with COPD: A systematic review. *Respiratory Care, 58*(5), 858–866.

Zwart, J. A., Dyb, G., Hagen, K., Ødegård, K. J., Dahl, A. A., Bovim, G., & Stovner, L. J. (2003). Depression and anxiety disorders associated with headache frequency. The Nord-Trøndelag Health Study. *European Journal of Neurology, 10*(2), 147–152.

Index

C. Charis, G. Panayiotou (eds.), *Somatoform and Other Psychosomatic Disorders*,
https://doi.org/10.1007/978-3-319-89360-0

C

D

E

The manufacturer's authorised representative in the EU is Springer Nature Customer Service Centre GmbH, Europaplatz 3, 69115 Heidelberg, Germany. If you have any concerns regarding our products, please contact ProductSafety@springernature.com

Printed and bound by CPI Group (UK) Ltd, Croydon, CR0 4YY

30/09/2026

02225643-0004